Environmental Health Risk IV

WIT*PRESS*

WIT Press publishes leading books in Science and Technology.
Visit our website for new and current list of titles.
www.witpress.com

WIT*eLibrary*

Home of the Transactions of the Wessex Institute.
Papers presented at Environmental Health Risk IV are archived in the
WIT eLibrary in volume 11 of WIT Transactions on
Biomedicine and Health (ISSN 1743-3525).
The WIT eLibrary provides the international scientific community with immediate and
permanent access to individual papers presented at WIT conferences.
http://library.witpress.com

FOURTH INTERNATIONAL CONFERENCE ON
THE IMPACT OF ENVIRONMENTAL FACTORS ON HEALTH

ENVIRONMENTAL HEALTH RISK IV

CONFERENCE CHAIRMAN

C.A. Brebbia
Wessex Institute of Technology, UK

INTERNATIONAL SCIENTIFIC ADVISORY COMMITTEE

Organised by
Wessex Institute of Technology, UK

Sponsored by
WIT Transactions on Biomedicine and Health

Environmental Health Risk IV

Editor

C.A. Brebbia
Wessex Institute of Technology, UK

WIT*PRESS* Southampton, Boston

Editor:

C.A. Brebbia
Wessex Institute of Technology, UK

Published by

WIT Press
Ashurst Lodge, Ashurst, Southampton, SO40 7AA, UK
Tel: 44 (0) 238 029 3223; Fax: 44 (0) 238 029 2853
E-Mail: witpress@witpress.com
http://www.witpress.com

For USA, Canada and Mexico

Computational Mechanics Inc
25 Bridge Street, Billerica, MA 01821, USA
Tel: 978 667 5841; Fax: 978 667 7582
E-Mail: infousa@witpress.com
http://www.witpress.com

British Library Cataloguing-in-Publication Data

A Catalogue record for this book is available
from the British Library

ISBN: 978-1-84564-083-5
ISSN: 1747-4485 (print)
ISSN: 1743-3525 (on-line)

The texts of the papers in this volume were set individually by the authors or under their supervision. Only minor corrections to the text may have been carried out by the publisher.

Printed in Great Britain by Cambridge Printing

PREFACE

This book contains most of the papers presented at the Fourth International Conference on the Impact of Environmental Factors in Health (Environmental Health Risk 07). It is part of a successful series that started at the University of Cardiff in 2001, followed by a second meeting in Catania (2003) and the last one in Bologna (2005).

Health problems related to the environment continue to be a major source of concern all over the world. Society needs to develop measures that will eliminate or considerably reduce hazardous factors from the environment that can result in health risk to humans. The Conference aimed to foster the development of better experimental and modelling tools to achieve these objectives.

This interaction between environmental risk and health is usually complex and involves a substantial number of factors. This resulted in an interdisciplinary meeting in which diverse aspects of the impact of environmental factors in health were discussed.

The papers published in this book are divided into the following sections:

- Air pollution
- The built environment and health
- Occupational health
- Water quality issues
- Risk prevention and monitoring
- Social and economical issues

The Editor is indebted to all members of the Scientific Advisory Committee who have helped to select the papers presented in this book. He is also grateful to all contributors for their excellent presentations.

The Editor
Malta, 2007

Contents

Section 3: Occupational health

Section 4: Water quality issues

Section 1
Air pollution

Indoor exposure associated risk for eczema in early childhood

O. Herbarth[1,2], G. J. Fritz[2], M. Rehwagen[1], M. Richter[1], S. Röder[1] & U. Schlink[1]
[1]*Department of Human Exposure Research and Epidemiology, Helmholtz-Centre for Environmental Research – UFZ, Germany*
[2]*Environmental Medicine and Environmental Hygiene, Faculty of Medicine, University of Leipzig, Germany*

Abstract

In the development of allergic disorders other factors besides a genetic disposition seem to play a role. Exposure to risk factors such as indoor air pollution is becoming increasingly interesting, especially during early childhood.

Within an epidemiological study involving 2536 children the effect of indoor exposure on allergic symptoms and physician-confirmed eczema has been investigated. The exposure situation has been characterised on hand of the redecoration activities before birth and in the first years of life.

Highly exposed children showed a significant effect on allergic disorders. The lifetime prevalences without any vs. of all three redecoration activities (painting, floor covering and new furniture) were for allergic symptoms 9.3 vs. 17.2% and for eczema 11.5 vs. 20.4%. Adjusted for confounders, the redecoration associated burden led to odds ratios of 1.8 (95%CI: 1.3-2.6) for allergic symptoms and 1.9 (95%CI: 1.4-2.7) for eczema.

Exposure emissions due to redecoration activities seem to be associated with the risk of eczema and allergic symptoms. Thus, prevention of allergic disorders should include the avoidance of such activities around birth and in the first year of life.

Keywords: indoor exposure, allergic disorders, children.

1 Introduction

Besides a genetic predisposition and the controversially-discussed hygiene hypothesis (Strachan [1, 2]), other factors influence the development of allergies

WIT Transactions on Biomedicine and Health, Vol 11, © 2007 WIT Press
www.witpress.com, ISSN 1743-3525 (on-line)
doi:10.2495/EHR070011

in early childhood: food, pollens, etc. and as lately described also indoor chemical pollutants, particularly volatile organic compounds (VOC) (Herbarth and Rehwagen [3], Wolkoff and Nielsen [4]). Important VOC sources are, e.g., smoking and emissions from building materials and furnishings (Samet et al. [5, 6], Cooke [7]). During and following home renovation activities, e.g., painting and/or floor covering, indoor exposure levels can be high. These exposure situations have been found to affect inflammatory processes as well as allergic disorders (Harving et al. [8], Koren et al. [9], Ware et al. [10], Norback et al. [11], Wieslander et al. [12] Diez et al. [13]). Moreover, it remains largely unclear whether a time window exists within which the organism may be especially sensitive to these specific environmental influences. Several studies have investigated the existence of a time period and whether varying factors of influence early in a child's life does lead to an increased incidence of sensitization later in life, including whether prenatal exposure via the mother may have an impact on the offspring. Until now these investigations have been restricted to environmental factors which are able to cause allergies directly above all to allergen exposure (Warner [14] Warner et al. [15, 16]). The effect of possibly indirectly affecting factors – trigger factors – is to a great extent unknown except for smoking. First attempts to clear up the role of indoor chemicals were given by Diez et al. [13] but restricted to risk groups.

The present study is intended not only to contribute to the debate of the extent of chemical noxes being involved in triggering allergen-induced processes but also address the question of timing by examining the influences of pre- and postnatal exposure due to renovation activities.

2 Material and methods

2.1 Study population

The presented investigation is based on the data of an epidemiologic cross-sectional study (LISS study - **L**eipzig **i**nfection, allergy and airway diseases study among **s**chool **s**tarters). The LISS study was carried out during the fall and winter 1997-1998 (birth cohort 1991/92) and included all children of the City of Leipzig and its surrounding county (n=3919) eligible to enter first grade in the fall of 1998 (Table 1). Participation was on a voluntary basis, requiring an informed written consent by both parents/guardian of the children. The study was approved by the ethics committee of the University of Leipzig.

The parents completed a detailed self-administered questionnaire on indoor exposure as well as their family medical history (e.g., physician-diagnosed diseases and symptoms of allergic disease). 2950 parents agreed to fill out this questionnaire. For this investigation, 2536 complete data sets were available (86% of self administered questionnaires).

The study design and methodology have been described in detail elsewhere (Krumbiegel et al. [17], Herbarth et al. [18]).

2.2 Disorders (target variables)

The target variables were lifetime prevalences of physician-diagnosed eczema and physician-diagnosed allergy-associated symptoms. Eczema was selected separately from the allergic symptoms since this manifestation is the earliest sign of an allergic disorder in children's life. The following questions were entered into the analyses: "Has a physician ever diagnosed eczema / endogenous eczema / atopic dermatitis / neurodermatitis in your child? and "At what age was this diagnosis made for the first time?" In addition to these eczema questions, a question pertaining to physician-diagnosed allergic diseases was included: "Has a physician ever diagnosed an allergy in your child?" This question corresponds with questions about the kind of allergy and allergic symptoms and the age at what these symptoms occur at the first time.

2.3 Predisposition

A predisposition was positive when either mother or father suffered from at least one of the following disorders: hay fever, eczema and/or asthma.

2.4 Exposure

To avoid a misclassification of the total exposure the outdoor pollution had been included in the statistical analysis. The main source of outdoor pollution in the investigated area is traffic. Considering earlier experience from epidemiological studies in the same city (Herbarth et al. [19], Fritz and Herbarth [20]) the traffic related exposure in the area of residence was estimated for each participant.

Indoor exposure was assessed based on questionnaire-based information focusing on type of home renovations, time of redecoration, i.e., prenatal (during pregnancy) as well as postnatal (during the first six years of the child's life), with special emphasis on the timing of renovations and the onset of the first overt of allergic symptoms. Exposure maxima are of special interest. Such maximum of indoor exposure is marked by a high emission of potential sources. Temporary sources originate from renovating activities. These activities are associated with high emissions of volatile organic compounds (VOCs). To assess the exposure maximum, three main types of renovations [painting, new floor covering, new furniture] were summed up in a variable called "reno_max". This means that all 3 activities have to be carried out at the same time, then the "reno_max" variable get "yes" otherwise "no".

The time of renovation was given by the parents in the questionnaire. With all this information it was possible to realize whether the activities took place before or after the first onset of the described diseases or symptoms.

2.5 Statistical analysis

The data analysis was performed using Statistica (Statsoft, Inc. 2004, STATISTICA for Windows Vers. 6 [26]). The χ^{2}-test was used to determine the statistical significance of the exposure-associated differences in prevalences.

Logistic regression analyses were applied to calculate the odds ratios (OR) for the association between target variables and indoor exposure linked activities. Odds ratios were adjusted for the following confounders: family history of atopy (FHA defined above), gender, contact to cats, number of older siblings, mother's smoking during pregnancy, smoking in the presence of the child, outdoor exposure (characterised by traffic density in the area of residence) (Fritz and Herbarth [20, 21]).

3 Results

At time of investigation (mean age of children 6.3 ± 0.6 years) (Table 1), the lifetime prevalences were 16.9% for eczema and 12.7% for allergic symptoms manifestations They are shown in Table 2 together with the frequencies of pertinent study parameters.

The control group has been selected considering all families who have not carried out any redecoration activities neither around the birth nor afterwards in the later life time. This concerns 537 study participants (21.2% of the study population). Table 3 shows the frequencies of redecoration activities and the link between different activities, divided in painting, floor covering and new furniture. The reno_max group comprises 936 study participants (36.9% of the study population).

Table 1: Study parameter description.

	N	%
study area		
population	656,878	
total no of 6 to 7 years old children in the area (one birth year)	3,919	
number of involved schools	119	
response		
(A) questionnaire	2,950	75.3 related to 3,919
(B) complete data set concerning all questions relevant for analysis	2,536	85.9 related to (A)
study participants		
mean age [a]	6.3	
female / male	1,257 / 1,279	49.6 / 50.4
participants with older siblings	1,051	41.4

Table 4 shows significantly higher prevalences of both allergic symptoms and diagnosed eczema associated with "reno_max" activities at any time. All cases are counted which take place after reno_max within the first 6 years of life and compared with the control group. The association between "reno_max" and allergic symptoms after adjustment for other possible allergy risk factors are shown in Table 5.

Table 2: Lifetime prevalences of allergic disorders and frequencies of some covariates (data referred to the age of 6.3 years).

ALLERGIC SYMPTOMS and DISEASES		prevalence [%]	n/2536
allergic symptoms (physician diagnosed)		12.7	321
eczema		16.9	428
EXPOSURE		frequency [%]	
OUTDOOR	traffic influenced area	35.7	903
INDOOR	renovation activities		
	painting	49.4	1252
	floor covering	68.8	1775
	new furniture	60.1	1524
no renovation activity of any sort		21.2	537
"reno-max" only: just before birth		22.0	557
	during the 1st year of life	6.5	164
	during the 2nd and 3rd year of life	5.2	131
	from the 4th year of life	3.3	84
PREDISPOSITION	family atopy history	33.8	857

Table 3: Frequencies of redecoration activities.

painting	floor covering	new furniture	
		No	Yes
No	No	21.2 (537) control group	4.7 (119)
No	Yes	10.2 (258)	14.6 (370)
Yes	No	3.4 (86)	3.2 (82)
Yes	Yes	5.8 (148)	36.9 (936) reno_max group

% (N); % refer to the total number of participants (N=2536).

As far as 'timing' of renovations was concerned, the data suggest that the strongest effect was observed when renovations took place just around birth (Figure 1). Only "reno_max" data have been considered in these logistic models adjusted for those variables called in Table 5. Included were 1473 cases (see Table 3, control group and reno_max group). All cases with one or two redecoration activities have been excluded. Apart from the adjusting variables in each of both models 4 variables were included to characterize the redecoration time (before birth, in the first, in the second / third year, in the fourth year of life and later). Both models, for allergic symptoms as well as for eczema, are significant with $p<0.0001$. It should be mentioned again that starting with birth only those cases have been considered for which the exposure takes place before first health effects were seen. In fact, timing showed a definite trend, the earlier in a child's life the renovations were carried out, the greater is the risk to develop allergic disorders later on (Figure 1).

Table 4: Prevalences of allergic disorders depending on extent of renovations (reno_max = wall painting + new floor covering + new furniture).

	prevalence [%]		
	never redecorated[1]	reno_max	p (χ^2)
allergic symptoms	9.3	16.8	<0.0001
eczema	11.5	20.3	<0.0001

[1]never redecorated means not any activity, neither painting nor floor covering nor new furniture; this group of participants is used to be the control group

Table 5: Adjusted Odds Ratios (OR) for allergic disorders depending on at most renovation activities (only cases included without any redecoration activity – internal control group - and with reno_max" activity, not included cases with one or two activities out of painting, floor covering and new furniture; total remaining cases n = 1473 included in the models).

		allergic symptoms		Eczema	
		OR	p	OR	p
parental predisposition		**2.53**	<0.0001	***1.30***	0.0705
sex		**0.71**	0.0251	**0.74**	0.0360
older siblings		1.13	0.4218	***0.76***	0.0594
smoking	during pregnancy	0.93	0.7861	1.28	0.2501
	ETS	1.23	0.2050	**1.49**	0.0073
pets (cat)		***1.33***	0.0590	1.21	0.1784
outdoor exposure (traffic)		1.15	0.3915	0.92	0.9169
indoor exposure (reno_max)		**1.85**	0.0004	**1.95**	<0.0001

Rem: ETS – environmental tobacco smoking (passive smoking); smoking in presence of the child, sex: 0 = male; 1 = female, both models high significant: $p_{model}<0.0001$, trend in italics.

To derive a kind of dose-response relationship the number of activities has been included in the model. The variable "indoor exposure (reno_max)" (Table 5) has been replaced by the number of renovation activities: no activity (control group), 1 or 2 activities and 3 activities (reno_max group). The risk increases per additional activity about 1.27 (95%CI: 1.14 … 1.41; p<0.0001) in the case of allergic symptoms and about 1.21 (95%CI: 1.10 … 1.33; p<0.0001) in the case of eczema. Both models are significant with p<0.0001 and base on n=2536 included cases.

A siblings and birth order effect as reported by Strachan and colleagues [22] was not observed in association with renovation activity among these study participants. Only a trend is visible for eczema and the number of older siblings within the logistic model. It can be suspected that with increasing birth number the renovation activity goes down. This is not the case. The ratio "number of no renovation activities/number of reno_max activities" within the group without older siblings (n=875) is 0.59 and within the group with older siblings (n=598) 0.55.

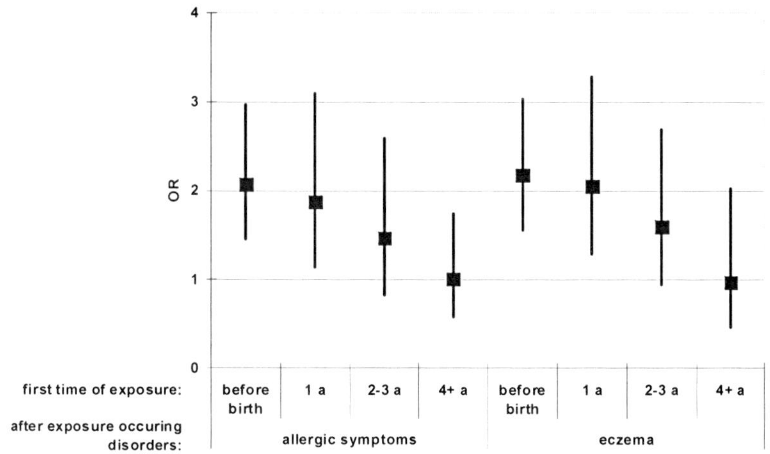

Figure 1: Odds Ratios (OR +/- 95%CI) for allergic disorders depending on the timing of the renovations – reno_max - (in years) and subsequent occurring disorders and symptoms (adjusted for parental predisposition, sex, older siblings, smoking in presence of the child in the first years of life (ETS), smoking during pregnancy, pets (cat), outdoor exposure characterised by traffic). (Rem: redecoration activities in the 1st, 2nd and 3rd, 4th year and later - 1a, 2-3a, 4+a; in both models ($p<0.0001$) considered only reno_max and control group, not considered cases with one or two redecoration activities (see Table 2, $N_{total}=1473$)).

4 Conclusion

This study suggests an influence of residential renovations on allergic disorders. The chemical indoor exposure levels seem to play an important role because of the frequency of renovations which were carried out in the investigated households. 78.8% of all parents in this study redecorate their apartment before birth and in early life of the children, 36.9% carry out all three activities, painting, floor covering and new furniture (Table 3), 28.5% of them before birth and in the first year of life (Table 2). Compared to other lifestyle behaviours, such as smoking (e.g., ETS - environmental tobacco smoking), renovation activities associated indoor exposure leads to the same or to a higher risk in terms of the increase of the odds ratio (Table 5).

The early manifestation of eczema and its role as predictor of respiratory allergic disorders later in life (Bergmann et al. [25]) allocates a special importance on this disorder in defining the timing of any adverse exposure effects, one reason to avoid redecoration associated exposure as well as their level of concentration during pregnancy and the first year of life (Figure 1 and Table 5).

The results of this study confirm the results of the LARS study (Diez et al. [13]). Whereas high risk children were involved in the LARS study the LISS study is population based on 75.3% of all children of one birth year living in the area (Table 1).

Considering the "hygiene-hypothesis" (Strachan [1, 2]) a strong sibling effect was not observed. A birth order effect on the frequency of the renovation activity was not observed as well.

Several limitations need to be considered. First, the presented results base on questionnaire data. The questions have been answered by the parents when the children were 6 years old. Secondly, regarding the symptoms and/or diseases the parents were asked to put down on the questionnaire physician diagnosed symptoms and/or diseases only. Results of newborn cohort studies which are carried out in the same area come to similar results concerning the frequency of redecoration activities and prevalence's (Herbarth et al. [23], Diez et al [13], Zutavern et al [24]). In these studies the information of redecoration activities and of health effects has been collected immediately.

However, the study has several notable strengths. First, the study sample size is very large. No comparative study with respect to the population size is known which addressed the topic we deal with especially concerning indoor air quality. Second, the study participants have been recruited from one birth year.

It can be concluded that extensive renovations during pregnancy, especially around the time of birth, and during the first year of life seem to affect the development of allergic disorders. These findings should be considered like active and passive smoking by general practitioners or specialists when they advice prospective parents, especially expectant mothers, on the "dos and don'ts" during and after pregnancy. Avoidance of such activities particularly by parents themselves affected by atopy would be an effective measure of prevention. In fact, in contrast to smoking (active and passive smoking), this prevention measure may be more effective, since the risk is greater, it is easier to achieve and avoidance of such activities (renovation, floor covering or painting) involve no personal consequences (e.g., habit and withdrawal symptoms).

The complexity of the problem will gain in importance since legislative measures to conserve energy will continue which indirectly will affect the air indoors. The reduction in air exchange between in- and outdoor will lead to elevated concentrations of noxious substances and an increasing indoor air problem.

Acknowledgements

The study was supported by the BMBF - Federal Ministry of Education and Research of Germany, the UFZ – Centre for Environmental Research Leipzig-Halle and the State Ministry of Family and Health of Saxony.

The authors wish to thank the children and their parents as well as the staff of the local public health departments for their excellent cooperation in carrying out the field study. We are also indebted to our co-workers of the LISS Study Team for the field work in the schools.

Parts of this paper have been published in Int J Hyg Environ Health 209 (2006) 241-247. The authors thank the publisher Elsevier for the possibility to republish parts of the published article.

References

[1] Strachan, D.P.: Hay fever, hygiene, and household size. B.M.J. 299, 1259-60 (1989).

[2] Strachan, D.P.: Family size, infection and atopy: the first decade of the "hygiene hypothesis". Thorax 55(Suppl 1), 2-10 (2000).

[3] Herbarth, O., Rehwagen, M.: VOCs - Investigation into Outdoor and Indoor Exposure: Initial results. Umweltmed. Forsch. Prax. 3:281-286 (1998).

[4] Wolkoff, P., Nielsen, G.D.: Organic compounds in indoor air - their relevance for perceived indoor air quality. Atmos. Environ. 4407-4417 (2001).

[5] Samet, J.M., Marbury, M.C., Spengler, J.D.: Health effects and sources of indoor air pollution. Part I. Am. Rev. Respir. Dis. 136, 1486-1508 (1987).

[6] Samet, J.M., Marbury, M.C., Spengler, J.D.: Health effects and sources of indoor air pollution. Part II. Am. Rev. Respir. Dis. 137, 221-242 (1988).

[7] Cooke, T.F.: Indoor air pollutants. A literature review. Rev. Environ. Health 9, 137-160 (1991).

[8] Harving, H., Dahl, R., Mølhave, L.: Lung function and bronchial reactivity in asthmatics during exposure to volatile organic compounds. Am. Rev. Respir. Dis. 143, 751-754 (1991).

[9] Koren, H.S., Graham, D.E., Devlin, R.B.: Exposure of humans to volatile organic mixture. III. Inflammatory response. Arch. Environ. Health 47: 39-44 (1992).

[10] Ware, J.H., Spengler, J.D., Neas, L.M., Samet, J.M., Wagner, G.R., Coultas, D., Ozkaynak, H., Schwab, M.: Respiratory and irritant health effects of ambient volatile organic compounds. The Kanawaha County Health Study. Am. J. Epidemiol. 137, 1287-1301 (1993).

[11] Norbäck, D., Björnsson, E., Janson, C., Widström, J., Boman, G.: Asthmatic symptoms and volatile organic compounds, formaldehyde, and carbon dioxide in dwellings. Occup. Environ. Med. 52, 388-395 (1995).

[12] Wieslander, G., Norback, D., Bjornsson, E., Janson, C., Boman, G.: Asthma and the indoor environment: the significance of emission of formaldehyde and volatile organic compounds from newly painted indoor surfaces. Int. Arch. Occup. Environ. Health 69, 115-124 (1997).

[13] Diez, U., Kroessner, T., Rehwagen, M., Richter, M., Wetzig, H., Schulz, R., Borte, M., Metzner, G., Krumbiegel, P., Herbarth, O.: Effects of indoor painting and smoking on airway symptoms in atopy risk children in the first year of life: results of the LARS-study. Leipzig Allergy High-Risk Children Study. Int. J. Hyg. Environ. Health 203:23-28 (2000).

[14] Warner, J.A.: Primary sensitization in infants. Ann. Allergy Asthma Immunol. 83(5), 426-30 (1999).

[15] Warner, J.A., Warner, J.O.: Early life events in allergic sensitization. Br .Med. Bull. 56(4), 883-893 (2000).
[16] Warner, J.A., Jones, C.A., Jones, A.C., Warner, J.O.: Prenatal origins of allergic disease. J. Allergy Clin. Immunol. 105, 493-498 (2000).
[17] Krumbiegel, P., Herbarth, O., Fritz, G.J., Schlink, U., Gutsmuths, F.-J., Kindler, A., Richter, T.: Helicobacter pylori prevalence in Leipzig's 1998 school entries: methodology and first results. Int. J. Hyg. Environ. Health 203:11-16 (2000).
[18] Herbarth, O., Fritz, G.J., Krumbiegel, P., Diez, U., Franck, U., Richter, M.: Effect of sulfur dioxide and particulate pollutants on bronchitis in children -- a risk analysis. Environ .Toxicol. 16(3), 269-276 (2001).
[19] Herbarth, O., Fritz, G.J., Diez, U., Rehwagen, M., Borte, M., Schulz, R., Richter, M., Krumbiegel, P., Müller, A.: Effect of volatile organic compounds in- and outdoors on allergies. 619-628. In Air Pollution VI. Ed. C.A. Brebbia, C.F. Ratto, H. Power. WIT Press Boston, Southampton (1998)
[20] Fritz, G.J., Herbarth, O.: Pulmonary function and urban air pollution in preschool children. Int. J. Hyg. Environ. Health 203, 235-244 (2001).
[21] Fritz, G.J., Herbarth, O.: Asthmatic disease among urban preschoolers: an observational study. Int. J. Hyg. Environ. Health 207, 23-30 (2004).
[22] Strachan, D.P., Harkins, L.S., Johnston, I.D., Anderson, H.R.: Childhood antecedents of allergic sensitization in young British adults. J. Allergy Clin. Immunol. 99, 6-12 (1997).
[23] Herbarth, O., Fritz, G.J., Behler, JC., Rehwagen, M., Puliafito, J.L., Richter, M., Schlink, U., sernaglia, J., Puliafito, E., Puliafito, C., Schilde, M., Wildführ, W.: Epidemiologic risk analysis of environmental attributed exposure on airway diseases and allergies in children. Centr. Eur. F. publ. Health 7, 2, 72-76 (1999)
[24] Zutavern, A., Brockow, I., Schaaf, B., Bolte, G., von Berg, A., Diez, U., Borte, M., Herbarth, O., Wichmann, H.E., Heinrich, J.: Timing of solid food introduction in relation to atopic dermatitis and sensitation considering reverse causality: results from a prospective birth cohort study. Pediatrics 117(2) 401-411 (2006)
[25] Bergmann, R.L., Edenharter, G., Bergmann, K.E., Forster, J., Bauer, C.P., Wahn, V., Zepp, F., Wahn, U.: Atopic dermatitis in early infancy predicts allergic airway disease at 5 years. Clin. Exp. Allergy 28(8), 965-970 (1998).
[26] StatSoft, Inc. STATISTICA für Windows [Software-System für Datenanalyse] Version 6. www.statsoft.com, 2001.

The case of atmospheric pollution using production waste in a building materials factory: an applied industrial case

F. Patania, A. Gagliano, F. Nocera, A. Galesi & A. D'Amico
Energy and Environment Division of DIIM,
Engineering Faculty of University of Catani, Italy

Abstract

The disposal of dangerous or special waste by combustion represents significant global atmospheric pollution even though emission limits do tend to curb greenhouse gases.

The hazardous industrial waste must be treated, stored or disposed of utilizing a large amount of energy and petroleum. So the use of such waste as a 'raw material' in the production of building materials not only reduces the waste to dispose of, but also the emission of atmospheric pollutants.

On this basis, research into the facilities of the DB Group (a large brick producer) has brought about a change in the raw materials used in production by using about 20% waste products without any significant variation in the end product.

Considering the above, this study wants to show: 1. the plant modifications to allow mixed raw material input; 2. the environmental control techniques used; 3. the beneficial results for atmospheric pollution.
Keywords: pollution, reuse, waste production.

1 Generality

The DB Group is a brick producer and utilizes low volumes of fly ash generated from the Enel Power Station as a raw material to substitute for a part of the clay and shale, which are the two main raw materials of a conventional brick

The development and marketing of commercial bricks that contain dry and pond fly ash and other waste should benefit the Enel Power Station and the brick

WIT Transactions on Biomedicine and Health, Vol 11, © 2007 WIT Press
www.witpress.com, ISSN 1743-3525 (on-line)
doi:10.2495/EHR070021

manufacturer by reducing the disposal of waste by-products and providing an economical brick ingredient

Although the incorporation of waste in fired brick has previously been studied worldwide using various formulations and different fly ash, there are no reported studies on using Enel Power Station fly ash.

So the authorities wanted to know the environmental impacts of the technology that was adopted by the DB Group brick industry. They were especially interested to know how the raw material influenced the atmospheric emissions of the brick manufacture stacks.

We know that models are useful tools to utilize when estimating environmental impacts from development projects and setting up proper mitigation policies of the Environment Impact Assessment.

Especially with regard to air quality, models are indispensable tools for evaluation. Thus, the selection and application of proper models is one of the most important factors for making reliable and accurate assessments.

The purpose of this study is to quantitatively evaluate the impacts and the atmospheric emissions of a brick manufacture both with the application of the US-EPA Industrial Source Complex Model (ISC) and measurements campaign.

2 The investigated area

The DB Group is located in the industrial area of Adrano, which is a little town in Sicily. It is situated around 41 km northwest of Catania, which is also the capital of the province to which Adrano belongs. It lies near the foot of Mount Etna, at the confluence of the Simeto and Salso Rivers.

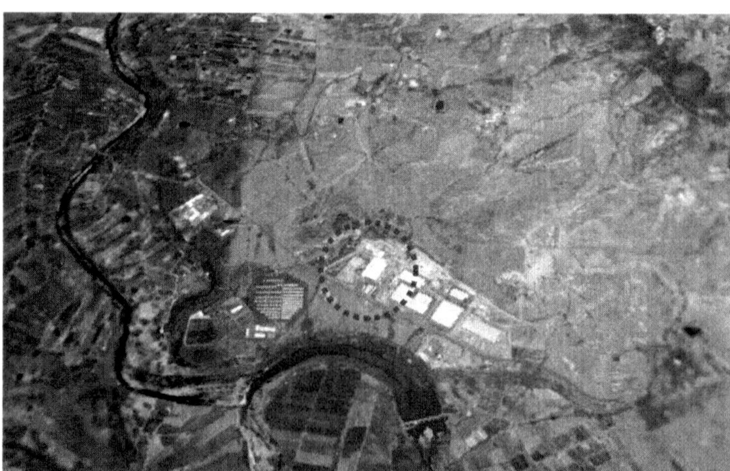

Figure 1: Investigated area.

3 Process description

Although the basic principles of manufacture are fairly uniform, individual manufacturing plants tailor their production to fit their particular raw materials and operation. Essentially, bricks are produced by mixing ground clay with water, forming the clay into the desired shape, and then drying and firing the bricks. In our case the manufacturing process has six general phases: mining and storage of raw materials, preparing raw materials, forming the brick, drying, firing and cooling and de-hacking and storing finished products.

Surface clays, shales and some fire clays are mined in open pits with power equipment. Then the clay or shale mixtures, with other non-dangerous waste coming from other industries, are transported to an open plant storage area bordered by trees. Furthering that, raw materials are wet by several sprinklers to avoid the dispersions of particulate matters in the atmosphere. The hazardous fly ash is transported from the Power Station to a closed plant area where the bad smells are controlled by suitable filters.

Bricks are made of 65% clay, 25% non-dangerous waste and 10% hazardous fly ash. Before the firing process begins, most of the water, contained in the bricks, is evaporated in dryer chambers at temperatures ranging from 38°C to 204°C. The dryer chambers are heated with waste heat from the kiln cooling zone and have supplemental gas burners that produce small amounts of NOx, CO, and CO_2 emissions. It is important to evaluate emission concentration coming from n.13 stacks of dryer chambers because they could exceed the Air Quality Standards. Bricks are then fired in a tunnel kiln heated by a 2 MW CHP plant.

4 Emissions

Emissions from brick manufacturing facilities include particulate matter (PM), PM less than or equal to 10 microns in aerodynamic diameter (PM-10), PM less than or equal to 2.5 microns in aerodynamic diameter (PM-2.5) sulfur dioxide (SO_2), sulfur trioxide (SO_3), nitrogen oxides (NOx), carbon monoxide (CO), carbon dioxide (CO_2), metals, total organic compounds (TOC) (including methane, ethane, volatile organic compounds (VOC), and some hazardous air pollutants (HAP)), hydrochloric acid (HCl), and fluoride compounds.

Factors that may affect emissions include raw material composition and moisture content, kiln fuel type, kiln operating parameters, and plant design. The primary sources of PM, PM-10, and PM-2.5 emissions are the raw material grinding and screening operations and the kilns. Combustion products, including SO_2, NOx, CO, and CO_2, are emitted from fuel combustion in brick kilns and some brick dryers. Organic compounds, including methane, ethane, VOC, and some HAP, are emitted from both brick dryers and kilns. Hydrogen fluoride (HF) and other fluoride compounds are emitted from kilns as a result of the release of the fluorine compounds contained in the raw material.

Fluorine typically is present in raw brick materials in the range of 0.01 to 0.06 percent. As the green bricks reach temperatures of 500°C to 600°C, the fluorine in the raw material forms HF and other fluorine compounds. Much of the fluorine is released as HF. Because fluorine content in clays and shales is highly variable, emissions of HF and other fluoride compounds vary considerably depending on the raw material used.

5 ISC3-model

The US-EPA Industrial Source Complex Model (ISC), originally developed over 20 years ago by the US-EPA, is now in its third version (ISC3). There are two versions of ISC3, a short-term model (ISCST3) and a long-term model (ISCLT3). The models differ in the averaging times available for calculation, available terrain and deposition options, and the format of input meteorological data. The ISC3 algorithm is regularly updated by the US-EPA and can be obtained free via the Internet from the US-EPA's website. The basic "free to all" ISC3 model is not as easy to use in terms of the user interface and digitisation of input data, but several software companies have produced proprietary programmes that incorporate the ISC3 model with a user-friendly GUI that simplifies the data entry and checking procedures. An example is the Breeze Air ISC3 model, by Trinity Consultants Inc. (USA), which is utilized to evaluate the atmospheric emissions of the brick manufacture.

An interesting feature of ISC3 is the characterisation of a new source type "Open Pit Sources", for modelling dry deposition of particulates from open pit sources. ISC3 also includes both states of the science dry and wet deposition algorithms. This kind of feature of ISC3 is useful to evaluate the emissions of the plant storage area of the brick manufacture. Dispersion models require a number of user specified input parameters. Some of these may vary with each type of model scenario; others rarely require alterations and shouldn't be changed from the model default. The most significant and commonly used model parameters include the following:

- Dispersion coefficients (i.e. land use classification, rural or urban)
- Plume rise
- Building wake effects
- Terrain effects
- Surface roughness
- Wind direction and wind speed
- Receptor grids.

The type of dispersion coefficient used can have a significant impact on dispersion model predictions. The standard procedure for determining whether rural or urban classification is more appropriate to classify the land use within a 3 km radius circle about the source. If more than 50% of this area is urban then urban dispersion coefficients should be used, otherwise rural coefficients should be used. In our case then rural coefficients was used. The effects of plume rise, which can be simulated by ISC3 include:

- No buoyancy induced dispersion
- Gradual plume rise

- Partial penetration of inversion layers
- No stack tip downwash.

We have taken into account both gradual plume rise and partial penetration of inversion layers. ISC3 have inbuilt algorithms to simulate the effects of building wakes and we have utilized a programme called BPIP (available on the Internet at the US-EPA's website) to determine the necessary parameters for downwash algorithms. This programme works out what obstacle dimensions are appropriate as a function of wind direction. Output from BPIP was incorporated into both ISC3

6 The simulation data

As shown in figure 2 the chosen domain of calculus, in Cartesian coordinates, has the following dimensions:

X direction	Y direction	Z direction
3.300 m	3.300 m	150 m

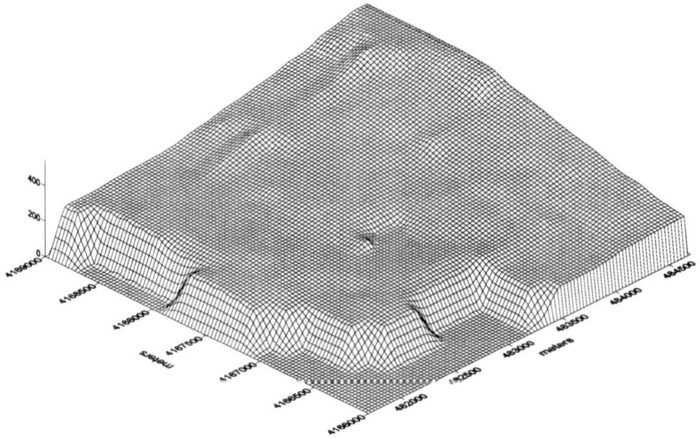

Figure 2: 3D-domain.

The domain is characterized by a grid with dimensions of 150m x 150m, n.158 buildings, n.16 point sources emissions and n.1 area source emission.

People modelled terrain and buildings both by the available cartography at scale 1:2000 and by inspections carried out in the area. Authors adopted particulate matter (PM) and sulfur dioxide (SO_2) as tracer gases, to valuate the atmospheric emissions and the air quality impacts. ISC3 requires hourly meteorological data to estimate plume dispersion. According to EPA's *Guideline on Air Quality Models*, five years of adequately representative data should be used (when available) to account for year-to year variation. The model simulation has been done with the data coming from the Agrometereological Station of Sicily Environmental Department that is located 5 kilometers (km) west of Adrano. The meteo input is based on hourly data of flow vector, wind speed, ambient temperature, stability class, rural mixing height and urban mixing height recorded by the Meteoclimatic Station from 1st January 2006 to 15th November 2006

The authors take into account three possible scenarios: the bricks are made without fly ash; with 10% hazardous fly ash; and with the maximum rate of hazardous fly ash allowed by air quality regulation. The emission sources characteristics are shown in tables 1, 2 and 3.

Table 1: Emission sources scenario without fly ash.

	Air Flow Nm^3/h	SO_2 mg/Nm^3	PM C mg/Nm^3	Temp K	Velocity m/s
Stack n.1 – 13 (dryer chambers)	15679	100	7	313	17.4
Stack n.14 (kiln)	34650	100	5	378	9.5
Stack n.15-16 (preparing raw materials)	-	-	-	288	5

Table 2: Emission sources scenario with 10% hazardous fly ash.

	Air Flow Nm^3/h	SO_2 mg/Nm^3	PM mg/Nm^3	Temp K	Velocity m/s
Stack n.1 – 13 (dryer chambers)	15679	100	7	313	17.4
Stack n.14 (kiln)	34650	100	5	378	9.5
Stack n.15-16 (preparing raw materials)	18000-	-	5	288	5

Table 3: Emission sources scenario with the maximum rate of hazardous fly ash.

	Air Flow Nm^3/h	SO_2 mg/Nm^3	PM mg/Nm^3	Temp K	Velocity m/s
Stack n.1 – 13 (dryer chambers)	15679	500	50	313	17.4
Stack n.14 (kiln)	34650	500	50	378	9.5
Stack n.15-16 (preparing raw materials)	18000-	-	50	288	5

7 Results

Figures 3 through 8 are maps that show examples of results of calculations of the maximum hourly concentration of PM and SO_2.

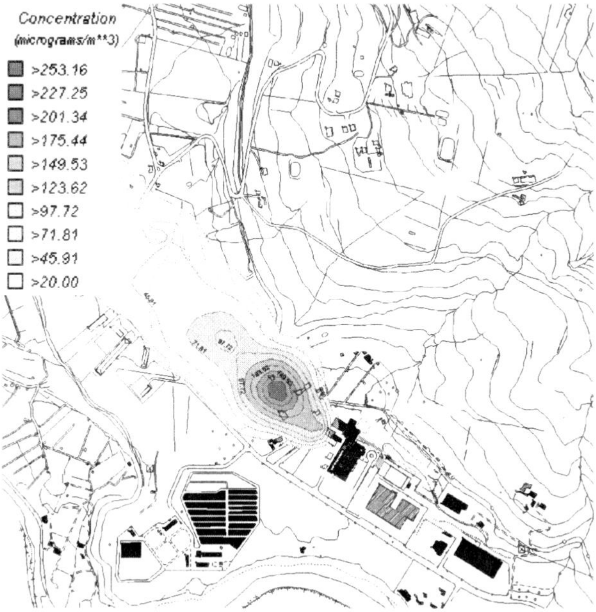

Figure 3: Scenario 1 – iso-concentration - SO_2 – V= 1.3 m/s – Dir: 135°.

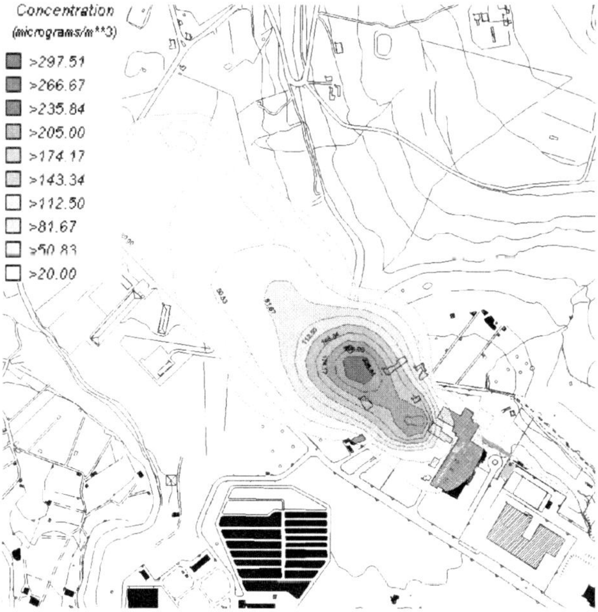

Figure 4: Scenario 2 – iso-concentration - SO_2 – V= 1.3 m/s – Dir: 135°.

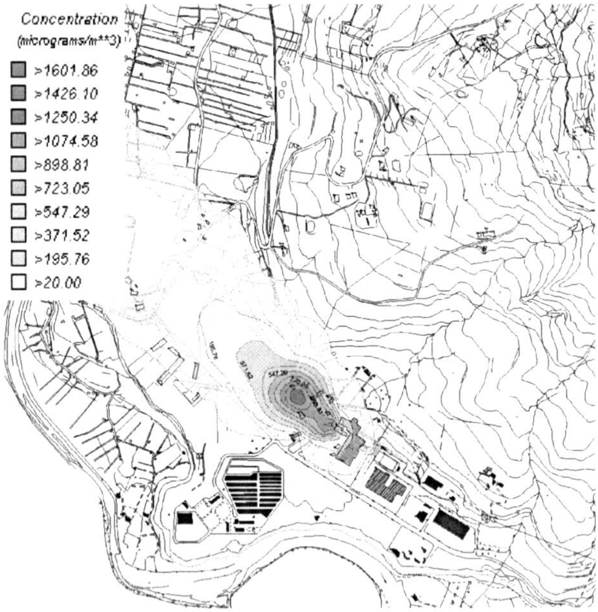

Figure 5: Scenario 3 – iso-concentration - SO_2 – V= 1.3 m/s – Dir: 135°.

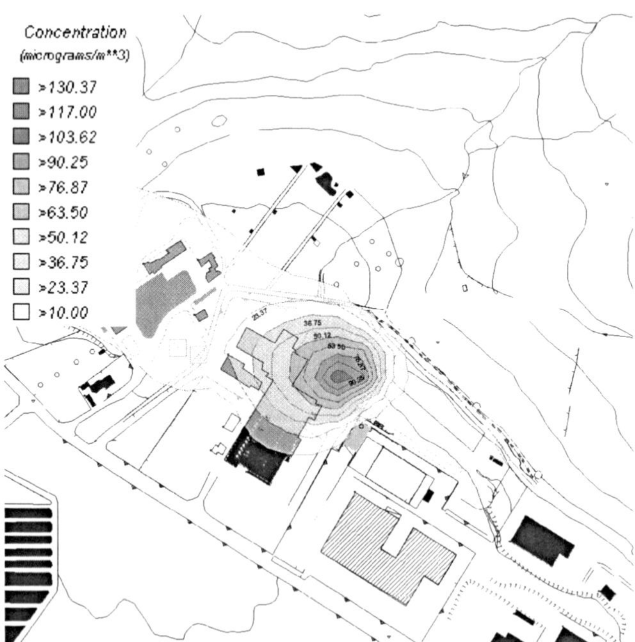

Figure 6: Scenario 1 – iso-concentration - PM– V= 1.3 m/s – Dir: 135°.

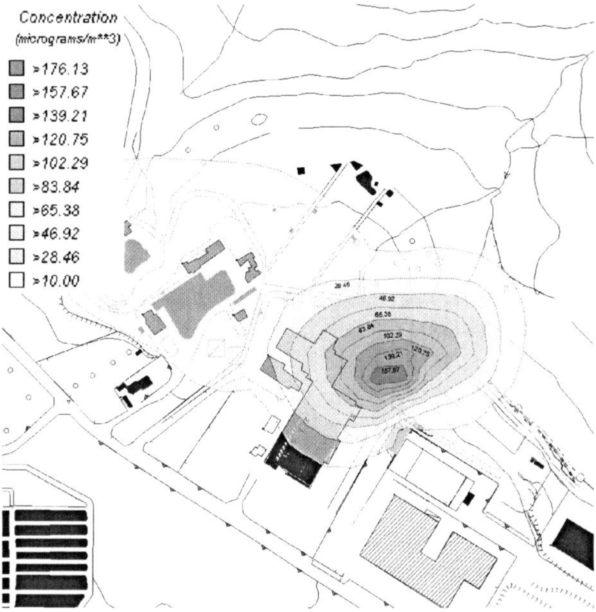

Figure 7: Scenario 2 – iso-concentration - PM – V= 1.3 m/s – Dir: 135°.

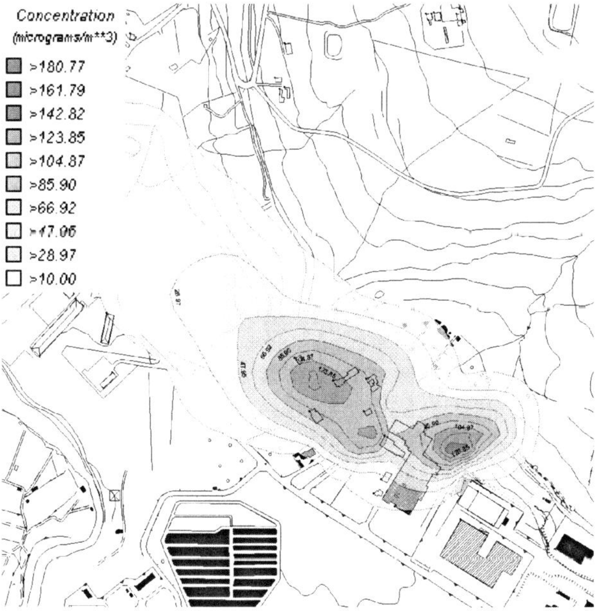

Figure 8: Scenario 3 – iso- concentration - PM – V= 1.3 m/s – Dir: 135°.

8 Control systems

So in the case of the maximum rate of hazards utilized by manufacture it needs to apply a variety of control systems, which may be used to reduce emissions from brick manufacturing operations. Grinding and screening operations must be controlled by fabric filtration systems. Particulate matter emissions from fugitive sources such as paved roads, unpaved roads, and storage piles can be controlled using wet suppression techniques (sprinklers). Dry scrubbers that use limestone as a sorption medium may be used to control HF emissions. Applying the previous control systems the values of polluting emissions, also utilizing maximum rates of hazardous fly ash, may be re-established to the acceptable values with the reference to an industrial area

9 Conclusions

From analysis of the plot of the concentration value it is possible to underline the following results:

- The reusing of low volumes of fly ash in the amount reported by the manufacture doesn't significantly increase the emission of SO_2 in atmosphere.
- The PM emission in the atmosphere, due the raw material grinding and screening operations and the kilns, indeed it increases by about 25%, however below the limit allowed by air quality regulation
- If the brick's manufacture process utilizes the maximum rate of hazardous fly ash allowed by air quality regulation, certainly the SO_2 and PM concentrations will achieve values upper than those ones tolerable by human health. In that case it needs to apply a variety of control systems to reduce emissions from brick manufacturing operations, such as: grinding and screening operations must be controlled by fabric filtration systems; particulate matter emissions coming from fugitive sources such as paved pr unpaved rods, storage piles and so on must be carefully controlled by wet suppression techniques (sprinklers); control of HF Emissions must be done by dry scrubbers using limestone as sorption medium.

Applying the previous control systems the values of polluting emissions, caused by application of maximum rates of hazardous fly ash, may be reestablished to the acceptable values with the reference to an industrial area. Moreover, and in a more simple way, the use of "raw materials", in building materials production, could be done without dangerous effects to human health if the local authorities consent such kind of processes only underneath the conditions to fix the rate of hazardous materials that can be utilized in the function of both the real status of air pollution in the situ of factory and the more unfavorable meteoclimatic condition for gas dispersion.

References

[1] Industrial Source Complex (ISCST3) model, EPA modeling guidelines

[2] F. Patania, A. Gagliano, F. Nocera, A. Galesi, A. Belluardo, The environmental control of air pollution by emission of gases coming from refineries through flow-dynamics modeling: an experimental feasibility test Air Pollution XIII, Editors C.A. Brebbia. L.C. WIT Press (UK). (2005) pp 22-33

Indoor air quality in old and new schools

K. Rumchev, R. Ourangui, D. Bertolatti & J. Spickett
School of Public Health, Curtin University of Technology, Perth, Australia

Abstract

It has been demonstrated that air pollution is associated with a wide variety of health impacts in humans, especially among the elderly and children. In this preliminary study the exposure levels of formaldehyde, particulate matter with a size less than 2.5 μm in diameter ($PM_{2.5}$), number of ultra fine particles as well as indoor temperature and relative humidity were measured in six primary schools (three old and three new schools). A total of 20 classrooms were monitored twice a week, at the beginning and at the end of the week. The aim of this study was to compare exposure levels to selected indoor air pollutants between old and new schools located within the Perth metropolitan area, Western Australia. According to the findings the formaldehyde levels were higher than maximum permissible levels recommended by NHMRC in 45% of samples in old schools and 67% of the samples in new schools. In regards to $PM_{2.5}$ concentrations, most samples were lower than the WHO guideline value of 25 μg/m^3 (24 hour exposure). In terms of ultra fine particles, generally old schools had a higher number of ultrafine particles.
Keywords: indoor air quality, formaldehyde, particulate matter, school.

1 Introduction

Indoor air quality has become a matter of growing global concern over the last thirty years. Recent research indicates that there is a relationship between respiratory disease including asthma and indoor air pollution [1]. Children are generally more susceptible to the effects of air pollution [2] especially particulate pollution [3], because their bodies are growing, and their developmental processes, especially in the lungs, may well be affected by air pollution [1]. Children experience higher exposures to environmental pollutants than adults because, per kg of body weight, they breathe a greater volume of air and ingest

WIT Transactions on Biomedicine and Health, Vol 11, © 2007 WIT Press
www.witpress.com, ISSN 1743-3525 (on-line)
doi:10.2495/EHR070031

more material than adults. Children also absorb contaminants more readily. Indoor air quality (IAQ) problems in schools are a significant public health concern. Apart from the home, school is the most important indoor environment for children aged 6-16 in determining pollutant and allergen exposure, as they would spend a significant portion of their lives (about one third or more) in school buildings. Some children may stay in a school setting up to 10 hours per day, at least 1100 hours per year. By the time they finish high school, they would have spent at least 14000 hours breathing the air inside school buildings [2,4]. This may indicate that indoor air quality in schools could have a substantial impact on children's health, thus preventing or reducing exposure to pollutants and allergens in school environment plays an important role in the health of school age children [5].

2 Methodology

Environmental monitoring study was conducted in randomly selected government primary schools located within the Perth Metropolitan area. The old schools are defined as those built in the late 1800s to early 1900s and the new schools built post 1985. In each school 3 or 4 classrooms were selected and all were used frequently and were occupied most of the day by the same group of students aged between 4 and 8. All rooms were monitored twice (once at the beginning and once at the end of the week) for 8 hours which would allow detection of any variations through out the day. A total of 20 classrooms were monitored for formaldehyde, particulate matter with size 2.5 mn in diameter ($PM_{2.5}$) and number of ultrafine particles per cubic centimetre. Temperature, relative humidity and air velocity were also measured. Information on heating, air conditioning and ventilation system was collected for each school and studied classrooms. Size and volume of classrooms were also measured and information related to the presence of furniture, materials, fabrics and shelves were collected. All classrooms were also examined for the presence of damp, mould or any unpleasant smell. Information regarding cleaning routines was collected from cleaning staff. Information about ambient temperature and relative humidity was obtained from the Australian Bureau of Meteorology.

2.1 Indoor air monitoring

Measurements of formaldehyde were conducted using the passive sampling method described by Levin et al., which utilizes passive diffusers containing acidified 2, 4-dinitrophenylhydrazine (DNPH) followed by analysis using the high-performance liquid chromatography (HPLC) [6].

$PM_{2.5}$ was measured using the Model 8520 DUST TRAK™ Aerosol Monitors with 2.5 μm inlet conditioner with corresponding impactor plate. Measurements from the DUSTTRAK™ were recorded as a mass concentration ($\mu m/m^3$).

P-TRAK Ultra fine Particle Counter (UPC) Model 8525 was used to measure the number of ultra fine particles per cubic centimetre (pt/cc).

Tinytag-ultra Data Logger which is a battery operated device was used to measure indoor temperature and relative humidity for 8 hours periods.

AIR VELOCITY METER MODEL 441M was used to measure air flow through open doors and windows. Kurz Instruments Series 400 is highly accurate instruments for measuring air velocity and static pressure in heating, ventilation, and air-conditioning (HVAC) applications.

AIR FLOW DVA 30VT anemometer was used to measure the air flow through open doors and windows. This instrument is a rotating vane anemometer with digital readout of air velocity.

3 Statistical consideration

Statistical analyses were performed with SPSS for Windows, version 14. Transformations were applied when the data did not follow normal distributions. Student t-tests, bivariate correlation and Chi-square test were employed to explore differences and associations between variables. In all statistical analysis, two-tailed tests were used and a 5% level of significance was applied.

4 Results

4.1 General

Six primary schools within the Perth Metropolitan area participated in this study.

All classrooms had air conditioning, gas heaters, ceiling fans and a number of natural vents on walls or the ceiling. Old schools had floor boards, mostly carpeted. The floor covering in new schools was a combination of vinyl and carpet ranging from 25% to 100% carpeting. However, there was a higher percentage of carpeting in old schools with over 90% of floor areas were fully carpeted while in new schools just over 70% of the floors were carpeted.

The results showed that the classrooms in new schools had larger room area than the old schools and the difference was significant ($p<0.01$). Also, it appeared that old school had bigger black board areas in comparison to new schools ($p<0.05$).

4.2 Indoor air quality in classrooms

The median concentration of formaldehyde in new schools was 148 $\mu g/m^3$ and was higher than those measured in old schools of 103 $\mu g/m^3$ although the difference was not statistically significant. In old schools 45% of the samples had higher formaldehyde levels than the maximum permissible level in Australia of 120 $\mu g/m^3$, while in new schools 67% of the samples were over these levels (Table 1).

In regards to particulate matter, the median concentrations of $PM_{2.5}$ in both schools were low and didn't exceed the WHO guideline value of 25 $\mu g/m^3$ (24h exposure) (Table 1). Only one classroom from the new and one from the old schools had values higher that 25 $\mu g/m^3$.

Table 1: Median (range) levels of formaldehyde (HCHO), $PM_{2.5}$, RH (%) and T°C for old and new schools.

	HCHO μg/m^3	$PM_{2.5}$ μg/m^3	RH (%)	T (°C)
New	148.37 (12.92-287.87)	10 (4 – 42)	55.0 (38.7-73.5)	23.0 (19.95-24.1)
Old	103.16 (5.67-305)	11 (4-37)	51.9 (39.4-62.7)	19.7 (17-22.1)
p value	**0.302**	**0.164**	**0.634**	**0.000**

Table 2: Median (range) levels of formaldehyde (HCHO), $PM_{2.5}$, RH (%) and T°C in classrooms with open and closed windows.

Windows and doors	**HCHO μg/m^3**	**$PM_{2.5}$ μg/m^3**	**UFP/cc**	**RH (%)**	**T (°C)**
closed	**108.4 (5.7-213.7)**	**10 (4 – 22)**	**12945**	**55.0 (38.7-73.5)**	**23.0 (19.95-24.1)**
open	**158.3 (9.5-305)**	**14.8 (5-42)**	**14263**	**51.9 (39.4-62.7)**	**19.7 (17-22.1)**
p value	**0.04**	**0.05**	**0.44**	**0.35**	**0.80**

As can be seen from Table 1, the indoor temperature and relative humidity were higher in new schools when compared with those in old schools and the difference was significant for temperature.

The number of UFP was higher (14158/cc) in the afternoon when compared to the number recorded in the morning (11748/cc). Additionally, the number of UFP was higher in old schools 16922/cc when compared to new schools 12128/cc and the difference was marginally significant ($p=0.06$). This is in agreement with the measured outdoor number of UFP as the number was higher outside the old schools (22790/cc) when compared with the new schools (9000/cc). Furthermore, the results show that children were exposed to higher number of UFP at the beginning of the week (14481/cc) when compared to the end of the week when the number of UFP dropped to 12770/cc.

4.3 Factors contributing to the concentrations of indoor air pollutants

In the present study exposure levels of $PM_{2.5}$ were significantly correlated with the number of UFP ($r=0.34$; $p<0.05$) and also with indoor relative humidity ($r=0.553$; $p<0.01$). Further to this, concentrations of $PM_{2.5}$, and formaldehyde were significantly increased when windows and doors were open (Table 2).

Although relative humidity, temperature and number of UFP were also affected by open windows and doors the differences were not significant when compared with rooms with closed windows and doors.

Indoor concentrations of $PM_{2.5}$ were significantly affected by the size of the blackboard as larger blackboard increased significantly the measured levels of $PM_{2.5}$ ($p=0.05$). It appears that old schools had a significantly ($p<0.01$) larger blackboard surface area (4.6 m^2) compared to those in new schools (1.6 m^2). In addition, significantly ($p<0.01$) more classrooms in old schools (90%) had carpet compared to 70% in new schools. However, the presence of carpet in classrooms didn't affect the measured levels of formaldehyde and particulate matter.

There was a significant correlation between formaldehyde levels and the average air exchange rate ($r=0.310$, $p=0.050$), with air velocity through openings ($r=0.334$, $p=0.035$).

The median indoor relative humidity in new schools was higher at 55% (38.7-73.5) when compared to the old schools at 51.8% (39.4-62.7). The median indoor temperature was 23°C (19.9-24.1) for new schools and 19.7°C (17.0-22.1) for old schools with a significant difference ($p=0.000$). However, both the temperature and relative humidity were within the recommended values suggested by ASHRAE [7].

5 Discussion

Indoor air pollution has been identified to be affecting children's health worldwide. Air pollutants usually enter the body through the respiratory tract. Environmental irritants such as formaldehyde have been associated with respiratory symptoms including asthma [8,9].

The current study was carried out in schools as children spend a large portion of their daily life at school where they come in contact with air pollutants through their lungs, eyes and skin. Good air quality in classrooms not only favours children's learning ability but also affects teacher and staff's productivity [10]. Concentrations of particulate matter and formaldehyde were compared between old and new schools located in Perth, Western Australia. Relative humidity, temperature and the number of ultrafine particles were also measured in each classroom. Due to time and resource restrictions, the number of schools which participated in the study was limited which is considered as a limitation of the study and it is acknowledged by the authors.

In order to reduce selection bias, the school locations were chosen within the same distance from the coast, all with a reasonable proximity to each other, with brick structures, containing the same furniture, have similar cleaning agents and routines, and all have similar activities performed as all were government schools. All schools were located away from industry and busy road.

Overall the formaldehyde concentrations measured in the present study were high as the median formaldehyde levels in some classes were higher than 120 $\mu g/m^3$ in both old and new schools, which is the current National Health and Medical Research Council (NHMRC) recommended guideline value for formaldehyde [11], and higher than the WHO threshold of 100 $\mu g/m^3$ [12].

These findings are not consistent with the findings established in the study of Seppänen et al [13] where the formaldehyde levels were below the detection limit of 5 $\mu g/m^3$, and in a study of Lee and Chang [14] where the formaldehyde levels ranged from undetectable to 27 $\mu g/m^3$. In the present study, higher number of new schools (67%) had higher concentrations of formaldehyde compared to the old schools (45%) which is consistent with the findings of Newton [15]. This may be due to a number of factors including the new materials and furniture in the new buildings.

Indoor concentrations of $PM_{2.5}$ were low as in new schools it ranged between 4-42 $\mu g/m^3$ and in old schools between 4-37 $\mu g/m^3$. These findings are consistent with that reported by Rumchev et al [16].

Guidelines for particulate matter have been undergoing a period of revision, as information regarding potential health impacts at lower levels has emerged. The current USEPA standard for PM_{10} (24 hr) is set at 150 $\mu g/m^3$, however proposed revisions aim to revoke this standard and replace it with a new standard for particles with size between 2.5 and 10 microns in diameter. WHO have recently updated the guideline values for exposure to $PM_{2.5}$ as 25 $\mu g/m^3$ (24-hour mean). In the present study exposure levels of $PM_{2.5}$ did not exceed the WHO guideline value of 25 $\mu g/m^3$.

In regards to the number of ultrafine particles, when comparing old and new schools, there was no significant difference in morning or afternoon measurements. The number of UFP measured in classrooms was similar to those found in a study by Rumchev et al [16].

There was a positive correlation between indoor and outdoor ultra-fine particles for both morning and afternoon measured levels (r=0.000, p=0.000). This may indicate that number of ultra fine particles outdoors strongly influence the number of those fine particles indoors.

The median indoor relative humidity in new schools was higher of 55% (38.7-73.5) when compared to those in old schools of 51.8% (39.4-62.7). Indoor temperatures suggested by ASHRAE [7] should be 19-23°C in winter. The median indoor temperature was 23°C (19.9-24.1) for new schools and 19.7°C (17.0-22.1) for old schools with a significant difference ($p=0.000$). The temperatures in the monitored classrooms were within the recommended temperatures.

Some studies determined that improved ventilation rate above 10 Ls^{-1} per person, and up to approximately 20 Ls^{-1} per person, were associated with significant improvements in perceived air quality [17]. In this study the exchange rate was more than adequate in both schools. The ventilation rate was more than 700 Ls^{-1} per person in old schools and over 3000 Ls^{-1} per person in new schools.

6 Conclusion and recommendations

In our daily lives we are exposed to various chemicals, some of which are suspected to pose significant health risks. A quantitative evaluation of risk is considered to be essential for developing rational methods for managing environmental chemicals. Investigation of air quality in classrooms helps us to characterise pollutant levels and implement corrective measures to improve air quality as required. The most efficient strategy to maintain indoor air quality is to remove the source of contamination or to minimise the levels of air pollutants which can be achieved by good ventilation.

A follow up study is recommended to be carried out in winter and summer when mechanical ventilation is in use to identify any differences between old and new buildings.

References

[1] CARB (California Air Resources Board): California office of environmental health hazard assessment 2000, *Particulate matter and sulphate: evaluation of current California air quality standards with respect to protection of children*, by G.D. Thurston, Nelson Institute of Environmental Medicine, Tuxedo.

[2] Kumar, R. & Eng, P. 1999, 'Indoor air quality solutions for school buildings', *Indoor Air*, vol. 2, pp. 590-595.

[3] Pope-III, C.A. 2000, 'Epidemiology of fine particulate air pollution and human health: biologic mechanisms and who's at risk?', *Environmental Health Perspectives,* vol. 108, pp. 713–723.

[4] Leickly, F.E. 2003, 'Children, their school environment, and asthma', *Annals of Allergy, Asthma and Immunology*, vol. 90, no. 1, pp. 3-5.

[5] Zhang, G., Spickett, J., Rumchev, K., Lee, A.H. & Stick, S. 2004, 'A low allergen school has improved indoor environmental quality in classrooms', School of Public Health, Curtin University of Technology, Perth.

[6] Levin, J.-O., Andersson, K., Lindahl, R. & Nilsson, C.A. 1985, 'Determination of sub-part-per-million levels of formaldehyde in air using active or passive sampling on 2,4-dinitrophenylhydrazine-coated glass fiber filters and high performance liquid chromatography', *Analytical Chemistry*, vol. 57, pp. 1032-1035.

[7] ASHRAE (American Society of Heating, Refrigerating and Air Conditioning Engineers) 1989, ASHRAE Standard 62-1989: Ventilation for Acceptable Indoor Air Quality, Atlanta.

[8] Rumchev, K.B., Spickett, J.T., Bulsara, M.K., Phillips, M.R. & Stick, S.M. 2002, 'Domestic exposure to formaldehyde significantly increases the risk of asthma in young children', *European Respiratory Journal*, vol. 20, no. 2, pp. 403-408.

[9] Rumchev, K., Spickett, J., Bulsara, M., Phillips, M. & Stick, S. 2004, 'Association of domestic exposure to volatile organic compounds with asthma in young children', *Thorax*, vol. 59, pp. 746-751.

[10] US EPA (United States Environmental Protection Agency) 1996, Indoor air quality basics for schools, U.S. Environmental Protection Agency.

[11] NHMRC (National Health & Medical Research Council) 1995, Interim national indoor air quality goals, the 115th NHMRC Session, Australian Department of Health and Aged Care.

[12] WHO (World Health Organisation) 1999, 'Air Quality Guidelines'.
[13] Seppänen, O.A., Fisk, W.J. & Mendell, M.J. 1999, 'Ventilation Rates and CO_2 Concentrations with Health and Other Responses in Commercial and Institutional Buildings', *Indoor Air*, vol. 9, no. 4, p. 226.
[14] Lee, S.C. & Chang, M. 2000, 'Indoor and outdoor air quality investigation at schools in Hong Kong', *Chemosphere*, vol. 41, no. 1-2, pp. 109-113.
[15] Newton, P.W. 2001, *Human Settlements*, Theme Report: Australia State of the Environment Report, CSIRO Publishing on behalf of the Department of the Environment and Heritage, Commonwealth of Australia.
[16] Rumchev, K., van den Broeck, V. & Spickett, J. 2003, 'Indoor air quality in university laboratories', *Environmental Health*, vol. 3, no. 3, pp. 11-19.

Relation between ambient air and breath volatile organic compounds

H. Dhondt[1,2], E. Goelen[1], G. Koppen[1] & L. Verschaeve[1,2]
[1]*Flemisch Institute of Technological Research, VITO, Belgium*
[2]*University of Antwerp, UA, Belgium*

Abstract

Breath analysis is a non-invasive tool that can be used to measure body impact following exposure to air pollutants. A method for collecting and analyzing exhaled breath was developed and used to compare individual exhaled breath volatile organic compounds (VOCs) with ambient air VOCs. Exhaled breath was collected in Teflon bags and analyzed using thermal desorption gas chromatography – mass spectrometry. The repeatability of this method was examined following analysis of 10 breath samples of each of three subjects. An environmental health study including 56 3-year-old children in Flanders examined abundances of VOCs in exhaled breath in relation to the presence of these VOCs in ambient air. It was demonstrated that a number of VOCs were either significantly retained or cleared by the body.
Keywords: exhaled breath, volatile organic compounds, ambient air.

1 Introduction

Monitoring the influence of environmental pollution on human health has increased remarkably during the past decades. So far, methods to evaluate exposure to or impact of these environmental pollutants mainly involved the collection and analysis of biological media such as blood or urine. Measuring biomarkers in breath, however, is a very attractive approach to monitoring environmental impact because it is non-invasive and makes repeated sampling possible [1]. Breath contains valuable information because the pulmonary alveolar membrane consists of a thin barrier separating the air in the alveoli of the lung from the blood in the capillaries.

WIT Transactions on Biomedicine and Health, Vol 11, © 2007 WIT Press
www.witpress.com, ISSN 1743-3525 (on-line)
doi:10.2495/EHR070041

The structure of this membrane allows diffusion of many volatiles. Consequently, inhalation of VOCs – present in the ambient air – will result in absorption of these VOCs by the pulmonary blood supply followed by subsequent distribution of these VOCs throughout the body. Following exhalation, the alveolar air will subsequently be enriched by the VOCs contained within the pulmonary blood to an extent determined by the concentration of the VOCs in the blood and blood-gas partition coefficients [2]. This blood – gas exchange model has resulted in extensive research with regard to the breath content and the potential to use breath analysis as a diagnostic tool able to link breath components with pathologies and their early onset. Almost 30 years ago Pauling and co-workers [3] reported that normal human breath contains a mixture of several hundred volatile organic compounds (VOCs). Since then new techniques have been developed and explored that allow detection of > 1000 volatiles in human exhaled breath [4]. Most studies, however, focus rather on singular compounds in exhaled breath as a potential biomarker for specific biological effects. Recently, profiling of VOCs in exhaled breath is gaining interest in the field of biomarker research [5, 6]. Metabolic profiling considers a set of compounds, their combinations and specific relations as a potential biomarker rather than increase or decrease of singular compounds. The aim of this study is to develop a method for collecting and analyzing exhaled breath of a variety of human subjects (children, patients, healthy controls) using gas chromatography – mass spectrometry. The method will be used firstly to compare individual exhaled breath VOCs with ambient air VOCs and secondly to find exhaled breath VOC patterns specific for oxidative stress.

2 Methodology

In order to find suitable combinations of compounds or specific ratios of volatile organic compounds that relate to specific health effects (metabolic VOC profiles), analytical methods are required that are able to detect, identify and possibly quantify as many VOCs as possible in exhaled breath. Such screening methods, however, often require large sample volumes because of the low concentrations of most VOCs present in the exhaled breath. For this reason a thermal desorption gas chromatography – mass spectrometry (GC-MS) method was further developed using sorbent tubes to preconcentrate large amounts of exhaled breath.

2.1 Sampling and sample preparation

Exhaled breath of study subjects was collected in Teflon bags. A 3-way valve was used to facilitate the collection of breath for children and for patients with severe airway obstruction. A Gillian® personal sampler was used to draw the breath content of this sampling bag over a sorbent tube containing 3 cm Carbograph 1TD/ 3 cm Carbopack X. For each breath test an equivalent amount of ambient air – present in the room which the subjects occupied during the breath test – was sampled on a sorbent tube. Although breath consists of a relatively ‘clean’ sample matrix compared to urine or blood, the high CO_2 content and humidity can turn out to be a serious challenge to GC-MS analysis. Because the moisture trapped onto the sorbent tubes was found to interfere with GC-MS output, sorbent tubes were purged with 500 mL Helium (50 mL/min) prior to analysis to expel the moisture.

2.2 Thermal desorption gas chromatography: mass spectrometry

Sampled VOCs were recovered from the adsorbent traps by thermal desorption (Markes International Ltd.). Analysis was performed by GC (HP 6890 series) – MS (HP 5973 Mass Selective Detector). The column was an RTX 502.2 column with a Crossbond phenyl methyl polysiloxane phase (105 m long, 0.32 mm ID and 1.8 μm film thickness). Thermal desorption, gas chromatography and mass spectrometry parameters are summarized in Table 1.

Table 1: Analytical settings of thermal desorption unit, gas chromatograph and mass spectrometer.

Parameter Desorption Unit	Setting
Primary desorption flow	20 mL/min
Primary split	Splitless
Primary desorption temperature	250 °C
Primary desorption time	15 min
Cold trap volume	0.02 mL
Cold trap temperature	-10 °C
Cold trap packing	Carbograph 1TD/Carbograph 2TD
Trap heating rate	MAX
Secondary desorption temperature	325 °C
Secondary desorption time	3 min
Prepurge time	1 min
Prepurge flow	20 mL/min

Parameter Gas Chromatograph	Setting
Column pressure	140 kPa
Initial temperature held 1 min	35 °C
Final temperature	270 °C
Temperature ramp	5 °C/min → 35-200 °C; 70 °C/min → 200-270 °C

Parameter Mass Spectrometer	Setting
Scan mode	EI
Temperature	230 °C
Transfer line temperature	175 °C
Scan range	25-200 amu
Scan frequency	2.14 scans/s

3 Results and discussion

3.1 Repeatability experiment

Repeatability of this method was evaluated by determining coefficients of variance for 56 VOCs present in exhaled breath of 3 subjects. Three subjects were asked to fill a 56 L Teflon bag with exhaled breath. 10 x 5 L of exhaled breath of each of the 3 subjects was captured on sorbent tubes and samples were subsequently analyzed. Coefficients of variance for these 56 VOCs are summarized in table 3. Coefficients of variance for these VOCs were well within acceptable range with 89% of the coefficients being ≤ 30%. Multiple ANOVA indicated that coefficients of variance were both subject ($p < 0.00$) and component ($p < 0.00$) dependent (Table 2).

Table 2: Multiple ANOVA results for coefficients of variance.

Source	Sum of Squares	Df	Mean Square	F-ratio	P-value
Subject	4086	2	2034	16.3	**0.00**
VOC	18334	71	258	2.1	**0.00**
Residual	17690	142	125		
Total (corrected)	40092	215			

Table 3 also shows abundances for VOCs in exhaled breath and ambient air for 2 non-smoking subjects and 1 smoker. VOCs for which areas under the curve (AUC) in exhaled breath were at least twice these in ambient air are marked. These compounds represent VOCs which are most likely to be metabolites produced by the body. Some of these well known metabolites include 2-methyl-1,3-butadiene, acetone, dimethyl sulfide, dimethyl disulfide, ethanol and 1-propanol. AUCs for VOCs in ambient air that exceed twice the amount of VOC in exhaled breath are also marked and represent those substances that are most likely to be retained by the body.

Data for subject 3 are somewhat different to these of subjects 1 and 2 as it seems that most VOCs are rather produced by the body than retained. A possible explanation could be that smokers are more exposed to these substances and that build-up of these VOCs leads to a release of these compounds rather than a steady state situation. Of course a larger sample is needed to test this hypothesis more fully and to gain more certainty concerning this indication.

3.2 Environmental health study

An environmental health monitoring study performed in Flanders allowed for collection and analysis of 7 L exhaled breath of 56 three-year-old children living in urban and rural areas in Flanders.

Table 3: Coefficients of variance and mean AUCs for 56 VOCs present in ambient air and exhaled breath of 3 subjects.

VOC	subject 1 (non-smoker) CV (%)	Mean AUC[1] (counts x 10^4)	Mean AUC[2] (counts x 10^4)	subject 2 (non-smoker) CV (%)	Mean AUC[1] (counts x 10^4)	Mean AUC[2] (counts x 10^4)	subject 3 (smoker) CV (%)	Mean AUC[1] (counts x 10^4)	Mean AUC[2] (counts x 10^4)
1-pentene	9.2	11.1	12.1	10.8	7.3	5.8	9.3	84.2	27.8
pentane	6.9	36.0	39.9	13.1	12.0	10.9	9.3	35.8	23.6
2-methyl-1,3-butadiene	2.0	11889.4	203.7	5.1	6205.2	33.1	1.7	16190.6	217.5
1-hexene	3.6	6.3	6.8	16.5	3.9	3.6	5.2	30.7	4.2
hexane	3.6	3.2	14.1	14.9	9.9	9.0	20.5	26.3	18.1
ethyl acetate	19.0	249.4	1348.0	45.3	104.6	318.6	4.0	14806.3	137.8
2-methyl hexane	12.0	13.7	41.5	10.0	32.0	24.8	19.8	171.1	78.3
3-methyl hexane	5.1	25.3	25.0	9.5	32.0	28.6	18.0	118.7	82.7
1,1,1-trichloroethane	6.0	5.1	6.5	5.5	10.0	10.0	27.5	4.9	19.6
cyclohexane	3.2	46.6	52.8	10.5	49.9	43.9	16.6	79.4	65.5
2,2,4-trimethyl pentane	2.3	51.7	51.9	12.2	75.8	67.0	17.2	106.6	0.0
heptane	1.8	12.3	14.9	8.1	7.8	6.5	13.0	23.2	14.2
benzene	3.4	273.8	483.9	15.5	327.5	449.1	5.1	5020.9	463.2
trichloroethylene	2.9	3.0	4.7	8.9	5.9	8.6	8.5	25.9	8.9
methylcyclohexane	2.5	31.6	39.2	9.3	20.1	17.2	16.6	36.1	25.8
octane	1.7	31.0	41.7	16.4	9.3	6.1	11.5	34.2	9.8
toluene	3.0	8[illegible]5.1	1292.1	13.9	504.7	685.4	10.2	7752.0	2049.8
tetrachloroethylene	1.4	22.0	13.6	9.5	15.5	14.6	21.7	43.6	15.3
nonane	3.2	53.6	64.0	21.0	7.4	5.2	12.8	16.6	7.4
ethylbenzene	6.2	107.9	223.1	18.2	62.3	127.0	10.4	547.2	196.5
m/p-xylene	6.3	220.0	453.7	19.2	115.8	255.5	12.4	940.3	423.7
o-xylene	6.3	94.8	196.4	20.3	41.9	89.4	17.3	202.1	143.4
styrene	9.3	42.3	196.4	21.3	13.8	29.0	4.3	202.7	56.1
a-pinene	4.5	210.9	325.4	12.3	63.8	20.3	23	77.3	74.2
decane	2.0	237.2	316.8	16.4	32.9	25.4	13.7	78.8	50.1
propylbenzene	4.2	7[illegible].4	170.9	35.4	23.0	33.7	15.3	80.0	50.5
1-ethyl-2-methyl benzene	3.9	9[illegible].5	218.9	21.7	22.3	36.2	20.0	55.1	53.6
1,2,4-trimethyl benzene	5.1	325.9	804.7	25.5	65.6	108.5	27.7	130.3	168.9
1,2,3-trimethyl benzene	5.0	9[illegible].2	210.7	24.4	17.0	28.3	18.6	45.3	43.1
ethanol	10.4	1495.4	2443.2	16.8	1085.1	182.3	10.2	28124.7	126.7
acetone	3.0	43052.3	2673.7	6.3	148773.2	420.2	2.9	52176.3	285.4

Table 3: Continued.

VOC	subject 1 (non-smoker) CV (%)	subject 1 Mean AUC[1] (counts x 10^4)	subject 1 Mean AUC[2] (counts x 10^4)	subject 2 (non-smoker) CV (%)	subject 2 Mean AUC[1] (counts x 10^4)	subject 2 Mean AUC[2] (counts x 10^4)	subject 3 (smoker) CV (%)	subject 3 Mean AUC[1] (counts x 10^4)	subject 3 Mean AUC[2] (counts x 10^4)
dimethyl sulfide	9.8	67.8	8.6	8.9	29.3	0.0	8.3	160.7	0.0
1-propanol	8.7	449.0	28.7	17.3	166.6	10.0	1.4	1406.4	2.4
2-butenal	13.4	510.3	18.9	23.9	36.4	9.8	6.9	219.4	12.5
2-butanone	7.6	214.4	243.8	9.3	94.6	74.8	1.9	1111.8	11.1
2-methyl furan	11.6	96.1	6.1	16.2	42.5	2.1	10.5	149.9	4.8
thiophene	64.3	5.0	1.6	8.9	5.3	3.5	6.5	36.2	2.5
2-pentanone	3.1	278.6	28.9	8.4	87.7	9.3	3	1753.9	13.2
1-methylthiopropane	8.2	57.4	0.6	10.8	3.7	0.0	6	207.9	0.0
3-penten-2-one	46.2	167.6	4.8	40.7	4.9	1.1	28.4	87.1	2.0
dimethyl disulfide	31.1	105.3	14.3	43	8.9	1.7	30.4	83.8	1.8
3-methylthiophene	60.5	271.0	3.1	27.9	72.7	3.3	48.1	64.6	3.3
hexanal	27.9	27.9	462.8	66.1	9.6	2.6	42	17.3	17.1
4-methyl octane	4.9	34.1	41.5	15.1	9.3	8.7	18.2	7.6	5.5
3-furaldehyde	30	15.4	1.4	31.3	3.4	0.4	23.2	13.1	0.3
2,6-dimethyl octane	3.8	28.7	28.4	11.2	5.9	5.0	23.1	11.0	6.8
2-heptanone	10.9	18.0	32.4	51.2	6.9	1.1	9.9	25.2	1.2
2-methyl nonaan	6.4	20.9	22.4	14.9	5.0	4.5	17.3	9.9	8.2
camphene	8.5	28.9	59.2	23.4	14.7	9.8	4.8	72.1	18.2
1-ethyl-3-methyl benzene	5.4	292.9	677.2	22.6	14.7	20.3	22	179.9	17.3
b-pinene	10.4	47.0	168.5	34	17.1	0.9	17.2	17.8	5.2
dimethyl sulfone	21.8	318.2	7.8	53.5	59.2	0.0	29.9	271.7	1.8
phenol	18.5	572.7	113.4	37.6	58.2	3.8	18.6	161.8	0.0
D-limonene	4.9	434.6	840.5	9.9	155.4	11.1	4.7	691.9	70.6
eucalyptol	11	10.3	16.5	31.3	6.8	0.0	13.5	3.7	0.0
methyl-ethenyl benzene	13.1	78.0	157.1	29.4	24.7	5.7	17.5	47.7	15.4

(dark shading) mean AUC breath ≥ 2 x mean AUC ambient air

(light shading) mean AUC ambient air ≥ 2 x mean AUC breath

CV (coefficient of variation) > 30 %

[1] breath

[2] ambient air

A standard gas mixture containing 52 VOCs of the 189 hazardous air pollutants mentioned in 1990 Clean Air Act Amendment [7] was used as a means to monitor these compounds in human breath. Of these 52 VOCs, 43 could be identified in the breath of these 3-year old subjects. Abundance of these 43 VOCs was compared to corresponding abundances of these VOCs in the ambient air the children inhaled previous to the breath test. A logarithmic (with base 2) transformation was applied to normalize both ambient air and breath abundance data. A paired student t-test at significance level of 0.01 was performed taking differences between abundances of VOCs in ambient air and exhaled breath. Table 4 shows the results of this t-test. A negative t-value indicates production or release of this VOC by the body. A positive t-value indicates retention of the VOC by the body.

Table 4: Retention / release of VOCs by the body.

VOC	t	p-value	VOC	t	p-value
isobutane	3.76	0.000	chlorobenzene	-2.80	0.007
2-methyl butane	4.20	0.000	butane	2.76	0.008
2-methyl-1,3-butadiene	-24.46	0.000	2,2,4-trimethyl pentane	-1.82	0.074
dichloromethane	14.93	0.000	heptane	-1.76	0.084
chloroform	5.32	0.000	propylbenzene	-1.71	0.093
3-methyl hexane	-4.64	0.000	3-methyl heptane	-1.63	0.108
1,1,1-trichloroethane	6.51	0.000	hexane	-1.54	0.130
cyclohexane	-3.88	0.000	methylcyclohexane	-1.45	0.153
octane	-4.19	0.000	2-methyl heptane	-1.43	0.157
tetrachloroethylene	-5.39	0.000	2-methyl pentane	-1.20	0.235
nonane	-4.19	0.000	trichloroethylene	-1.18	0.245
styrene	-14.57	0.000	ethylbenzene	1.15	0.256
decane	-6.13	0.000	1,3-Butadiene	0.88	0.381
1-hexene	-3.47	0.001	3-methyl pentane	-0.62	0.536
2-methyl hexane	-3.21	0.002	benzene	-0.50	0.622
1,2-dichloroethane	3.28	0.002	methylcyclopentane	-0.48	0.631
α-pinene	3.07	0.003	pentane	0.46	0.648
carbon Tetrachloride	3.01	0.004	toluene	-0.32	0.754
m/p-xylene	3.02	0.004	1,2,3-trimethyl benzene	-0.20	0.842
1-pentene	2.92	0.005	m-methyl toluene	0.15	0.882
o-xylene	2.86	0.006	1,2,4-trimethyl benzene	-0.13	0.900
ethylacetate	2.78	0.007			

4 Conclusion

A sampling and thermal desorption gas chromatography – mass spectrometry method was developed that allows monitoring of C_5-C_{12} VOCs in exhaled breath of subjects as young as 3 years old. A repeatability experiment demonstrated that the method can be considered reliable for at least 56 VOCs present in exhaled breath with 89% of the coefficients of variance being less than 30% (and 85% ≤

20%). Bearing in mind that coefficients of variance of 20% are normal for standard chemical analysis methods and that we are evaluating a screening method rather than a method optimized to monitor a small selection of compounds, we can conclude that coefficients of variance up to 30% are acceptable and even better than a lot of other whole organism bioassays [8]. The abundances of 43 VOCs in inhaled and exhaled air were compared for 56 3-year-old children and revealed that for this study group certain compounds were significantly retained in the body while the clearance rate for other compounds was systematically larger than the absorption.

The non-invasive nature of breath sampling makes this test more convenient than monitoring blood; however several factors, including the high concentration of water vapor and the short biological half-lives of many absorbed vapors make screening methods difficult to validate. In these experiments issues such as breakthrough, background, stability of compounds on sorbent material and stability of mass detector signal over time were avoided by comparing samples of ambient air and exhaled breath samples, prepared and analyzed at the same time, following the same procedure and correcting for background. However, before a fully validated method can be presented, there are still important issues about stability, variability and sensitivity that need to be addressed.

References

[1] Kharitonov, S.A. & Barnes, P.J., Exhaled markers of pulmonary disease. *Am. J. Respir. Crit. Care. Med.* **163**, pp. 1693 – 1722, 2001.

[2] Kharitonov, S.A., Alving, K. & Barnes, P.J., ERS Task Force Report. Exhaled and nasal nitric oxide measurements: recommendation. *Eur. Respir. J.* **10**, pp. 1683 – 1693, 1997.

[3] Pauling, L., Robinson, A.B., Teranishi, R. & Cary, P. Quantitative analysis of urine vapour and breath by gas-liquid partition chromatography. *Proc. Natl. Acad. Sci. USA.* **68**, pp. 2374 – 2376, 1971.

[4] Amman, A. & Smith, D., (eds). *Breath analysis for clinical diagnosis and therapeutic monitoring.* World Scientific, 2005.

[5] Basanta, M., Koimtzis, T., Singh, D., Wilson, I. & Thomas, C.L.P. An adaptive breath sampler for use with human subjects with an impaired respiratory function. *The Analyst.* **132**, pp. 153 – 163, 2006.

[6] Phillips, M., Cataneo, R.N., Greenberg, J., Gunawardena, R., Naidu, A. & Rahbari-Oskoui, R. Effect of age on the breath methylated alkane contour, a display of apparent new markers of oxidative stress. *J. Lab. Clin. Med.* **136 (3)**, pp. 244 – 249, 2000.

[7] United States Environmental Protection Agency (USEPA). 1990 Amendments to the Clear Air Act, www.epa.gov/oar/caa/caaa.txt

[8] Rymer, J.C., Sabatier R., Daver, A., Bourleaud, J., Assicot, M., Bremond, J., Rapin, J., Salhi, S.L., Thirion, B., Vassault, A., Ingrand, J. & Pau, B. A new approach for clinical biological assay comparison and standardization: Application of principal component analysis to a multicenter study of twenty-one carcinoembryonic antigen immunoassay kits. *Clin. Chem.* **45 (6)**, pp. 869 – 881, 1999.

A dynamic model of mobile source air pollution and its properties

V. Rumchev & L. Caccetta
Department of Mathematics and Statistics, Curtin University of Technology, Australia

Abstract

Air pollution has been recognised as a serious concern in modern society. Various adverse effects have been analysed with exposure to air contamination. In this paper, a (discrete-time) dynamic model of mobile source air pollution (DMSAP) to predict the emission levels from a vehicle population within a monitoring system over time is developed. An essential feature of the model is the dynamics of vehicle population. The vehicle population is structured into different interconnected "age" groups (cohorts). It is assumed that vehicles of the same group have similar physical characteristics and behaviour such as engine types, engine conditions, emissions amounts, travelling habits and depreciation factors. Therefore, the model is suitable for large cities or metropolitan areas, where small group characteristics do not affect the aggregate behaviour of the vehicle population. Because of the nature of mobile source air pollution process, the DMSAP model exhibits positive linear systems (PLS) behaviour. Two important properties of DMSAP model with direct impact on the decision making process are discussed in this paper, namely maintainability and controllability. Maintainability is a property of the system to maintain (preserve) desired emission levels of pollution. Controllability is a property that shows the ability of the system to achieve desired emission levels from given ones. Maintainability and controllability are strong intrinsic properties of the system. For example, if the system is controllable it can be "moved" from any initial to any other (terminal) desired emission levels. In this paper some very recent advances of control theory for positive systems are used to study maintainability and controllability properties of DMSAP model.
Keywords: environmental modelling, air pollution, mobile sources, dynamic models, positive linear systems, maintainability, null-controllability, reachability, controllability.

www.witpress.com, ISSN 1743-3525 (on-line)
doi:10.2495/EHR070051

1 Introduction

Mobile source air pollution as a percentage of total air emissions has dramatically increased over the past few decades. Motor vehicles are primary sources of air pollution today. For example, in the USA in 1995, according to Deaton and Winebrake [1], only highway vehicles contributed 64% of national CO emissions, 35% of national NO_x emissions and 27% of national volatile organic compound (VOC) emissions. Millions of vehicles (automobiles, trucks, buses etc.) are on the road and most of them operating four-stroke, spark ignition internal combustion engine (ICE) technology. The components of the exhaust gas such as CO and NO_x create air quality problems in urban areas throughout the world. These components, as well as some others are a major cause of lung cancer and a variety of respiratory illnesses.

In order to better understand the role of mobile source emission in urban areas models, which help to predict the emissions from such sources over time, are needed. The purpose of this paper is to develop a simple dynamic model of mobile source air pollution (DMSAP), which can be used to predict the emissions of the total vehicle population. The vehicle population is structured into different interconnected "age" groups (cohorts). It is assumed that vehicles of the same group have similar physical characteristics and behaviour such as engine types, engine conditions, emissions amounts, travelling habits and depreciation factors. Therefore, the model is suitable for large cities or metropolitan areas, where small group characteristics do not affect the aggregate behaviour of the vehicle population. Two important properties of DMSAP are also studied in the paper namely maintainability and controllability. Maintainability is a property of the vehicle population to maintain (preserve) desired emission levels of pollution. Controllability is a property that shows the ability of the system to achieve desired emission levels from given ones.

The paper is organised as follows. A discrete-time dynamic model of mobile source air pollution is developed in section 2. Section 3 is devoted to its maintainability property. Controllability of the system described by DMSAP is studied in section 4. The paper is concluded with some final remarks on how to achieve and maintain a desired emission levels.

2 The model

2.1 Evolution of vehicle population

Consider a vehicle population on the road in a given area (large city, metropolitan area, etc.). The total vehicle population can be divided into n different cohorts (categories, groups) C_i, $i = 1, 2, \ldots, n$, on the basis of the attribute "age", the cohort C_1 being the youngest and C_n the oldest.

Let $x_i(t)$, $t = 0, 1, 2, \ldots$, denote the number of vehicles of cohort C_i at the beginning of time period t, where a single time period corresponds to the time between the samplings of the system (normally a year). Clearly, $x_i(0)$ is the initial number of vehicles in the ith cohort. It is assumed in this paper that the cohort span is one year. During year t, $t = 0, 1, 2,\ldots$, a fraction α_i of the vehicles constituting the ith cohort will progress to $(i + 1)$-st cohort, whilst some of the vehicles will be scrapped due to accidents or breakdowns, or because of long lifetime. All vehicles $u_i(t)$ (new and used) purchased from outside the system (that is the total vehicle population) during year t are related to the beginning of the period. They can be used as decision (control) variables, which are, obviously, non-negative, $u_i(t) \geq 0$ for $t = 0, 1, 2,\ldots$, and $i = 1, 2,\ldots, p$, where $p < n$, assuming that vehicles are delivered into the first p cohort only.

The evolution of the vehicle population can, then, be modelled by the simple system of difference balance equations

$$x_1(t + 1) = u_1(t), \tag{1}$$

$$x_{i+1}(t + 1) = \alpha_i x_i(t) + u_{i+1}(t), \quad i = 1, 2, \ldots, n - 1; t = 0, 1, 2, \ldots, \tag{2}$$

where $x_i(t)$ is the number of vehicles (state variables) in cohort C_i at the beginning of year t, $u_i(t)$ is the number of vehicles (decision variables) purchased from outside the system into C_i during year t, and $\alpha_i \in (0, 1)$, $i = 1, 2, \ldots, n - 1$, is the progression fraction of the ith cohort, which is strictly positive and less than unity under the realistic assumptions that (i) some, but not all, vehicles are disposed because of long lifetime or (ii) due to accidents or breakdowns.

The difference balance equations (1) and (2) together constitutes a discrete-time dynamic model of the vehicle population. It is a simple cohort-type model, see Rumchev, Caccetta and Kostova [2].

The system (1)-(2) can be rewritten in the following vector form

$$\boldsymbol{x}(t + 1) = \boldsymbol{A}\, \boldsymbol{x}(t) + \boldsymbol{B}\, \boldsymbol{u}(t), t = 0, 1, 2, \ldots, \tag{3}$$

with

$$\boldsymbol{A} = \begin{bmatrix} 0 & 0 & 0 & \cdots & 0 & 0 \\ \alpha_1 & 0 & 0 & \cdots & 0 & 0 \\ 0 & \alpha_2 & 0 & \cdots & 0 & 0 \\ \vdots & \vdots & \vdots & \ddots & \vdots & \vdots \\ 0 & 0 & 0 & \cdots & 0 & 0 \\ 0 & 0 & 0 & \cdots & \alpha_{n-1} & 0 \end{bmatrix} \geq 0, \; 0 < \alpha_i < 1, i = 1, 2, \ldots, n - 1, \tag{3a}$$

$$\boldsymbol{B} = [\boldsymbol{e}_1\, \boldsymbol{e}_2 \ldots \boldsymbol{e}_p] \geq 0, \tag{3b}$$

where $\boldsymbol{e}_i$, $i = 1,\ldots, p$ $(p < n)$, are the unit basis vectors, $\boldsymbol{x}(t) = (x_1(t),\ldots, x_n(t))'$ is named a state vector and the decision (control) vector is non-negative, i.e.

$$\boldsymbol{u}(t) = (u_1(t),\ldots, u_p(t))' \geq 0, \tag{3c}$$

assuming that the decision (control) variables $u_j(t)$ affect directly the first p cohort only and '$'$' denotes the transpose.

Throughout this paper nonnegative real matrices, respectively vectors, are denoted as $\boldsymbol{A} \geq 0$, respectively $\boldsymbol{x} \geq 0$, where the inequality is component-wise; that is $a_{ij} \geq 0$, respectively, $x_j \geq 0$, for all i and j. The notation $\boldsymbol{A} > 0$ ($\boldsymbol{x} > 0$) is used for matrices (vectors) with all its entries positive, i.e. $a_{ij} > 0 \quad (x_j > 0)$ for all i and j.

An $n \times n$ matrix A is said to be nil-potent with index of nil-potency $k \leq n$ if $\boldsymbol{A}^s \neq 0$ for $s = 1,2,\ldots, k\text{-}1$ but $\boldsymbol{A}^s = 0$ for $s = k, k+1,\ldots, n$. An immediate consequence of Cayley-Hamilton theorem is that all eigenvalues of a nilpotent matrix are equal to zero, see, for example, Goldberg [3] and for more information about the properties of nil-potent matrices Bru and Johnson [4]. It is not difficult to find out that the cohort matrix (3a) is a nilpotent matrix and, therefore, all its eigenvalues are zeros.

The state vector $\boldsymbol{x}(t)$ represents the distribution of vehicles (population distribution) among the cohorts whilst the size of the vehicle population at the beginning of year t is given by $X(t) = \sum_{i=1}^{n} x_i(t)$.

The system (3) with (3a), (3b) and (3c) is a discrete-time positive linear dynamic system - see Kaczorek [5] or Farina and Rinaldi [6]. The state variables $x_i(t)$ of such systems are always positive (or at least non-negative in value) whenever the initial state and the controls are non-negative. This is a common property of positive systems.

2.2 Emission levels

Let m_i be the average annual distances (in *km* or *miles*) travelled by one vehicle of cohort C_i during one time period and e_{ji} (called emission level or factor) be the average emission (in *g/km* or *g/miles*) of pollutant type j, $j = 1, 2, \ldots, k$, from one vehicle of the ith cohort. Note that $e_{ji} > 0$ for all i, j. Then the total emission level $\varepsilon_j(t)$ for the jth type of pollutant during time period t is given by the following expression

$$\varepsilon_j(t) = \sum_{i=1}^{n} x_i(t) m_i e_{ji} \,. \tag{4}$$

Let, now, the total emission vector be denoted as $\boldsymbol{\varepsilon}(t) = (\varepsilon_1(t),\ldots, \varepsilon_k(t))$, the matrix of emission levels as $\boldsymbol{E} = \left\lfloor \varepsilon_{ji} \right\rfloor_{k \times n}$ and the average distances matrix as $\boldsymbol{M} = \text{diag}\{ m_1,\ldots, m_n\}$. The total emissions vector then can be represented as

$$\boldsymbol{\varepsilon}(t) = \boldsymbol{EM}\,\boldsymbol{x}(t) \tag{5}$$

The emission levels and the average annual distances as well as the progression fractions are usually known from demographic and engineering studies, and there are (at least in the developed countries) accepted standards for the emissions from mobile sources. These standards, indeed, are upper limits $\bar{\varepsilon}_j$ on total pollution of type j, $j = 1, 2,\dots, k$, i.e. the total emissions are subject to the following restrictions:

$$\varepsilon_j(t) \le \bar{\varepsilon}_j, \quad j = 1, 2,\dots, k, \tag{6}$$

or, in vector form,

$$\boldsymbol{EM}\,\boldsymbol{x}(t) \le \bar{\varepsilon}, \tag{7}$$

where $\bar{\boldsymbol{\varepsilon}} = (\bar{\varepsilon}_1,\dots,\bar{\varepsilon}_k)'$ is the vector of standards (allowed limits) for the total emissions.

Formulas (4)-(5) express the relationship between the vehicle population and the emissions of various pollutants while (6)-(7) introduce restrictions on the population (state variables) and, consequently, on the numbers of new purchases (decision variables, controls) from outside the vehicle population.

As a matter of fact the dynamic model of mobile air pollution includes (3)-(3c) (or, equivalently, (1)-(2)) and (5) (or, equivalently (4)) because any implementation of the decisions $u_j(t)$ affects the states $x_j(t)$ and, consequently, the emission levels $\varepsilon_j(t)$. At the same time the dynamics of the model is concentrated in the vehicle population and that is why in the following sections the main attention is on the equation (3) with (3a)-(3c).

3 Maintainabilty

Definition 1. The state $\boldsymbol{x}_e \ge 0$ of the system (3) (or (1) - (2)) is said to be maintainable at time t if and only if there exists a control $\boldsymbol{u} \ge 0$ such that $\boldsymbol{x}(t + 1) = \boldsymbol{x}(t) = \boldsymbol{x}_e$.

It readily follows from (3) that a state $\boldsymbol{x}_e \ge 0$ is maintainable at time t if and only if there exists a control vector $\boldsymbol{u} \ge 0$ such that

$$\boldsymbol{x}_e = \boldsymbol{A}\,\boldsymbol{x}_e + \boldsymbol{Bu} \qquad \text{with} \quad \boldsymbol{u} \ge 0 \text{ and } \boldsymbol{A}, \boldsymbol{B} \ge 0. \tag{8}$$

Equation (8) tells us that if the state $\boldsymbol{x}_e$ of the time-invariant system (3) is maintainable at time t it is maintainable for all t, i.e. it is maintainable at all times. Therefore, it is called simply a maintainable state.

Equation (8) is referred to as maintainability equation (equilibrium equation) and its solutions as maintainable or equilibrium states (points). In the case of time-invariant systems the maintainable states are also equilibrium states of the system but we prefer to use the term maintainability since equilibrium states are associated with the stability of the motion, which is an asymptotic notion (James and Rumchev [7]), while maintainability is a short term concept.

Equation (8) can be rewritten in the form

$$(\boldsymbol{I}-\boldsymbol{A})\,\boldsymbol{x}_e=\boldsymbol{Bu} \qquad \text{with} \quad \boldsymbol{u}\geq 0 \text{ and } \boldsymbol{A},\boldsymbol{B}\geq 0. \tag{9}$$

Definition 2. The set X_e of all maintainable (equilibrium) states $\boldsymbol{x}_e$

$$X_e=\{\boldsymbol{x}_e \mid (\boldsymbol{I}-\boldsymbol{A})\,\boldsymbol{x}_e=\boldsymbol{Bu} \text{ with } \boldsymbol{u},\boldsymbol{A},\boldsymbol{B}\geq 0\} \tag{10}$$

is called a maintainable (equilibrium) set or a set of maintainable states.

A square matrix $\boldsymbol{C}$ is an M-matrix (see, for example, Berman and Plemmons [8]) if there exists a non-negative matrix $\boldsymbol{D}\geq 0$ with dominant (maximal) eigenvalue $\rho(\boldsymbol{D})\geq 0$ such that $\boldsymbol{C}=c\boldsymbol{I}-\boldsymbol{D}$, where $c\geq\rho(\boldsymbol{D})$ and $\boldsymbol{I}$ is the $n\times n$ identity matrix. The M-matrix is non-singular if $c>\rho(\boldsymbol{D})$ and singular if $c=\rho(\boldsymbol{D})$. Moreover, when $\boldsymbol{C}$ is non-singular the inverse exists and is nonnegative, i.e. $\boldsymbol{C}^{-1}=(c\boldsymbol{I}-\boldsymbol{D})^{-1}\geq 0$. Thus, $\boldsymbol{C}^{-1}$ exists and is nonnegative if and only if $c>\rho(\boldsymbol{D})$.

All eigenvalues of the cohort matrix $\boldsymbol{A}$ given by (3a) are zeros. Therefore the matrix $(\boldsymbol{I}-\boldsymbol{A})$ is a non-singular M – matrix and its inverse exists and is non-negative, $(\boldsymbol{I}-\boldsymbol{A})^{-1}\geq 0$, so that the maintainable set (10) can be represented as

$$\begin{aligned} X_e &= \{\boldsymbol{x}_e \mid \boldsymbol{x}_e=(\boldsymbol{I}-\boldsymbol{A})^{-1}\boldsymbol{Bu} \text{ with } \boldsymbol{u},\boldsymbol{B}\geq 0\} = \\ &= \{\boldsymbol{x}_e \mid \boldsymbol{x}_e=\sum_{j=1}^{p} u_j\, col_j(\boldsymbol{I}-\boldsymbol{A})^{-1}\boldsymbol{B},\ u_j\geq 0\} \end{aligned} \tag{11}$$

The maintainable set (11) is a polyhedral cone called cone of maintainable states or maintainable cone. The vectors $col_j\,(\boldsymbol{I}-\boldsymbol{A})^{-1}\boldsymbol{B}\geq 0$ are named edges (minimal generators, extreme rays) of the polyhedral cone. Let us specify the cone of maintainable states for the dynamic model of mobile source air pollution (3) – (3c). It is not difficult to obtain given (3a) that

$$(\boldsymbol{I}-\boldsymbol{A})^{-1}=\begin{bmatrix} 1 & 0 & 0 & \cdots & 0 & 0\\ \alpha_1 & 1 & 0 & \cdots & 0 & 0\\ \alpha_1\alpha_2 & \alpha_2 & 1 & \cdots & 0 & 0\\ \vdots & \vdots & \ddots & \ddots & \vdots & \vdots\\ \alpha_1\ldots\alpha_{n-2} & \alpha_2\ldots\alpha_{n-1} & \cdots & \alpha_{n-2} & 1 & 0\\ \alpha_1\ldots\alpha_{n-2}\alpha_{n-1} & \alpha_2\ldots\alpha_{n-1} & \cdots & \alpha_{n-2}\alpha_{n-1} & \alpha_{n-1} & 1 \end{bmatrix} \tag{12}$$

So, in this case, the first $p\leq n$ columns of (12) are the edges of the cone of maintainable states (11). Notice also that $\boldsymbol{B}'\boldsymbol{B}=\boldsymbol{I}$ for $\boldsymbol{B}$ given by (3b). Now, if a given state (distribution of vehicles among the different cohorts) $\boldsymbol{x}^*$ is in the maintainable cone (11) – (12) then there exists a decision vector

$$u^* = (B'B)^{-1}B'(I - A)x^* = B'(I - A)\,x^* \tag{13}$$

such that this state can be maintained. If the state x^* does not belong to the maintainable cone then there is no admissible decisions that can keep that state and the desired distribution of vehicles among the vehicle population cannot be preserved to the next time period.

To see better that the set of maintainable states is not that large consider a vehicle population for which only the purchase of new vehicles is allowed, so $u_1 \geq 0$ but $u_j = 0$ for $j = 2,\ldots, p$. In this case the maintainable cone is a ray in the nonnegative orthant with the origin as its initial point (vertex).

$$X_e = \{x_e \mid x_e = u_1(1,\alpha_1,\alpha_1\alpha_2,\ldots,\alpha_1\ldots\alpha_{n-2},\alpha_{n-1})',\, u_1 \geq 0\} \tag{14}$$

Only states that are on the ray (14) are maintainable; all the other nonnegative states cannot be maintained by admissible decision $u_1 \geq 0$ and, consequently, the corresponding desired emission levels cannot be maintained.

4 Controllability

Definition 3. The positive system (3) (and the nonnegative pair (A, B)) is said be (Rumchev and James [9])

(a) *reachable* (or controllable-from-the-origin) if for any state $x_f \geq 0$ but $x_f \neq 0$, and some finite t there exists a non-negative decision sequence $\{u(s), s = 0, 1, 2,\ldots, t-1\}$ that transfers the system from the origin $x(0) = 0$ to the state $x(t) = x_f$;

(b) *null-controllable* (or controllable-to-the-origin) if for any state $x_0 \geq 0$ and some finite t there exists a non-negative decision sequence$\{u(s), s = 0, 1, \ldots, t-1\}$that transfers the system from the state $x_0 = x(0)$ to the origin $x(t) = 0$;

(c) *controllable* if for any non-negative pair $x_0, x_f \geq 0$ and some finite t there exists a non-negative decision sequence$\{u(s), s = 0, 1, \ldots, t-1\}$ that transfers the system from the state to $x_0 = x(0)$ the state $x_f = x(t)$.

Controllability is a fundamental property of dynamical systems that shows their ability to move in space. It has direct implications in many control problems such as optimal control, feedback stabilization, nonnegative realizations and system minimality among others.

Definition 4. The matrix

$$\mathcal{R}_t(A, B) = [\, B \mid AB \mid A^2B \mid \ldots \mid A^{t-1}B \,] \geq 0 \tag{15}$$

is called t - step *reachability matrix*.

A column vector with exactly one non-zero entry is called *monomial*. The product of a non-singular diagonal matrix and a permutation matrix is called *monomial matrix*, see Berman and Plemmons [8]. A monomial matrix consists of linearly independent monomial columns. A monomial vector is called *i*-monomial if the non-zero entry is in the *i*th position. A selection of n non-zero entries, one from each row and column of a square matrix is called a *diagonal*. The non-zero entries of a monomial matrix always form a diagonal.

Proposition 1. The discrete-time positive linear system (3) (and the nonnegative pair $(\boldsymbol{A}, \boldsymbol{B}) \geq 0$) is

- **(a)** *reachable* if and only if the n – step reachability matrix $\mathcal{R}_n(\boldsymbol{A}, \boldsymbol{B})$ contains an $n \times n$ monomial submatrix;
- **(b)** *null-controllable* if and only if $\boldsymbol{A}$ is a nil-potent matrix;
- **(c)** *controllable* (in finite time) if and only if it is reachable and null-controllable.

The proof of Proposition 1 is given by Rumchev and James [9]. It is used in this paper to study controllability property of the vehicle population and, consequently, the controllability property of discrete time dynamic model of mobile source air-pollution (3) with (3a)-(3c) and (5).

Let us first see whether (3) with (3a)-(3c) is reachable. It is not difficult to prove that

$$A^k = \begin{bmatrix} 0 & 0 & 0 & 0 & \cdots & 0 & 0 \\ 0 & 0 & 0 & 0 & \cdots & 0 & 0 \\ \vdots & \vdots & \vdots & \vdots & \vdots & \vdots & \vdots \\ 0 & 0 & 0 & 0 & \cdots & 0 & 0 \\ \alpha_1\alpha_2\ldots\alpha_k & 0 & 0 & 0 & \cdots & 0 & 0 \\ 0 & \ddots & 0 & 0 & \cdots & 0 & 0 \\ 0 & 0 & \alpha_{n-k}\alpha_{n-k+1}\ldots\alpha_{n-1} & 0 & \cdots & 0 & 0 \end{bmatrix}, \qquad (16)$$

for $k = 1,\ldots, n$-1, and

$$A^n = \mathbf{0}. \qquad (17)$$

Since, by hypothesis, $\alpha_i \in (0, 1)$, $i = 1, 2, \ldots, n - 1$, the first $(n - k)$ columns of A^k are monomial that is scalar multiples of the unit basis vectors $\boldsymbol{e}_{k+1} = (0,\ldots,0,1,0,\ldots, 0)'$, $k = 1,\ldots, n$-1; as a matter of fact they are $(k + 1)$ – monomials.

Consider, now, the reachability matrix (15) for the system (3)-(3c). The matrix $\boldsymbol{B}$ given by (3b) consists of the unit basis vectors $\boldsymbol{e}_i$, $i = 1, 2,\ldots, p$, and, hence, the first p columns ($p \leq n$) of reachabilility matrix $\mathcal{R}_t(\boldsymbol{A}, \boldsymbol{B})$ are i – monomials, $i = 1, 2,\ldots, p$. Since the first $(n - k)$ columns of A^k are $(k + 1)$ –

monomials for $k = 1,\ldots, p,\ldots, n$-1 and the matrix $\boldsymbol{B}$ is of the form (3b), the first $(n - p)$ columns of the block $\boldsymbol{A}^p\boldsymbol{B}$ in reachability matrix of (3)-(3c) are i – monomials, that is scalar multiples of $\boldsymbol{e}_i$ for $i = p$+1,..., n. Therefore, the reachability matrix of dynamic model of mobile source air pollution contains n linearly independent monomial columns, which form a monomial matrix, and by Proposition 1(a) the system is reachable. On the other hand, the nil-potency of the matrix $\boldsymbol{A}$ given by (3a) implies, according to Proposition 1(b), the null-controllability of the system. So, the dynamic model of mobile source air pollution is reachable and null-controllable and, therefore, by Proposition 1(c) it is controllable. Thus, the following result has been proved.

Proposition 2. The dynamic model of mobile source air pollution (3) – (3c) (or, equivalently (1) – (2)) is controllable.

It is also not difficult to see from the proof of Proposition 2 that the system (3)-(3c) is controllable only if the matrix $\boldsymbol{B}$ contains $\boldsymbol{e}_1$, which means that *new vehicles must be allowed* into the system; it is controllable even when $\boldsymbol{B} = \boldsymbol{e}_1$ that is only new vehicles are allowed into the system. This is the necessary condition for controllability of the dynamic model of mobile source air pollution.

Proposition 3. The dynamic model of mobile source air pollution is controllable only if new vehicles are allowed into the vehicle population.

5 Final remarks

Although, in practice, desired emission levels have to be achieved first and then maintained, this paper treats first the maintainability problem because of its relative simplicity. Now, let the desired emission levels $\boldsymbol{\varepsilon}^*$ be given. Then, to determine the corresponding system state $\boldsymbol{x}^*$ the following linear programming (LP) problem can be solved

$$\text{Min}\ \{\boldsymbol{wx} \mid \boldsymbol{EM}\,\boldsymbol{x} = \boldsymbol{\varepsilon}^*, \boldsymbol{x} \geq \underline{\boldsymbol{x}} \geq 0\} \tag{18}$$

where the weight coefficients vector $\boldsymbol{w} \geq 0$ can be chosen as $\boldsymbol{w}$ = (0,..., 0, $w_{p+1},\ldots,w_n)'$ with $\sum_{i=p+1}^{n} w_i = 1$ to minimise the number of old vehicles in the population. The solution $\boldsymbol{x}^*$ to LP (18) is the distribution of vehicles among the cohorts that produces the desired emission levels $\boldsymbol{\varepsilon}^*$. The state $\boldsymbol{x}^* \geq 0$ then is to be reached first from the current (initial) state $\boldsymbol{x}(0) \geq 0$ and then maintained; the state $\boldsymbol{x}^*$ can always be achieved only if there is an inflow (purchases) of new cars into the vehicle population and maintained if it is in the maintainable cone. To determine the corresponding decision policies, the implementation of which leads to the desired emission levels, one has to formulate and solve some specific decision (control) problems; these problems will be discussed in another paper.

References

[1] Deaton M.L. & Winebrake J.J., *Dynamic modelling of environmental systems*, Springer-Verlag: NewYork, etc., pp. 144&152-153, 2000.

[2] Rumchev V.G., Caccetta L. & Kostova S., Positive linear dynamic model of mobile source air pollution and problems of control. *Systems Science*, **20(1)**, pp. 31-46, 2003.

[3] Goldberg, J. L., *Matrix Theory with Applications*, McGraw-Hill: New York, p. 247, 1992.

[4] Bru, R. & Johnson, C. R. Nilpotence of products of nonnegative matrices. *Rocky Mountain Journal of Mathematics*, 23 (1), pp.5-16, 1993.

[5] Kaczorek T., *Positive 1D and 2D Systems*, Springer: London, 2002

[6] Farina L. & Rinaldi S., *Positive Linear Systems: Theory and Applications*, Wiley: New York, 2000.

[7] G. James & V. Rumchev, Stability of Positive Linear Discrete-Time Systems, *Bulletin of The Polish Academy of Sciences. Technical Sciences.* **53** (1), pp. 1 – 8, 2005.

[8] Berman A. & Plemmons R., *Non-negative matrices in Mathematical Sciences*, SIAM: Philadelphia, 1994.

[9] Rumchev, V. & James, D.G., Controllability of positive linear discrete-time systems. *International Journal of Control*, **50** (**3**), pp.845-857, 1989.

Section 2
The built environment and health

Daylight, architecture and people's health

M. Boubekri
School of Architecture, University of Illinois at Urbana-Champaign, USA

Abstract

While the evidence linking light to a plethora of health issues is plentiful, building industry and its regulatory bodies are yet to address this issue in a manner that reflects its saliency. It has been suggested that one way to cultivate support for daylighting legislation is to underscore its health effects. Though these may be long term ones, they are, nonetheless, real and should be taken into serious consideration. Many cities around the world have now zoning ordinances that legislate public access to sunlight in streets and public parks, but this legislation still doesn't go far enough to command the presence of sunlight inside people's homes and workplaces. For the most part, sunlight (or daylight) is still considered as an amenity in our living and workplaces. The question that remains unanswered is whether it is really only an amenity? This paper examines the relationship between light and human health and discusses daylighting standards in light of this relationship.
Keywords: sunlight health vitamin D lighting standards.

1 Introduction

Neither current lighting design guidelines nor the illumination standards address health issues related to light and building occupants despite the large body of evidence connecting light to range of health issues. Lighting standards have been largely based on visual performance as the sole criterion for prescribing lighting quantities (Boubekri [1]). The use of visual performance as the single criterion for prescribing illuminance levels, concerns about energy efficiency and consumption and improvement in lighting technologies have caused requirements for light levels to decrease over the last fifty or sixty years (IES [2, 3]). Research indicates that electric lighting alone cannot address health needs of the occupants. In fact, electric light may be the cause of several health problems. If one must address the health issues, it becomes necessary to look at daylighting

WIT Transactions on Biomedicine and Health, Vol 11, © 2007 WIT Press
www.witpress.com, ISSN 1743-3525 (on-line)
doi:10.2495/EHR070061

not only to provide sufficient light levels to perform visual tasks or as an energy saving solution but also to be a therapeutic and healing agent for building occupants.

The effects of light may be positive or negative depending on quantities and duration of exposure. Overexposure to sunlight, for example, may cause skin cancer; underexposure, on the other hand, can cause insufficient amounts of vitamin D and subsequently a whole range of other illnesses.

It is also generally accepted that people feel better under daylight conditions. Although we may not yet know or understand all the psychological causes of the positive or "feel good," effects of natural light, medical science has provided ample information that sheds light on the causal relationships between light and some physical aspects of human health.

2 Population groups underexposed to sunlight

Inadequate exposure to sunlight and low dietary intake is usually the cause for the development of clinical vitamin D deficiency. Rickets, a long cured illness in most developed countries can still be found in some tropical countries because infants are swaddled and women are confined to the home. Elderly persons who are dependent on care providers for mobility, bed-ridden people, people living or working in windowless environments, and people living or working in highly dense areas with limited sunlight exposure may be at risk of underexposure to sunlight and vitamin D deficiency. A medical study in Australia examined the association between changes of seasons, high incidence of hip fracture and vitamin D levels in a population of elderly, not very mobile patients in the Tasmania region (Inderjeeth et al [4]). Of these patients, 68% either lived in institutional care or were dependent on a care-provider for mobility. Of these patients, 48% indicated going outdoors less than once a week. The results of this survey found no statistically significant seasonal variations in vitamin D concentration among these patients, and this lack of variation was attributed to the fact that patients were mostly bed-ridden or housebound. This Australian study underscores the absolute necessity of sunlight in people's lives. No matter what these patients diet was, it was not sufficient to overcome vitamin D deficiencies, which was the cause of bone frailty in these patients.

3 Sunlight and health

3.1 Synthesis of Vitamin D

The healing effects of vitamin D were observed at the beginning of the 20th century, when researchers were trying to understand the causes of rickets and find a cure for it. It was found that an antirachitic dietary factor was found in cod liver oil and named vitamin D. In 1921 the same healing effect was also observed not only in cod liver oil but also in UV radiation. The dual source of diet and light as antirachitic agents became then established. Today we know that there are two forms of vitamin D: vitamin D2 (ergocalciferol) and vitamin

D3 (cholecalciferol). D2 is the result of UV light irradiating a yeast sterol, ergosterol (provitamin D2); the second results from the irradiation of 7-dehydrocholesterol (provitamin D3), a sterol naturally found in several skin layers.

About 90% of Vitamin D of our bodies' needs comes from casual exposure to UVB (290-315 nm) portion the visible spectrum (Reichrath [5]). When skin is exposed to UV-B radiation, it converts a pro-hormone form found in the skin (7-dehydrocholesterol) into vitamin D. This compound travels to the liver, where it is converted to the serum (25-dehydroxyvitamin D or 25-OHD) (Glerup [6]). This serum is present in the blood serum and is the compound tested to assess vitamin D levels. It has been estimated that under normal conditions the skin can produce 80-100% of the body's required vitamin D (Glerup [6]).

3.2 Vitamin D deficiency and health problems

Vitamin D deficiency is linked to other serious illnesses in addition to bone frailty. Vitamin D deficiency can cause serious healthy problems for the elderly (Holick [7]) especially at the end of winter (Webb [8]) causing risks of hip fractures among older people. The principal causes of vitamin D deficiency are dietary imbalance and lack of exposure to sunlight. Supplementation of vitamin D with calcium in elderly women and men is shown to alleviate the problem of hip fractures (Dawson-Hughes *et al* [9], Chapuy *et al* [10], Trivedi *et al* [11], Bischoff-Ferrari *et al* [12]).

Studies have found that women in Arab countries of the Arabian Gulf region who cover totally their bodies suffer from vitamin D deficiency more than their western counterparts. Along with melanin content of the skin and a high number of pregnancies, low exposure of the skin to sunlight is believed to be one the major contributing factor to such deficiency (Ghannam *et a*l [13], Gannage-Yared *et al* [14], Saadi *et al* [15]). The fact that there is higher incidences of rickets cases (Dawodu *et al* [16]) and that circulating levels of bone resorption markers are higher (Gannage-Yared *et al* [14], Saadi *et al* [15]) and bone density of Arab women is low compared to their western counterparts is evidence that such deficiency has biological effects. Because bone remodeling is a dynamic process, reduction of bone resorption eventually results in a decrease in the degree of bone formation. Hypertension is supposed to be the most identifiable risk factor for heart failure. Factors causing hypertension may be genetic or environmental. Among the environmental factors, there is epidemiological evidence suggesting a link between insufficiencies of vitamin D with hypertension (Rostand [17]). UVB radiation was found to reduce arterial pressure in patients with mild hypertension (Krause et al [18]) while supplements of vitamin D reduced systolic blood pressure in elderly women who were diagnosed having low Vitamin D.

Vitamin D deficiency is believed to have multiple effects on various components of our cardiovascular systems. Its insufficiency can be harmful to the heart and blood vessels. Numerous reports suggest that Vitamin D deficiency causes heart failure, but such failure is reversible with vitamin D replenishment. Hypovitaminosis D is common amongst patients with heart failure

(Shane *et al* [19], Schleithoff [20]) but in general a causal relationship had been established between lack of vitamin D and heart malfunctions (Shane *et al* [19], Schleithoff [20]).

3.3 Does sunlight prevent cancer?

Numerous studies have established the favorable effect of vitamin D on our immune system. It is widely recognized now that the active vitamin D metabolite 1,25$(OH)_2$D is not produced only in the kidney as previously believed but in other tissues including colon, prostate, skin and osteoblasts cancer (Schwartz *et al* [21], Reichrath *et al* [22], Lehmann *et al* [23]). The vitamin D metabolite produced outside the kidneys is now considered to be an autocrine hormone (where the hormone acts on the same cell that produced it) or paracrine hormone (where the hormone acts locally by diffusing from its source to target cells in the neighborhood.) hormones, that regulate various cellular function in specific tissues including cell growth (Schwartz *et al* [21], Reichrath *et al* [22], Lehmann *et al* [23]). An association between vitamin D deficiency and various types of cancer including colon, breast and prostate cancer was found (Garland *et al* [24], Gorman *et al* [25], Grant [26]). Literature shows a latitudinal association between exposure to sunlight and decreased vitamin D serum levels has been demonstrated in the literature. Literature also indicates that there is an association between sun exposure and increased survival rate in various cancerous malignancies (Berwick *et al* [27], Moan *et al* [28]).

Vitamin D has a direct effect on drastic changes in blood pressure and renal osteodystrophy, an illness caused by chronic renal failure. One study found seasonal patterns in blood pressure variations amongst dialysis and renal transplant subject populations (Prasad et al [29]). Not only did patients register higher blood pressure in winter than during summer, but the length of daylight hours patients were exposed to also significantly affected blood pressure levels. The longer the exposure to daylight hours, the more normalized blood pressure became.

Decreased exposure to sunlight reduces vitamin D3 in our bodies. This has been established through the study of organ-transplant recipients who need to protect themselves from solar UV-exposure due to immunosuppressive medication they receive and the resulting risk to develop skin cancer. Renal transplant patients studied showed levels of serum 25(OH)D levels, a marker of vitamin D status, significantly lower than that of a control group of age and gender matched control group in a study (Querings and Reichrath [30]).

3.4 Sunlight vs Vitamin-D dietary supplements:

The debate about whether sunlight is more effective than dietary supplements in producing vitamin D in human bodies has been previously examined in two other studies, one in the United States and the other in Sweden. The results of the American study (Webb *et al* [31]) were congruous with the Australian study. Webb's investigation found that seasonal variation changes in serum 25(OH)D concentrations (Vitamin D) caused by sunlight exposure were highest in free-living subjects and declined substantially and proportionally as the subjects became less mobile, irrespective of vitamin D dietary supplements. The Swedish investigation also confirmed these findings (Landin-Wilhelmsen *et al* [32]). The Swedish study concluded that although helpful, dietary supplements could not supplant entirely the effects of sunlight on vitamin D levels in human bodies, and that adequate measures must be taken to guarantee access to sunlight, especially for subjects who may be less mobile or have minimal outdoor activity.

4 Discussion

There is ample evidence suggesting that inadequate exposure to proper light in our everyday lives can either be the cause of many health problems and that light could be used therapeutically to overcome health deficiencies or even perhaps as preventive medicine. Despite this knowledge, the building industry and its regulatory agencies has yet to address this issue in a manner that reflects its saliency. Building illumination codes do not address the issue of light and health, and are primarily concerned with visual performance criteria.

The illumination levels suggested for therapeutic purposes are several times higher than those currently required by standards for visual task performance in most types of buildings. It is evident that it would not be reasonable from a cost and energy consumption standpoint to suggest that buildings should be illuminated at such high illuminance levels using electric light. Natural light, however, and especially sunlight when available, can supply for a few hours each day and at almost no cost, these needed high illumination levels in most of geographical location and seasons. But since research has established that one may not always count on the idea that people will get the necessary exposure to high daylight illuminance levels by spending time outdoor, and given the fact that most people spend 80 to 90% of their lifetime indoors, it becomes imperative to the necessary daylight inside our buildings. As we have shown, medical research suggests that human beings need daylight and sunlight to live. Daylighting legislation should take into consideration not only the visual performance requirements for setting up lighting standards but also health and overall wellbeing criteria. Currently, architects aren't required by law to provide natural light for buildings. It is true that most inhabitable buildings are required to have windows, but the provision of windows is addressed in building codes mostly in terms of fire safety and means of egress rather than to supply natural light to the space.

A more comprehensive approach to daylighting legislation would be one that first creates an environment that allows sunlight to penetrate buildings to achieve certain daylight levels inside buildings.

References

[1] Boubekri Boubekri M., "An overview of current daylighting legislation:, Human-Environmental System, 7(2), 57-63, 2004

[2] Illuminating Engineering Society, IES Lighting Handbook, Vol. 53, No. 8, 422, 1958
[3] Illuminating Engineering Society, Selection of Illuminance value for interior lighting design (RQQ report no. 6), Journal of IES, 1980.
[4] Inderjeeth CA, Barett T, Al-Lahham, Mulford J, Nicklason F, Reberger C, Seasonal variation, hip fracture and vitamin D levels in Southern Tasmania, N Z Med 26(1152): 183-5, April 2002.
[5] Reichrath J., Sunlight, skin cancer and vitamin D: What are the conclusion of recent findings that protection against solar ultraviolet (UV) radiation causes 25-hydroxyvitamin D deficiency in solid organ-transplant recipients, xeroderma pigmentation, and other risk groups? J. Steroid Bioch. & Molec. Biol, doi: 10.1016/j.jsbmb.2006.12.029, 2006
[6] Glerup H. et al., Commonly recommended daily intake of vitamin D is not sufficient if sunlight exposure is limited, J. Internal Medicine: 260-268, 2000.
[7] Holick M. F. Mayo Clinic proc. 81 (2006) 353-373.
[8] Webb A. R., Pilbeam C., Hanafin N., Holick M. F., Am. J. Clin. Nutr. 51: 1075-1081, 1990.
[9] Dawson-Hughes B., Dallal, G.E., Krall E.A., Harris S., Sokoll L.J., Falconer G., Ann. Intern. Med. 115: 505-512, 1991.
[10] Chapuy M. C., Arlot M. E., Duboeuf F., New Engl. J. Med. 327: 1637-1642, 1992.
[11] Trivedi D. P., Doll R., Khaw K. T., BMJ 326: 469-475, 2003.
[12] Bischoff-Ferrari H.A., Giovannucci E., Willett W.C., Dietrich T., Dawson-Hughes B., Am J. Clin. Nutr. 84:(18-28, 20006.
[13] Ghannam N.N., Hammami, M. M., Bakheet B.A., "Bone mineral density of the spine and femur in Saudi females: relation to vitamin D status, pregnancy, and lactation" calcify Tissue Int.; 65:23-8, 1999.
[14] Gannage-Yared M.H., Chemali R., Yacoub N., Halaby G. "Hypovitaminosis D in a sunny country: relation to lifestyle and bone markers. J. Bone Miner res.; 15:1856-82, 2000.
[15] Saadi H., Dawodu A., "Vitamin D deficiency in Arabian women and children: time for action. In: Kinger I, Laura V editors. Trends in Lifestyle and Health Research, Nova Sciences Publishers, p. 163-74, 2005.
[16] Dawodu A., Khadir A., hardy D.J. Varady E. "Nutritional rickets in UAE: an unresolved cause of childhood morbidity. Middle east Paediatr.; 7:12-4, 2002.
[17] Rostand S.G., "Ultraviolet light may contribute to geographic and racial blood pressure differences' Hypertension; 30:150-6, 1997.
[18] Krause R., Buhring M., Hopfenmuller W., Holick M. F., Sharma A. M. "Ultraviolet B and blood pressure" lancet; 352:709-10, 1998.
[19] Shane E., Mancini D., Aaronson K., et al. "Bone mass, vitamin D deficiency, and hyperparathyroidism in congestive heart failure. Am. J. Med; 103:197-207, 1997.

[20] Schleithoff S. S., Zitterman A., Stuttgen B. et al., "Low levels of intact osteocalcin in patients with congestive heart failure" J. Bone Miner Metab; 21:247-52, 2003.

[21] Schwartz G.G., Whitlatch L.W., Chen, T.C., Lokeshwar B.L., Holick M.F., "Human prostate cells synthesize 1,25-dihydroxyvitamin D_3 from 25-dihydroxyvitamin D_3, Cancer Edidmiol. Biomarkers Prev 7: 391-395, 1998.

[22] Reichrath J., Rafi, L. Rech, M. Mitschele T., Meineke V. Gartner B.C., Tilgen W., Holick M. F., "Analysis of the vitamin D system in cutaneous squamous cell carcinomas (SCC), J Cut. Pathol. 31 (3): 224-231, 2004.

[23] Lehmann B, Querings K., Reichrath J., "Vitamin D and skin: new aspects for dermatology" Exp. Dermatol, 13 (s4): 11-15, 2004.

[24] Garland C.F. Comstock G.W. Garland F.C., et al, "Serum 25 hydroxyvitamin D and colon cancer: eight year prospective study" lancet 2: 1176-1178, 1989.

[25] Gorham E.D., garland F.C., garland C.F. "Sunlight and breast cancer incidence in the USSR" Int. J Epidemiol. 19 : 614-622, 1990.

[26] Grant W.B., "An estimate of premature cancer mortality in the U.S. due to inadequate doses of solar ultraviolet-B radiation", cancer 94: 1867-1875, 2002.

[27] Berwick M., Armstrong B. K. Ben-Porat L., Fine J. Kricker A., Eberle C., Barnhill R., "Sun exposure and mortality from melanoma" J. natl. Cancer Inst. 97 (3): 195-199, 2005.

[28] Moan J., Porojnicu A.C., Robsham T.E., Dahlback A., Juzeniene A., Tretli A. Grant W., "Solar radiation, vitamin D and survival rate of colon cancer in Norway" J. Photochem. Photobiol. B 78 (3): 189-193, 2005.

[29] Parasad GV, Nash MM, Zaltman JS, Seasonal variation in outpatient blood pressure in stable renal transplant recipients, Transplantation 72(11): 1792-4, 2001.

[30] Querings K., Reichrath J., 25-Hydroxyvitamin D deficiency in renal transplant recipients, J. Clin. End. Metab. 91 (2): 526-529, 2006.

[31] Webb AR, Pillbeam C, Hanafin N, Holick MF, An evaluation of the relative contribution of exposure to sunlight and of diet to the circulating concentration of 25-hydroxyvitamin D in an elderly nursing home population in Boston, American Journal of Clinical Nutrition 51(6): 1075-81, June, 1990.

[32] Landin-Wilhelmsen K, Wilhelmsen L, Wilske J, Lappas G, Rosen T, Lindstedt G, Lundberg PA, Bengtsson BA, Sunlight increases serum 25(OH)vitamin D concentration whereas 1,25(OH) 2D3 is unaffected. Results from a general population study in Goteborg, Sweden (The WHO MONICA Project), European Journal of Clinical Nutrition, 49(6):400-7, June, 1995.

Survey system for life styles of the elderly and to identify the consumption of food and drink

A. Sawada[1], T. Oyabu[1], S. Seto[2] & T. Katsube[3]
[1]*Graduate School of Regional Economic Systems, Kanazawa Seiryo University, Japan*
[2]*Kinjo University, Japan*
[3]*Faculty of Engineering, Saitama University, Japan*

Abstract

From the viewpoint of welfare costs, it is necessary to survey whether older people eat, drink and live their daily lives in safety. It is especially desired that an older person drinks green tea and/or coffee routinely and autonomously takes meals, namely breakfast, lunch and supper. In addition, it is better for an older person to eat fruits such as oranges and apples to prevent colds, Alzheimer's disease and other illnesses. In this study, a system to recognize the eating of a meal, the drinking of a beverage and the eating of a fruit was constructed using odor sensors. Three metal oxide odor sensors were adopted for this system. The system can identify behavior by analyzing characteristics of odor sensors. As for the results, the system recognizes this behavior successfully and also detects the level of fatigue of an older person. A high correlation coefficient (over 0.85) was obtained between the degree of fatigue due to bodily sensations and the output of the sensor. The sensor was highly sensitivity to hydrogen gas. When humans are fatigued or stressed, their exhaled breath contains hydrogen at high concentrations. Discriminating analysis was used to identify the kind of fruits eaten and teeth brushing behavior from odor sensor outputs.

Keywords: odor sensor, sensory system, aged people, welfare system.

1 Introduction

In Japan, birthrate is declining and the population is aging. Therefore, the labor force and manufacturing capabilities are also decreasing. Other advanced industrial countries are in the same situation. The fees for pensions and medical

WIT Transactions on Biomedicine and Health, Vol 11, © 2007 WIT Press
www.witpress.com, ISSN 1743-3525 (on-line)
doi:10.2495/EHR070071

treatment for the elderly are more than 1.0×10^6 million yen per year. The cost of the self-governing body has exerted additional pressure upon the fees. It is important to keep various costs down for the elderly with good services. It is necessary to consider various ideas and results from many branches of study to find reasonable means of settling issues arising from these subjects.

In this study, we examined whether the health condition and life pattern of the elderly can be identified by detecting breath odors. The breath odor changes according to human behavior, namely taking a meal, brushing teeth and drinking beverages. It would be very effective if a system could survey the patterns of daily life and some of diseases of the elderly. We developed a breath odor sensing system for this purpose. Humans generate strong breath odors when they have stress and are fatigued. In this paper, breath odor is defined as the odor generated from the human mouth. Breath odor is also generated when teeth are brushed. This is not bad breath. The main odor is due to menthol when teeth are brushed. On the other hand, breath odor decreases briefly when the subject drinks water, tea or milk.

In Japan, apples and oranges are very familiar to the general person, and these fruits are harvested in the greatest number. They are also effective to keep humans healthy. The Ministry of Agriculture, Forestry and Fisheries of Japan is recommending that fruits should be eaten everyday. Three metal oxide gas sensors were adopted to detect breath odor. This type of sensory system is very popular [1–5]. Daily patterns in the sensor outputs were examined, and the identification of the fruit eaten, and the relationship between the grade of fatigue and sensor output were examined. The system was constructed to survey the life style and fundamental behavior of a solitary elderly person [6]. In addition, the system could potentially identify diseases of the elderly in near future.

2 Experimental

Breath odor is generated according to the kind of meal, stress, teeth brushing and when amount of sputum is low. Usually, the breath contains mainly hydrogen and methane at a ratio of approximately 9:1. The percentage of hydrogen in exhaled air increases as the subject experiences stress. The offensive odor substances in the expiration are chiefly ammonia, amines, hydrogen sulfide, indoles and methyl mercaptan.

Breath odor is composed of mainly reducing gases. Therefore, the system adopts three metal oxide gas sensors that are highly sensitive to the reducing gases. The material of two sensors is tin oxide and the third is indium oxide. These three sensors are referred to as sensor 1, 2 and 3. Each sensor is connected to a load resistance and dc supply is applied to the circuit. The voltage at both ends of the resistance is called the sensor output. The output increases as the grade of breath odor becomes higher. When the sensor output is at high voltage, the resistance of the sensor is low. A photograph of the three sensors is shown in Figure 1. The sensors are installed on the reverse side of the lid of a glass bottle. The three sensor-outputs are directed to a mobile computer. The program for logging data was developed using C as the programming language.

A photograph of the system is shown in Figure 2. The three sensors are incorporated into a stuffed doll and exhaled air is introduced into the doll using a small motor in later units. However, a glass bottle was adopted in this experiment to carry this out easily. The stuffed doll was not used in the experiments. The stuffed doll generally has a comforting effect on human beings.

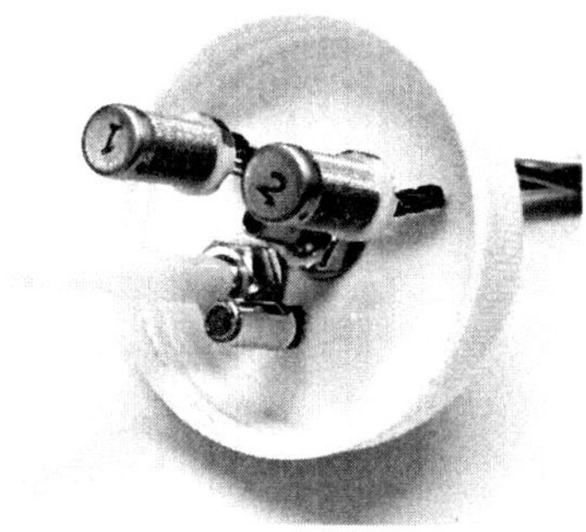

Figure 1: Three adopted sensors installed on the lid of the experimental bottle.

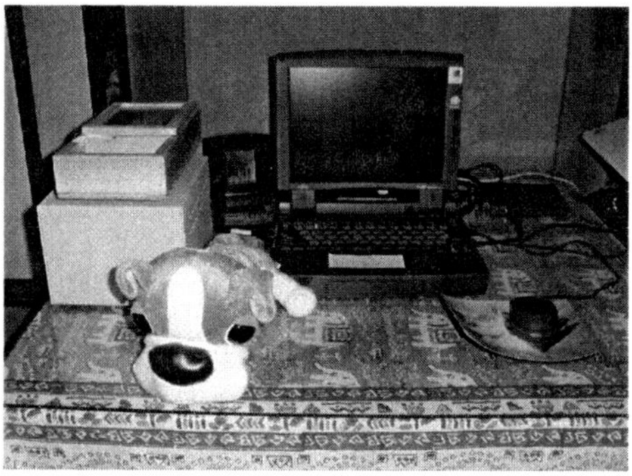

Figure 2: Experimental system for detecting breath odor.

Eating fruit, brushing teeth and the grade of fatigue are identified using sensor outputs. The glass bottle has an entry and exhaust vent. Its capacity is 150 *ml*. The measurement of breath odor was carried out as follows. The offset level of each sensor was measured for 30 seconds and the breath was introduced for 5 seconds. The breath also ran out via the vent at the same time. The sensor output increased according to the odor grade, and the characteristics could be approximated using an exponential function. The difference between the offset level and the output value at 120 seconds was adopted as the real output for analysis. The experiment was over in 120 seconds.

3 Results

3.1 Daily fluctuation of sensor output

The outputs of the sensors for 40 *ppm* of ethyl alcohol are shown in Figure 3. Sensors 1 and 2 (S1 and S2), which are made of tin oxide, have a high sensitivity. Sensor 3 (S3), which is made of indium oxide, has a low sensitivity. Examples of the odor sensor outputs for exhaled air are shown in Figure 4. The characteristics were measured after the subject ate Chinese noodle soup. The outputs of sensors 1 and 2 are high because the soup contains many odors. The three sensor outputs for each behavior are shown in Figure 5 as a bar chart. In the figure, the bars for the three sensors were high at breakfast, lunchtime and

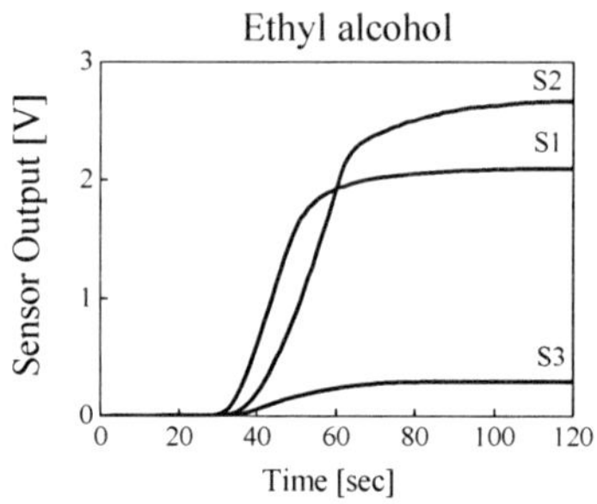

Figure 3: Characteristics of the three sensors for 40 *ppm* of ethyl alcohol.

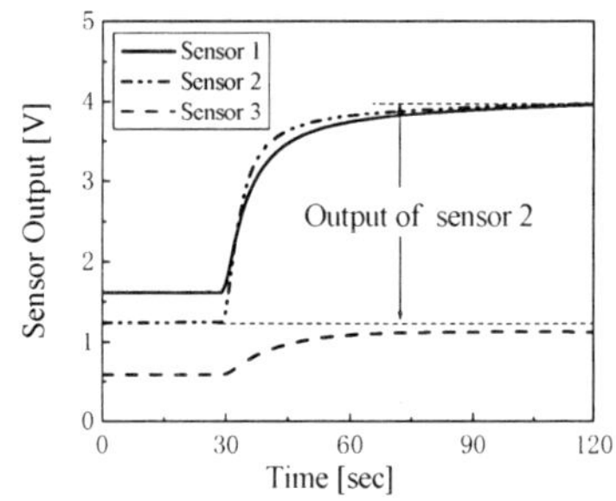

Figure 4: Characteristics of the three odor sensors for expiration after taking Chinese noodle soup.

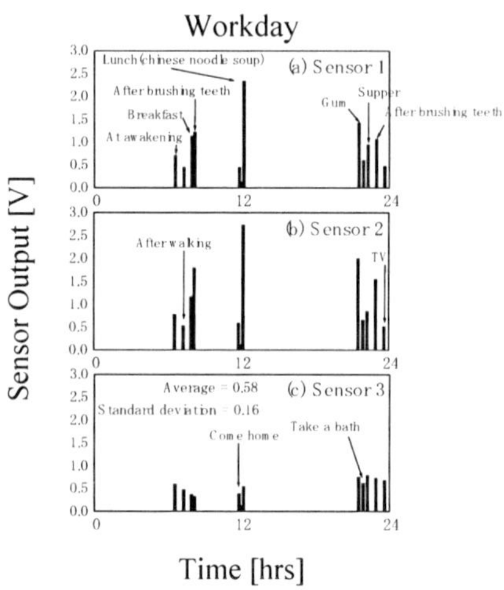

Figure 5: Daily patterns of the three sensor outputs displayed on bar graphs.

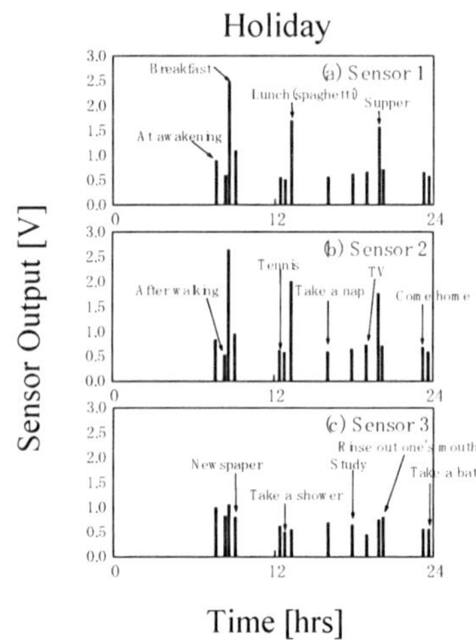

Figure 6: Daily patterns of the three sensor outputs displayed on bar graphs. The subject did not brush his teeth.

supper. The outputs of sensors 1 and 2 were higher than that for sensor 3. The output of sensor 3 did not change greatly due to meals. The subject was 54 years old. The outputs of sensors 1 and 2 also increased when the subject chewed gum containing menthol. When the subject ate soup, for example miso soup or noodle soup, the sensor outputs increased. Various kinds of stock are used in noodle soup and miso soup. The flavor is increased by these stocks. The average and standard deviations of sensor 3 output in Figure 5 are 0.58 and 0.16. The data were collected on a workday. The same characteristics were also measured on a holiday, as shown in Figure 6. Teeth were not brushed during the day. The experiment was carried out to remove the influence of teeth brushing. The subject ate a ham sandwich, fresh vegetables and yoghurt at breakfast. The outputs of sensors 1 and 2 are also high and the characteristics are similar to Figure 5. Sensor 3 output fluctuates less than the outputs of sensors 1 and 2. The averages (*ave*), standard deviations (*s*) and coefficients of variation (*cv*) of the three sensor outputs adopted are summarized in Table 1. The *cv* is derived by the equation: s / age × 100 [%]. The values of sensors 1 and 2 show almost the same tendency, while the value of sensor 3 is fairly different to those of sensors 1 and 2.

Taking a meal is important and fundamental behavior for humans, and especially breakfast and supper are important to maintain a healthy condition. We adopted a new coefficient to identify the normal grade of nutrition. The coefficient is introduced by the following calculation. Both sensor 1 outputs for breakfast (*mab*) and supper (*mas*) are added, the value is divided by two, and then multiplied 100. The system collected 14 values for 14 days. The data are indicated on a histogram in Figure 7. In the figure, the average of the coefficients is 6.9 and *s* is 3.4. The coefficient exceeded 12 when the subject ate garlic. We can identify that the subject has normal eating habits when the coefficient is close to the average.

Table 1: Average (*ave*), standard deviation (*s*) and coefficient of variation (*cv*) of the three sensor outputs.

	S1	S2	S3
ave	0.94	1.00	0.71
s	0.58	0.65	0.18
cv	62	65	25

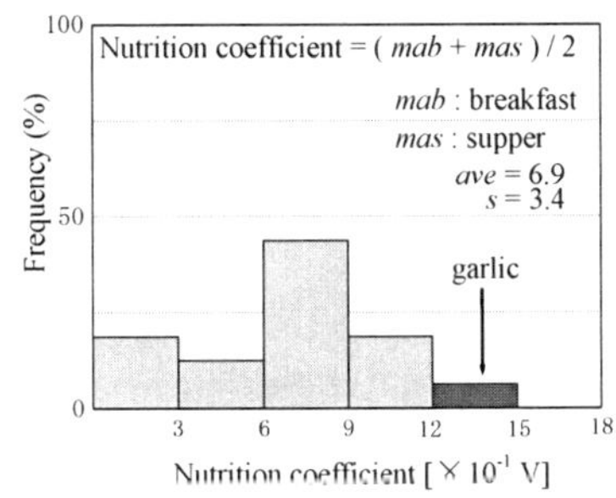

Figure 7: Histogram of sensor 1 output for breakfast and supper.

3.2 Sensor outputs at awakening and after walking

Humans generate various odors from their body as they age, and the odor grade becomes high. Breath odor grade also becomes higher. It may be possible to detect some diseases by examining breath odor at awakening. It is an odor for an inactive hour. The sensor output after a walk in the morning is considered as an offset level on the day. The system can recognize progress of disease or of a disorder of body by understanding breath odor characteristics statistically. The histograms of sensor outputs at awakening and after walking in the morning are shown in Figure 8. Figure (a) shows the histogram for sensor 1 output, (b) for sensor 2, and (c) is for sensor 3. The histogram at awakening is displaced toward the right and the histogram after walking is displaced toward at left side. Namely, the breath odor grade decreases as a result of washing the subject's face and walking. We consider the level as an offset level to recognize behavior and diseases. The levels are added according to daily behavior. If there was not an event to increase odor grade, the level was almost constant. The average, standard deviation and coefficient of variation of three sensor outputs at awakening and after walking are summarized in Table 2. The data for sensors 1 and 2 are similar. The data for sensor 3 are different from sensors 1 and 2. These characteristics correspond to the data on Table 1. There is a tendency for the odor grade after walking to become lower than the grade at awakening. It is effective to compare the breath odor grades for other behavior with this grade.

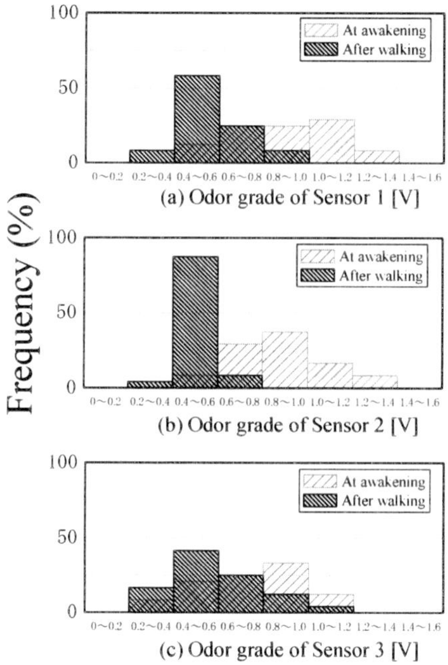

Figure 8: Histograms of sensor outputs at awakening and after walking in the morning.

Table 2: Average (*ave*), standard deviation (*s*) and coefficient of variation (*cv*) of the three sensor outputs at awakening and after walking in the morning.

	At awakening			After walking		
	S1	S2	S3	S1	S2	S3
ave	0.90	0.87	0.75	0.57	0.52	0.59
s	0.22	0.21	0.28	0.15	0.10	0.22
cv	25	25	28	26	18	38

3.3 The sensor output after brushing teeth

Brushing teeth is an autonomic human behavior. The behavior is necessary to keep a keen sense in the mouth and to prevent tooth decay and periodontal disease. It is also said that brushing teeth activates cerebral responses that stimulate the gums. It is very important for a person to have tasty meals throughout life, and brushing teeth is effective against the items. In this study, we identified brushing teeth as an important behavior using the odor sensor grades. Polishing materials, medicinal materials and menthol as a flavoring are contained in toothpastes. Consequently, the odor sensor system can detect teeth brushing by sensing menthol. The output characteristics of the odor sensors for brushing teeth are indicated in Figure 9. The output of sensor 2 is larger than that for sensor 1 after brushing. The system can identify brushing teeth from the sensor outputs, and the identification probability is over 90%.

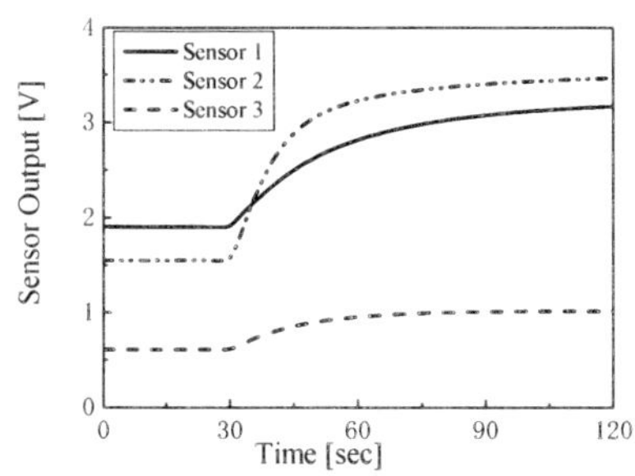

Figure 9: Characteristics of the three odor sensors for exhaled breath after brushing teeth.

3.4 Identification of eating fruit

For human beings, fruits have an important role in keeping humans healthy. Therefore, the Ministry of Agriculture, Forestry and Fisheries of Japan recommends the eating of fruit. Apples and oranges are very popular among Japanese because large amounts are harvested in Japan. Apples relieve physical fatigue and also to remove mental fatigue. They are a staple in the prevention of hyperlipidemia.

Oranges contain vitamin C and some mineral components. People sometimes bleed from the gums and the eyes when they are deficient in vitamin C. Oranges are good to prevent colds, aging, diabetes and heart disease. The breath odor characteristics were examined when a subject ate an apple, an orange and a Hassaku orange. Examples of the results are shown in Figure 10. Figure (a) shows the characteristics for apple, (b) for orange and (c) for Hassaku orange. In these figures, the output of sensor 2 is higher than that of sensor 1.

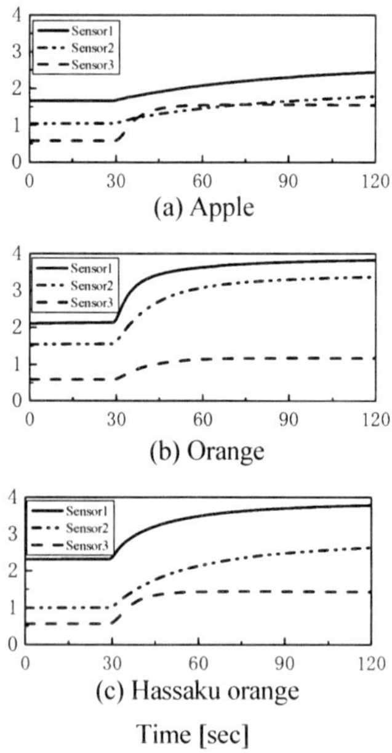

Figure 10: Characteristics of the three odor sensors for exhaled breath after eating fruit: (a) apple, (b) orange and (c) Hassaku orange. Vertical axis means sensor output [V].

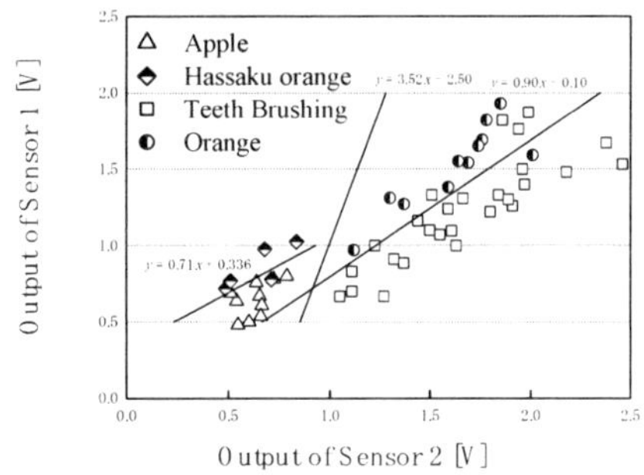

Figure 11: Relationship between sensor 1 and 2 outputs.

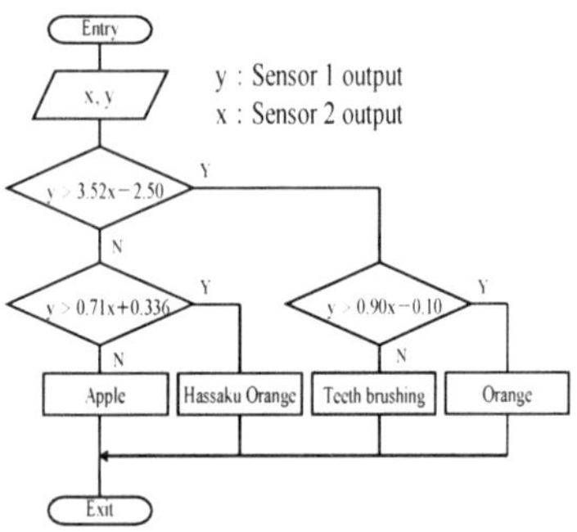

Figure 12: Flow chart for identifying teeth brushing and eating apples, oranges or Hassaku oranges.

3.5 Identification of fruit and teeth brushing using a scatter diagram

The identification of the eating of an apple, an orange and a Hassaku orange and teeth brushing as behavior is investigated using the three odor sensor outputs. The system adopted the outputs of three sensors when the identification was carried out. An example of a scatter diagram is shown in Figure 11. The figure shows the scatter diagram for sensors 1 (y) and 2 (x) when the subject has eaten fruit and brushed teeth. We can distinguish the apple–Hassaku orange group from the orange–teeth brushing group using a discriminant function, and the identification rate is 100%. The discriminant function derived is shown in eq. (1), in which y means sensor 1 output and x means sensor 2 output.

$$y = 3.52x - 2.50 \tag{1}$$

We can also distinguish the orange group from the teeth brushing group using a discriminant function, but the identification rate in that case is 85%. The function is indicated in eq. (2). The system can also distinguish the apple group from the Hassaku orange group using the same function, and the identification rate is over 90%. The function is shown in eq. (3). It is, however, better to gather more data to confirm these relationship.

$$y = 0.90x - 0.10 \tag{2}$$

$$y = 0.71x + 0.336 \tag{3}$$

The flow chart for the identification is shown in Figure 12. In the first place, the outputs (x, y) are entered into the system. The apple–Hassaku orange group and orange–teeth brushing group are classified. Then “orange” and “teeth brushing” are separated. After that, “apple” and “Hassaku orange” are separated.

3.6 Identification of stress and fatigue

Stress and fatigue are spread among human beings according to the progress of IT society. It is sometimes said that mental fatigue occurs more frequently than physical fatigue in the elderly population. The following conditions are caused by fatigue; headache, high blood pressure, angina and some intraoral diseases. If a person has intraoral diseases, the inside of the mouth dries and bad breath odor results. In this experiment, first the subject identified the grade of stress and fatigue due to bodily sensations. The grades were expressed in five stages. Sensor 3 output was then examined. The results are shown in Figure 13. Sensor 3 output, which is highly sensitivity to hydrogen gas, increases as the grade of mental and physical fatigue (*rmf*, *rpf*) based on bodily sensations of the subject increases. The output also became markedly higher when the subject had a cold and took a medicine. In this experiment, the system achieved a high correlation coefficient of about 0.9 (S3). There was dispersion in the data between the sensor output and the grade of fatigue.

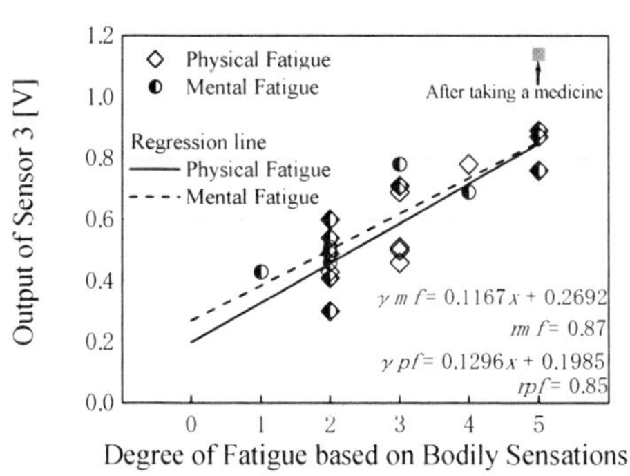

Figure 13: Correlation between degree of fatigue based on bodily sensations and output of sensor 3.

4 Conclusion

The pattern of life in the elderly and the grade of fatigue were examined by investigating breath odor using three metal oxide gas sensors. These sensors have different sensitivities to chemical substances. Sensor 3, an indium oxide type, has high sensitivity to hydrogen gas. The volume of hydrogen gas in exhaled breath increases when the subject is fatigued. The sensor outputs regarding breath odor show fluctuations in daily patterns. The patterns arise according to eating meals regularly. The odor after walking in the morning is lower than the one at awakening. Brushing teeth, which is an autonomous behavior, and eating three kinds of citrus fruits can be identified. The output level of sensor 3 is linear with respect to the grade of fatigue based on subjective bodily sensations. As sensor 3 is highly sensitivity to hydrogen gas, this observation supports the idea that hydrogen concentration in exhaled breath increases when the subject is fatigued.

The pattern of life in the elderly may be surveyed in detail without the invasion of privacy, and a survey system with high reliability for the aged may be constructed.

References

[1] Diamond, D., *Principles of Chemical and Biological Sensors*, New York, John Wiley & Sons, 1998.

[2] Gardner, J.W. & Bartlett, P.N., *Electronic Noses Principles and Applications*, Oxford, Oxford University Press, 1999.

[3] Gardner, J.W., *Microsensors*, New York, John Wiley & Sons, 1994.

[4] Joshi, R. & Sanderson, A.C., *Multisensor Fusion*, New Jersey, World Scientific, 1999.

[5] Mutambara, G.O., *Decentralized Estimation and Control for Multisensor Systems*, Boston, CRC Press, 1998.

[6] Oyabu, T., Okada, A., Manninen, O. & Lee, D.-D., Proposition of a survey device with odor sensors for an elderly person. *Sensors & Actuators B*, **96**, pp.239-244, 2003.

Building materials vs. fungal colonization – model experiments

E. Piecková[1], Z. Pivovarová[1], Z. Sternová[2] & E. Droba[2]
[1]*Slovak Medical University, Slovakia*
[2]*Research and Development Institute of Building Construction, NOVA, Slovakia*

Abstract

The antifugal potential of indoor building materials of 7 different types – without as well as with a paint or oily coating – was studied according to the ISO 846: 1997 E. Spore suspensions of micromycetes *Acremonium* sp., *Aspergillus ustus, A. versicolor, Cladosporium sphaerospermum, Penicillium* sp. and *Scedosporium apiospermum* were inoculated onto the materials' surface (clean and dusty – to simulate the real state in the indoor environment). Systems were kept under defined water activities (a_w) 0.94, 0.83 and 0.75 and incubated at 22–25°C for 3 months. Microbial growth was evaluated visually after the 1st, 2nd and 3rd months of the experiment. At the end of the period, the vitality of fungal propagules on the material surfaces was estimated by the printing method onto Sabouraud agar medium. All building materials with any lime composition or oily coating showed a certain resistance to the fungal colonization, even under very moist conditions (a_w = 0.94). Thus, their broader employment in the indoor environment could be emphasized. Representatives of the common airborne mycoflora – aspergilli, penicillia, and *C. sphaerospermum* – were able to develop visible growth on all materials tested with and without the house dust as well, although the colonization was of different degrees depending on the humidity. The fungi of *Acremonium* sp. and *S. apiospermum* favoured – as had been expected – the highest a_w = 0.94 the most. No building material showed fungicidal properties – micromycetes were capable of germinating when printed from the material surface onto the agar. The dust reduced the materials' antifungal properties only very moderately. *A. versicolor* – a producer of carcinogenic mycotoxin sterigmatocystin – could colonize materials under any experimental conditions. Wooden facings seemed to be the most resistant to the moulds.
Keywords: building materials, indoor environment, moulds, water activity, temperature, antifungal properties.

WIT Transactions on Biomedicine and Health, Vol 11, © 2007 WIT Press
www.witpress.com, ISSN 1743-3525 (on-line)
doi:10.2495/EHR070081

1 Introduction

Monitoring of exposure to indoor fungi is rather complicated due to lack of standard and exact practical methods to evaluate how indoor microclimate (temperature, relative humidity, dust, ventilation, constructing materials and furnishings), outdoor ambient, and microscopic fungi affect each other.

It was found that alternaria-propagules were predominant mainly in dwellings not heated sufficiently, aspergilli colonized houses and flats with wallpaper especially, while concrete surfaces favoured cladosporia [1]. The ability of *Penicillium* sp. and *Aspergillus* sp., the so-called first colonizers, to grow on/in common house-dust under a relative humidity of 76–80% can probably explain their dominant prevalence even in healthy buildings. The secondary (*Cladosporium* sp., *Alternaria* sp., *Chaetomium* sp., 85% relative humidity needed) and tertiary colonizers (*Fusarium* sp., *Acremonium* sp., yeasts, optimal relative humidity above 90%) are able to biodeteriorate any constructing material (plaster board, concrete, lime-cement and cement plasters, brick and ceramic tiles, paintings, wood, paper etc.) under optimal thermal and moist conditions. This was proved by several studies of mouldy dwellings in Slovakia [2–4].

The *Stachybotrys chartarum* isolates from moist schools and dwellings in Denmark produced trichothecenous mycotoxin trichodermol when cultivated onto cardboard [5] and vinyl ceiling [3]. Mutagenic and foetotoxic mycotoxins alternariol and its monomethylether adversely affecting mice were detected in cellulose tiles overgrown with *Alternaria alternata*. This isolate was also able to grow on cardboard [6]. The metabolite synthesis of fungi depends on the quality of constructing materials (e.g. [7, 8]). In our previous experiments on tracheal organ cultures of 1-d-old chicks, varying ciliostatic activity was found in chloroform extracts of biomass from building materials (mineral wool, plasterboard, cardboard) inoculated with pure isolates of some moulds of indoor origin (*Penicillium chrysogenum, P. palitans, Trichoderma viride, Stachybotrys* sp. and *A. versicolor*). Generally, extracts from growth on materials composed of finely divided cellulose were more active than those from growth on mineral wool [9].

2 Materials and methods

A testing method according to the modified ISO 846 was used [10]. It is possible to distinguish between the fungal resistance of a material on its own (growth test) and fungistatic/fungicidic properties of that material in the presence of the complex growth medium (fungicidic test) under defined conditions (23–25°C – growth of mesofili, relative humidity 95% min., 4 weeks, also with dusty materials – real conditions' simulation).

Samples of the following building materials – without as well as with a paint or oily coating – were evaluated for their antifungal properties: fine, grain and traditional lime plaster, traditional gypsum mortar, joint cement, ceramic tiles, wooden facings.

Spore suspensions of micromycetes *Acremonium* sp., *Scedosporium apiospermum* (belonging to tertiary indoor fungal colonizers as indicators of long-lasting dampness and depending on essential nutrients in the environment), *Aspergillus ustus, A. versicolor* – a toxic fungus, *Penicillium* sp. (so-called primary indoor colonizers, components of a common airborne mycoflora of any non-sterile environment) and *Cladosporium sphaerospermum* as a representative of secondary indoor colonizers commonly present in the outdoor fungi were inoculated onto materials' surface (clean or dusty). Systems were kept under defined water activities (a_w; processed by NaCl as given in the STN 56 0030 [11]) 0.94, 0.83 and 0.75 and incubated at room temperature (22–25°C) for 3 months. Microbial growth was evaluated visually after the 1st, 2nd and 3rd months of the experiment. At the end of the period, the vitality of fungal propagules on the material surfaces was estimated by the printing method onto Sabouraud agar medium.

3 Results and discussion

3.1 Building materials without house dust layer

Wood and lime plasters were shown to be the most resistant to fungal growth under given experimental conditions, while tiles and plaster mortars enabled all microfungi to growth.

No painting or coating changed this resistance, but:

- An oily coating appeared to be more antifungal than common watery painting,
- *Acremonium* sp. was able to growth on all materials tested only when cultivated at $a_w = 0.94$,
- *Aspergillus versicolor* and *Penicillium* sp. overgrew materials under all moisture conditions, except for wood and a fine lime plaster, when they grew only at $a_w = 0.94$ after 3 months,
- none of the materials tested showed any fungicidic potential as micromycetes remained cultivable after 3 months of the experiment under all moistures used, fig. 1–3.

3.2 Dusty building materials

Wood (naked as well as coated) was again the most fungal-resistant. Ceramic tiles and silicone cement with oily coating had a lower resistance and, finally, the cement with painting was proven, too. *Acremonium* sp. did not even colonize any of the wooden samples tested, and on the others grew only occasionally. *A. versicolor* colonized all systems of dusty building materials under the given moisture conditions. Thus, the house dust affected antifungal properties of the materials only very moderately, fig. 4–6.

Notes to figures

0 – no growth of moulds, 1 – microscopically visible colonization, 2 – visible growth, 25% surface, 3 - 50% surface, 4 – more than 50% surface, 5 – overrun.

A – fine lime plaster Terra R-605, B – traditional lime plaster, C – ceramic tiles, D – grain lime plaster Terra 141 P, E – joint cement (silicone), F – traditional gypsum mortar, G – wood

C. sphaerospermum, *Acremonium sp.*, *A. versicolor*, *A. ustus*, *Penicillium sp.*, *Scedosporium apiospermum*

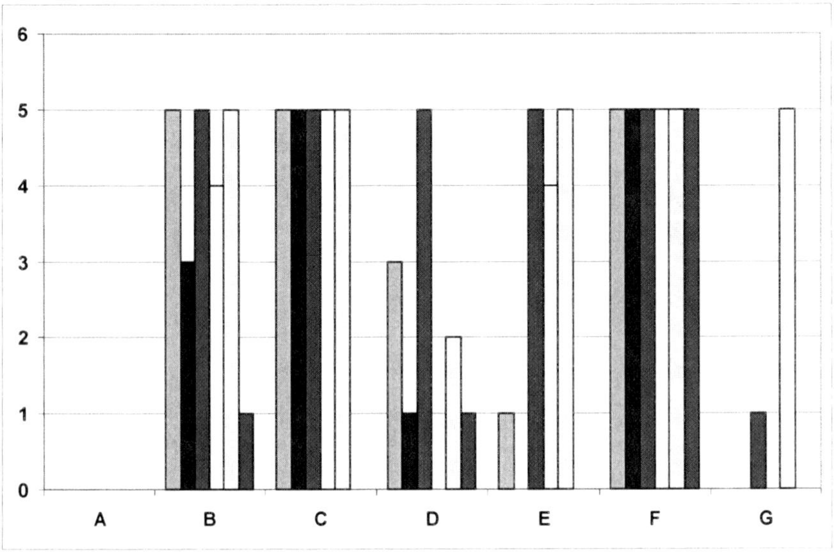

Figure 1: Fungal colonization of building materials under their water activity 0.94.

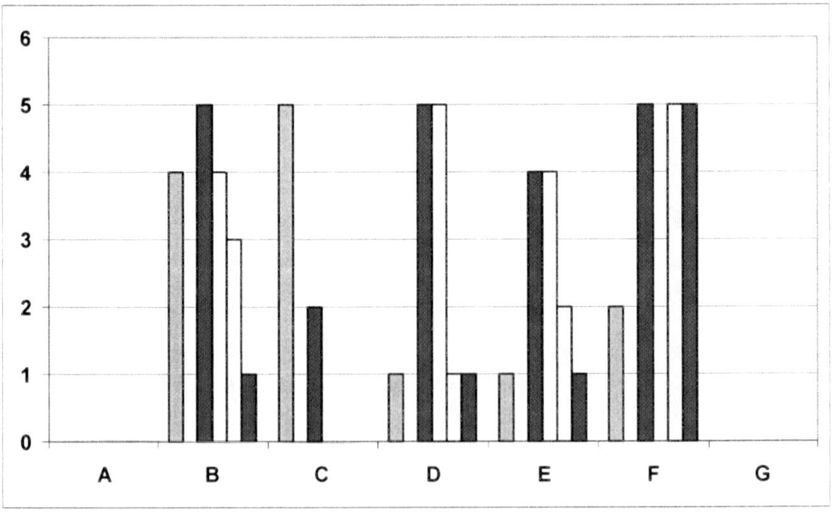

Figure 2: Fungal colonization of building materials under their water activity 0.83.

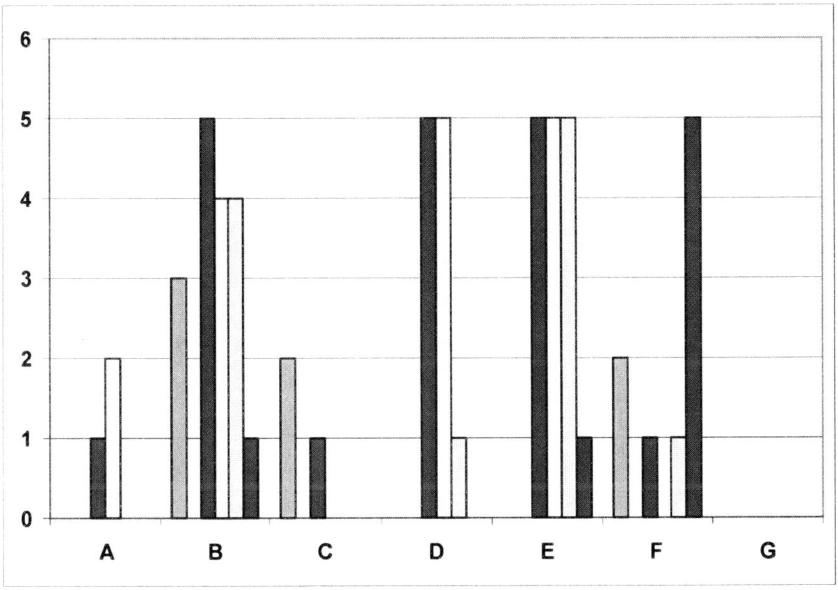

Figure 3: Fungal colonization of building materials under their water activity 0.75.

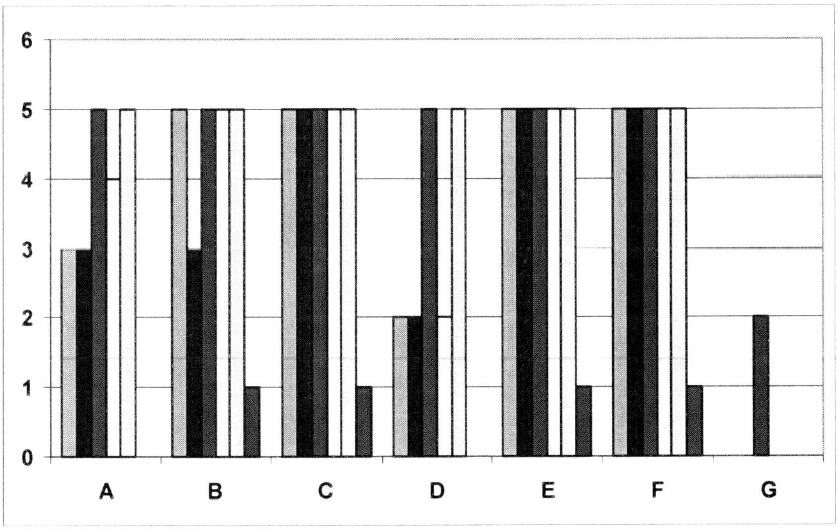

Figure 4: Fungal colonization of dusty building materials with water activity 0.94.

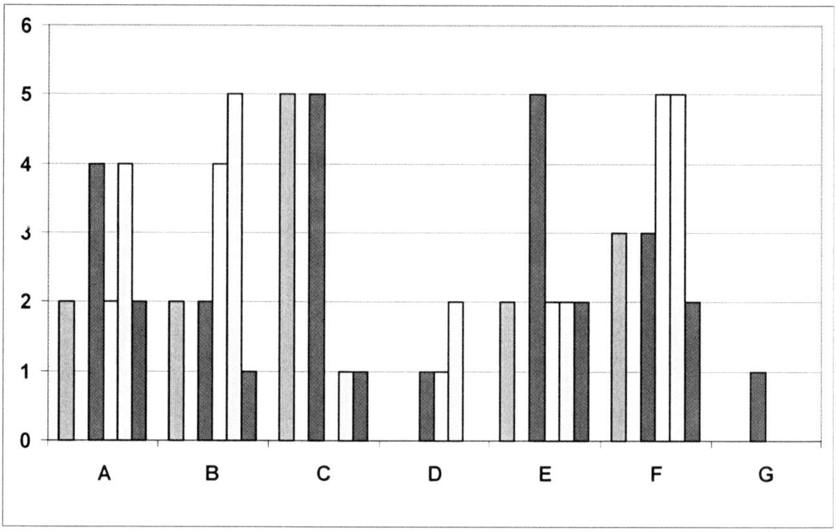

Figure 5: Fungal colonization of dusty building materials with water activity 0.83.

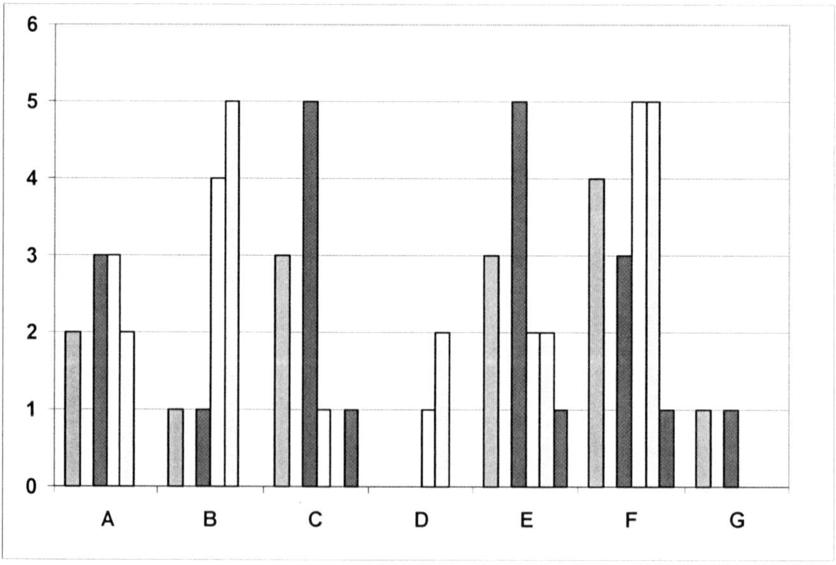

Figure 6: Fungal colonization of dusty building materials with water activity 0.75.

Actually, the results proved that – from the fungal colonization point of view – the physical characteristics (diffusion properties and moisture content) of the building materials used in the construction are the most potent factors affecting the appearance and development of the moulds. Finally, the presence of the house dust on the materials' surfaces did not promote their fungal colonization extremely. Less porous or materials that were easily dried were, generally, more resistant to the fungal colonization. The same could also be said about their coating types. Anyway, fungal growths depended on the particular moulds as well.

4 Conclusion

In the model of the 3-month experiments, all building materials with lime components or oily coating showed a certain antifungal resistance, including under very damp conditions ($a_w = 0.94$).

Representatives of common airborne fungi – the primary colonizers of the surfaces, aspergilli and penicillia, and the secondary one *Cladosporium sphaerospermum* visibly grew on samples tested – clean or dusty (simulation of real indoor "dirty" surfaces), although in particular extension due to given moisture conditions. The tertiary colonizers *Acremonium* sp. and *Scedosporium apiospermum* fulfilled the expectation – an especially, high $a_w = 0.94$ favoured their development on the materials.

No material seemed to be fungicidal – mould propagules kept their vitality expressed as the ability to germinate on a complete nutrient medium (Sabouraud agar) after 3 months of the experiment.

Wood, both naked and with coating, may be considered as the most fungal resistant building material – a possible effect of natural terpenes – but no celulolytic microorganisms were employed.

Antifungal properties of indoor materials' surfaces could be improved by coatings, even in very damp spaces ($a_w = 0.94$, bathrooms, kitchens). The traditional mortar materials were shown not to be proper mycologically even in the environment with the lowest $a_w = 0.75$, which is common in the rooms with a wrong household regime (e.g. too little or incorrectly ventilated and heated sleeping rooms).

References

[1] Peat, J. K., Dickerson, J. & Li, J., Effects of damp and mould in the home on respiratory health: A review of the literature. *Allergy* , **53**, pp. 120 – 128, 1998.

[2] Kalliokoski, P., Pasanen, A.-L., Korpi, A. & Pasanen, P., House dust as a growth medium for microorganisms. *Indoor air '96 – Proc. of the 7th Int. Conf. On Indoor Air Quality and Climate*: Nagoya, Japan, pp. 131 – 136, 1996.

[3] Hodgson, M. J., Morey, P. & Leung, W.-Y., Building-associated pulmonary disease from exposure to *Stachybotrys chartarum* and

Aspergillus versicolor. *Journal of Occupational and Environmental Medicine*, **40**, pp. 241 – 249, 1998.

[4] Piecková, E. & Jesenská, Z., Study of mycotic contamination of plasters *in vitro*. (In Slovak). *Hygiena*, **45**, pp. 37 – 41, 2000.

[5] Nielsen, K. F., Hansen, M. O., Larsen, T. O. & Thrane, U., Production of trichothecene mycotoxins on water damaged gypsum boards in Danish buildings. *International Biodeterioration and Biodegradation*, **42**, pp. 1 – 7, 1998a.

[6] Ren, P., Ahearn, D. G. & Crow, Jr., S. A., Mycotoxins of *Alternaria alternata* produced on ceiling tiles. *Journal of Industrial Microbiology and Biotechnology*, **20**, pp. 53 – 54, 1998.

[7] Nielsen, K. F., Thrane, U. & Larsen, T. O., Production of mycotoxins on artificially inoculated building materials. *International Biodeterioration and Biodegradation*, **42**, pp. 9 – 16, 1998b.

[8] Gravesen, S., Nielsen, P. A., Iversen, R. & Nielsen, K. F., Microfungal contamination of damp buildings – examples of risk constructions and risk materials. *Environmental Health Perspectives*, **107**, pp. 505 – 508,1999.

[9] Wilkins, K. & Piecková, E., Detection of ciliostatic activity in fungal growth on building materials. *Environmental Science and Pollution Research*, **9**, pp. 105 – 106, 2002.

[10] ISO 846: (E) prepared by Technical Committee ISO/TC 61 Plastics, Subcommittee SC6 Aging, chemical and environmental resistance, 1997.

[11] STN 56 0030: Measurement of the water activity in foods, 1999.

Use of the *in vitro* model for the evaluation of toxic effects of metabolites produced by fungi

Z. Kováčiková[1], E. Piecková[1], E. Tátrai[2], Z. Pivovarová[1] & M. Mataušic-Pišl[3]
[1]*Slovak Medical University, Bratislava, Slovakia*
[2]*National Institute of Environmental Health, Budapest, Hungary*
[3]*Institute of Medical Research and Occupational Health, Zagreb, Croatia*

Abstract

There are several reports about chronic intoxications, allergies or other pulmonary health problems of dwellers (especially babies) and workers from buildings contaminated with microfungi. Material from presented work was collected during the study of indoor fungal colonization of mouldy dwellings and public buildings in Slovakia. The isolated fungi were cultivated for 10 days in liquid media and their products – both endo- and exometabolites were isolated. The metabolites from four isolates of *Stachybotrys chartarum*, two of *Aspergillus versicolor* and one of *Penicillium chrysogenum* were used. Their effects were studied *in vitro* on rat alveolar epithelial type 2 cells, from the toxicological point of view one of the most important lung cells type. Type 2 cells were cultured for 20 hours in DMEM and then they were exposed for 24 hours to various concentrations of metabolites. The toxicity was evaluated by staining the cells for alkaline phosphatase which is a marker for this cell type. The toxic effect of metabolites from all isolates of *Stachybotrys chartarum* was dose dependent, there were differencies in the extent of cytotoxicity. From the tested microorganisms *Stachabotrys chartarum* and *Aspergillus versicolor* showed high toxic effects (*Stachybotrys* higher than *Aspergillus*), while *Penicillium chrysogenum* only minor toxic effects in this test.
Keywords: alveolar epithelial type 2 cells, Stachybotrys chartarum, Aspergillus versicolor, Penicillium chrysogenum, metabolites.

www.witpress.com, ISSN 1743-3525 (on-line)
doi:10.2495/EHR070091

1 Introduction

Exposure to microbes is recognized as a potential cause of inflammation related health problems among occupants of mouldy buildings. The current understanding is that the microbial growth affects the indoor air quality and occupants are exposed to biological pollutants but there are not information which components of the microbial flora are most harmful [1]. During a 5-year study of indoor fungal colonization of mouldy dwellings and public buildings in Slovakia, 147 wall scrapings, house dust and air samples were collected [2]. From recovered isolates of various microfungi 4 isolates of *Stachybotrys chartarum*, 2 isolates of *Aspergillus versicolor* and 1 of *Penicillium chrysogenum* were chosen for this study. As inhalation route is the possible entry of microorganisms or their products our attention must be focused on the lung. Lung is a very complex organ, it consists only in the bronchoalveolar region from more than 40 cell types [3]. Alveolar epithelial type 2 cells belong (from the toxicological point of view) to the most important cells. Type 2 cells are cuboidal cells with lamellar body structures that cover approximately 5% of alveolar surface area and play a critical role in preserving the functional integrity of the alveolar surface [4]. Histochemical staining revealed that in the bronchoalveolar region of lung alkaline phosphatase is uniquely associated with the apical portion of alveolar type 2 cells and therefore alkaline phosphatase is used as marker for this type of cells. In presented study we used this marker for studying the effect of metabolites produced by fungi on alveolar epithelial type 2 cells isolated from rats.

2 Materials and methods

2.1 Isolation of fungal metabolites

Stachybotrys chartarum, *Aspergillus versicolor* and *Penicillium chrysogenum* were inoculated on a liquid medium (2% yeast extract and 10% sucrose) and cultivated at 25°C for 10 days. The fermented cultures were filtered through Whatman paper No. 5 under reduced pressure. Both media and biomass filter cakes were collected. Separated biomass (endometabolites) and cultivation media (exometabolites) were extracted twice with chloroform, extracts were concentrated in vacuo to dryness (Buchi 461 Water Bath, Buchi RE 121 Rotavapor, Flavil, Switzerland).

2.2 Isolation and cultivation of alveolar epithelial type 2 cells

Male Wistar rats (Velaz, Prague, Czech Republic) of about 180-200 g were used in these experiments. Alveolar epithelial type 2 cells were isolated according to Richards et al. [5] and Hoet et al. [6]. Cells were cultivated under standard laboratory conditions in Dulbecco´s Modified Eagles´ Medium (DMEM) with 5% fetal bovine serum (FBS) for 20 hours in the atmosphere of 5% carbon dioxide in air at 37°C before exposure to metabolites. The metabolites were applied at various concentrations in fresh medium with 5% FBS and the cultivation continued for another 24 hours. After finishing the cultivation the medium was withdrawn, cells were washed twice with phosphate buffered saline and the staining for alkaline phosphatase was performed.

2.3 Alkaline phosphatase staining (APh)

The cells were stained by the adapted method of Bingle et al [7]. One tablet of naphtol AS-TR phosphate was dissolved in 10 ml deionised water and 3 tablets of Fast Red RC were dissolved in 5 ml TRIS-HCl buffer pH 8.5. Cells were stained in a mixture of 5 ml AS-TR and 5 ml Fast Red by incubation for 30 minutes at room temperature. Positive cells were stained bright red. Only cells with 4 or more lamellar bodies were considered to be type 2 cells.

3 Results

3.1 Comparing the number of alkaline phosphatase positive cells after exposure to metabolites from various *Stachybotrys chartarum* isolates

Staining of type 2 cells showed that endometabolites from *Stachybotrys chartarum* decreased the number of alkaline phosphatase positive cells dose dependently. The individual samples differ in the extent of changes. The greatest inhibition was seen in sample 3 (Figure 1).

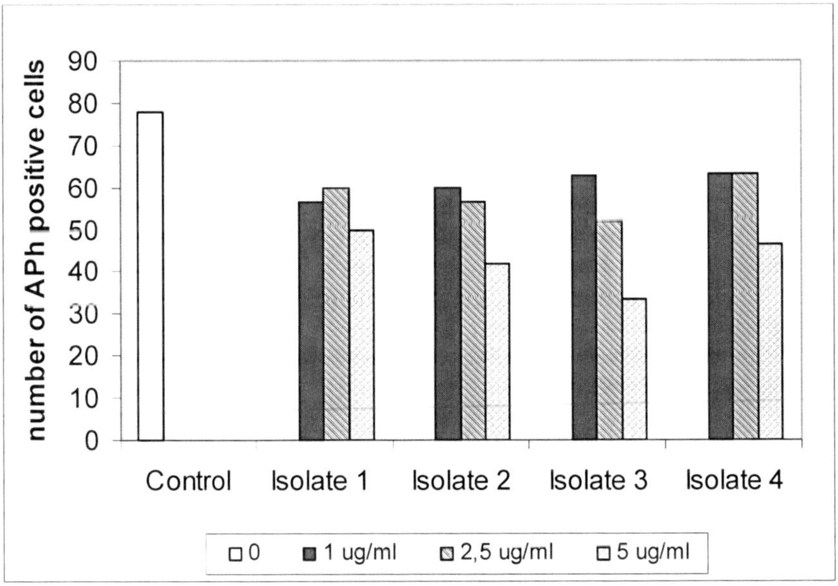

Figure 1: Effect of endometabolites from 4 isolates of *Stachybotrys chartarum* on alkaline phosphatase positivity of alveolar epithelial type 2 cells after 24 h *in vitro* culture.

3.2 Effect of metabolites from *Aspergillus versicolor* on alveolar epithelial type 2 cells

Results from 24 hours exposure of type 2 cells to metabolites isolated from *Aspergillus versicolor* are summarized in Figure 2. Both endo- and exometabolites of two isolates were tested. The higher dose (2μg/ml) of endometabolites showed greater toxicity than the same concentration of exometabolites but the exposure to lower doses exhibited similar effects of both types of metabolites.

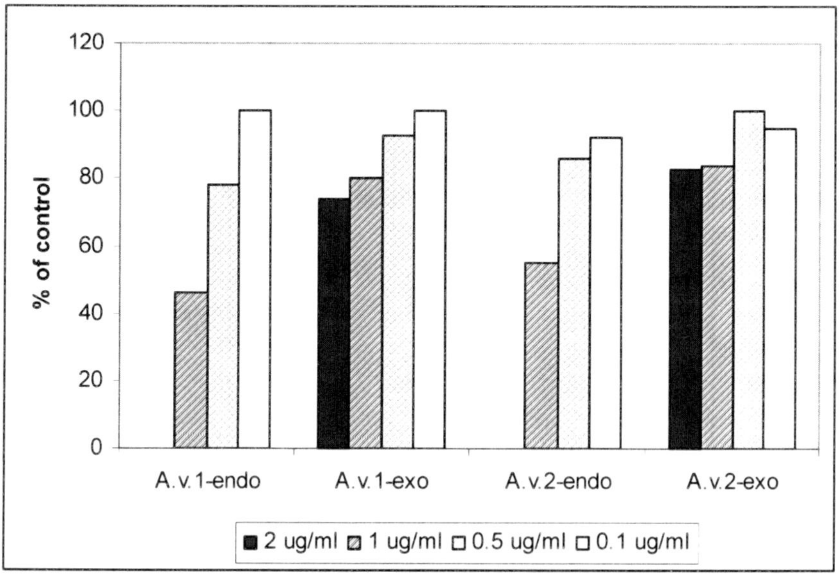

Figure 2: Effect of endo- and exometabolites from 2 isolates of *Aspergillus versicolor* on alkaline phosphatase positivity of lung epithelial type 2 cells after 24 h in *vitro* culture. (A.v.: *Aspergillus versicolor;* endo: endometabolites; exo: exometabolites.

3.3 Exposure of alveolar epithelial type 2 cells to metabolites produced by *Penicillium chrysogenum*

The pilot study of influence of both endo- and exometabolites from *Penicillium chrysogenum* on the type 2 cells at the concentration 0.1-2 μg/ml showed that the exposed cells exhibited 85-97% alkaline phosphatase positivity of the control value.

4 Discussion

The aim of the study was to compare the effect of metabolites produced by various fungi isolated from mouldy buildings. *In vitro* cultured alveolar epithelial type 2 cells isolated from rats were used for testing their effect. Metabolites from four different isolates of *Stachybotrys chartarum*, two of *Aspergillus versicolor* and one of *Penicillium chrysogenum* were studied. The effect decreased in order *Stachybotrys chartarum*, *Aspergillus versicolor*, *Penicillium chrysogenum*. The metabolites from all isolates of *S. chartarum* and *A. versicolor* exhibited similar results, their toxic effect was increased dose dependently, they differ only in their extent. There is evidence [8] that microfungi can concurrently produce mixture of metabolites, each of them has different effect and these metabolites may act synergistically what may be the possible explanation for differencies between individual isolates. Metabolites of *P. chrysogenum* showed only minor effect on the alkaline positivity of the type 2 cells. Figure 2 gives evidence that there are differencies between the effect of endo- and exometabolites of *A. versicolor:* the higher concentration of endometabolites were more toxic than the same concentration of exometabolites but at lower concentration (which are more near to the reality) there were not significant differencies. The results were same also in case of *S. chartarum* (unpublished results). There are differencies not only in the effect of particular isolates but also in response of particular lung cell type. In the previous study [9] we have proved that alveolar macrophages are more sensitive to the metabolites produced by *S. chartarum* than type 2 cells.

Acknowledgements

The study was supported by the Ministry of Health of the Slovak Republic under the project 2005/36-SZU-14 and by EC contract HEAR NAS QLK6-2002-90945.

References

[1] Huttunen, K., Hyvärinen, A., Nevalainen, A., Komulainen, H. & Hirvonen, M.R., Production of proinflammatory mediators by indoor air bacteria and fungal spores in mouse and human cell lines. *Environmental Health Perspectives* **111 (1)**, pp.85-92, 2003.

[2] Piecková, E., Hurbánková, M., Pivovarová, Z., Černá, S., Kováčiková, Z., Líšková, A., Wilkins, K. & Tátrai, E., Toxic effects of *Stachybotrys chartarum*. *Trends in Medical Mycology. 9th Congress of the European Confederation of Medical Mycology and 7th Trends in Invasive Fungal Infection*. Amsterdam, pp. 35-36, 2003.

[3] Sorokin, S.P., Properties of alveolar cells and tissues that strengthen alveolar defences. *Archives of Internal Medicine* **126**, pp. 450-163, 1970.

[4] Castranova, V., Rabovsky, J., Tucker, J.H. & Miles, P.R., The alveolar type II epithelial cell: a multifunctional pneumocyte. *Toxicology and Applied Pharmacology* **93**, pp.472-483, 1988.

[5] Richards, R.J., Davies, N., Atkins, J. & Oreffo, V.I.C., Isolation, biochemical characterisation and culture of lung type II cells of the rat. *Lung* **165**, pp. 143-158, 1987.

[6] Hoet, P.M.H., Lewis, C.P.L., Demedts, M. & Nemery, B., Putrescine and paraquat uptake in human lung slices and isolated type II pneumocytes. *Biochemical Pharmacology* **48**, pp.517-524, 1994.

[7] Bingle, L., Bull, T.B., Fox, B., Guz, A., Richards, R.J. & Tetley, T.D., Type II pneumocytes in mixed cell culture of human lung: a light and electron microscopic study. *Environmental Health Perspectives* **85**, pp. 71-80, 1990.

[8] Andersson, M.A., Nikulin, M., Koljalg, U., Andersson, M.C., Rainey, F., Reijula, K., Hintikka, E.L. & Salkinoja-Salonen, M., Bacteria, molds, and toxins in water damaged building materials. *Applied and Environmental Microbiology* **63**, pp. 387-393, 1997.

[9] Kováčiková, Z., Tátrai, E., Piecková, E., Tulinská, J., Pivovarová, Z., Mataušic-Pišl, M., Kuricová, M. & Wsolová, L., *In vitro* study of toxic effects of *Stachybotrys chartarum* metabolites on lung cells. *Alternatives to Laboratory Animals,* 2007 (in press).

Validation and implication of segmentation on Empirical Bayes for highway safety studies

R. R. Souleyrette, R. P. Haas & T. H. Maze
Iowa State University, SAIC and Iowa State University, USA

Abstract

Typically, crash frequency is modelled as Poison where the variation is the square root of the expected number. If the expected number of crashes is small, the variation is a large percentage of the expected number of crashes, and the observed number of crashes provides a crude estimate for the expected number. A better estimate is obtained when the expected number is large. For a specific location, there are two approaches for performing measurements where the expected number of crashes is large. One approach is to measure over a long period of time. However, data are not often available for long periods. Even if available, changes in conditions over time, such as increase in traffic volumes or improvement in infrastructure, may limit the useful time frame. Another approach is to perform measurements over a large number of similar locations, providing a relatively precise estimate for the distribution. Then, one can use the Empirical Bayes (EB) approach to combine the relatively precise estimate for the distribution with the less precise estimate for the expected number at the location of interest, resulting is an improved estimate for the expected number at that location. This paper explores the two approaches. It uses multiple years of data from the Highway Safety Information System for California intersections and highway links from the State of Iowa. Data from a single year is used to estimate the expected number of crashes at locations, following the EB approach. Data from multiple years at each location is then used to estimate the expected number of crashes at those locations, and the results from the two approaches are compared. No such large scale validation has yet been performed. The effect of *a priori* segmentation of the highway system is also explored. Longer, homogeneous sections are found both to improve the statistical validity of models and to improve the EB correction of one-year section crash estimates.
Keywords: count models, Empirical Bayes, crash frequency estimations, segmentation for crash sampling.

WIT Transactions on Biomedicine and Health, Vol 11, © 2007 WIT Press
www.witpress.com, ISSN 1743-3525 (on-line)
doi:10.2495/EHR070101

1 Introduction

The traditional methods for determining the benefit of roadway safety improvements can be divided into three types; before-after studies, cross-sectional studies, and regression studies. By far the most commonly used technique is before and after studies where one physical change is made to a location or locations and the analyst waits to see if crash trends at the location(s) are improved. The problem with this method is that it requires data for several years before and after the change and does not take into account temporal changes that occur in the after period (changes in stream composition, changes in automobile design, climate changes, etc.) Another traditional method is to use cross-sectional studies where one group of similar locations is treated with and another group of similar locations are not treated (sometimes called case/control studies). The problems with cross-sectional studies are that they ignore spatial differences (e.g., changes in land use, changes in traffic volumes, changes in enforcement policies, etc.) and place the safety engineer in the moral dilemma of specifically not applying a treatment to a control group where the engineer may believe the changes will improve safety.

To increase the number of data cases, cross-sectional data can be combined with case/control data, however, controlling for similarities in intersection geometry and volume is particularly critical. Often time there are a small number of very similar sites or a large number of sites with variations (traffic volume and geometry) which compromise the comparison.

Another common method is to model crash performance, typically using Poisson or Negative Binominal regression (commonly called a count model) to create Safety Performance Functions (SPFs). SPFs commonly include traffic volumes, traffic characteristics and patterns (e.g., percent trucks) and geometric differences in the highway. The regression model cannot take into account every variable that is responsible for a crash and there is a good deal of multi co-linearity between variables. As a result, typically regression models account for only a minority of the variance in crash counts and making them relatively inaccurate when it comes to estimating the benefits of a treatment.

The Empirical Bayes (EB) approach combines the strengths of before-after studies, cross-sectional studies, and regression methods when estimating the safety related benefits of an improvement. EB uses data from a group of similar control sites and pre-treatment data from the case site to determine the crash performance before the improvement is made. This allows comparison of the after treatment safety performance at a site to estimate the expected safety performance had the improvement not been made. The difference during this period is the "safety benefit" of the treatment. In other words, EB bases the expected safety performance (without the treatment at the site) on the performance observed at the site prior to treatment, and the performance at similar sites. EB reduces the variability of estimates of safety performance beyond traditional methods. (1)

EB also helps to diminish the impact of regression to the mean. Regression to the mean impacts estimates when treatments are applied to roadway segments or intersections that may be randomly experiencing poor safety performance. Even without the treatment, the safety performance is likely to improve. Because EB estimates rely on untreated locations, use of a safety performance sample from similar untreated sites tends to reduce the impact of regression to the mean.

2 Overview of Empirical Bayes

One of the challenges in working with traffic crash statistics is generating accurate estimates for the expected number of crashes per year at a location. The root of the difficulty is that the actual number of crashes follows a Poisson distribution with mean (λ) equal to the expected number of crashes, and this distribution is broad for the types of locations typically studied in transportation. As a rough estimate, the 95% confidence interval for λ is $\lambda \pm 2\sqrt{\lambda / N}$, where N is the number of years for which data are available. For a location where the expected number of crashes is 20, the 95% confidence interval has width 18 for a single year of crash data. A single year of data provides a very unreliable estimate for the expected number of crashes.

One way to improve the estimate for the expected number of crashes is to use multiple years of crash data. For five years of crash data, the width of the 95% confidence interval is 8. For ten years of crash data, the width is about 5.6. It is not practical to use longer periods because traffic conditions are likely to have changed so much over such long periods that the historical crashes are no longer good indicators of the number of crashes that would currently occur.

An alternate method for providing more accurate estimates for the expected number of crashes, would be to group together data from a large number of identical locations. Since the locations are identical, the expected number of crashes at each location would be the same, and the observations from these locations can be combined to estimate λ. In essence, one replaces a long time-series of crash data at a single location with crash data from a large number of identical locations.

While this is a good approach in theory, in the real world, there are no "identical locations". In the real world, the expected number of crashes for a collection of similar locations will be close to each other, but not exactly the same. The Empirical Bayes approach takes this into consideration by combining the distribution in the observed number of crashes that comes about because of the Poisson nature of crashes with the distribution for the expected number of crashes at similar locations. The Empirical Bayesian formula is:

$$\lambda = \left(\frac{1}{1 + \varphi / N\lambda_0} \right) \frac{n}{N} + \left(\frac{\varphi / N\lambda_0}{1 + \varphi / N\lambda_0} \right) \lambda_0$$

where λ_0 is the average number of crashes per year for the entire collection of locations, n is the number of crashes observed at the location of interest during N

years of observations, and φ is a parameter that indicates how much variation exists in the expected number of crashes for the locations in the collection. If φ is large, the variation in the expected number of crashes is small; if φ is small, the variation is large. One can see this in the formula above. If φ is large, the expected number of crashes is close to λ_0 for all the locations in the collection, so the formula weights the λ_0 term more strongly. If φ is small, the opposite occurs.

One can think of the collection of similar locations as providing a model for the location of interest. Thought of in this way, the Empirical Bayes formula generates an improved estimate for the expected number of crashes for a location by taking a weighted average of an estimate based on crash data for that location and an estimate based on the model. The value for the weight changes to place more emphasis on the more accurate of the two approaches.

This thought process points to another way to improve estimates for the expected number of crashes. In the above formula, the simplest model was used to estimate the expected number of crashes for locations in the collection – the average for the collection. One could further improve the estimate for the expected number of crashes at the location of interest by using a better model for the expected number of crashes in the collection. An improved model will result in lower unexplained variance in the collection, a higher value for φ, and greater weight for the model term in the Empirical Bayesian formula. Because the EB formula places more weight on the more accurate model, the resulting estimates for the expected number of crashes at the location of interest should be more accurate.

3 Research objective

The objective of this research is to explore the relationship between the effectiveness of the Empirical Bayesian formula at correcting estimates for the expected number of crashes at a location and the accuracy of the model for the expected number of crashes in the comparison group. To meet this objective, crash data were collected for both a large number of similar locations and for a number of years at each location. Comparisons were made between estimates for the expected number of crashes using, 1) a single year of data with different models and the Empirical Bayesian formula, and 2) several years of crash data at specific locations. These comparisons verify the value of the Empirical Bayesian approach at improving estimates for the expected number of crashes and emphasize the importance of an accurate model for the expected number of crashes in the comparison group. A second objective is to explore the relationship between segmentation and accuracy of estimates, as crash data must be aggregated to units of analysis prior to processing.

4 Description of the data used

Two types of data were used for this research. The first type of data was crash data and road inventory data from Iowa. Both the crash and road inventory data are maintained by the Iowa Department of Transportation (a USA state level agency) and are available to support safety analysts. For this analysis, five years of crash data were compiled for more than 7,000 miles of Iowa roads. The roads were classified into three primary categories: 2-lane roads, multi-lane and divided roads, and freeways and Interstates. The 2-lane roads were further subdivided into low, medium, and high volume roads based on average annual daily traffic (AADT).

To support this research, the roads were divided into segments. Analysis was conducted on the annual number of crashes for these segments. Three different sizes of segments were used: short segments with approximate length of 0.25 miles, medium segments with approximate length of 2.5 miles, and long segments with approximate length of 4 miles. All in all, this created fifteen collections of segments for which crash models were developed.

The second type of data was crash and road inventory data from the US Federal Highway Administration, Highway Safety Information System (HSIS). The HSIS data are collected from seven participating States and maintained by the Federal Highway Administration to support highway safety research. (More information is available from the HSIS website at http://www.hsisinfo.org/.) For this research, five years of crash and road inventory data were provided for the approximately 18,000 junctions (intersections) included in the California HSIS data. One limitation regarding the California HSIS data was noted – few of the cross street volumes had been recently updated.

The data were filtered to identify intersections for which key intersection attributes (i.e., intersection geometry and type of traffic control) were constant over the five-year period and the number of crashes per year was tallied for each of these intersections. As with the Iowa data, the intersections were then divided into groups based on the intersection geometry and the type of traffic control at the intersection, and crash models were developed for the different groups of intersections. This resulted in three datasets: multi-phase signal control (873 intersections), single-phase signal control (374 intersections) and two-way stop-control, aka through-stop control (3047 intersections).

5 Analysis approach

For each of the 15 road section datasets and for the three intersection datasets, negative binomial safety performance functions (SPFs) were fit using the R program (available at http://www.r-project.org/) While five years of crash data were available, only 2004 crash data were used to develop the models. This was to demonstrate the use of EB where several years of crash data may not be available. Road models (SPFs) are of the general form: Crashes = α Length $(AADT)^{\beta}$. Table 1 presents the road model parameters and descriptive statistics.

The intersection model (SPF) are of three forms: a) Crashes = $\alpha(ADTML)^{\beta}$, b) Crashes = $\alpha(ADTML)^{\beta}(ADTXS)^{\gamma}$, or c) Crashes = $\alpha\ (ADTML)^{\beta}(NXSL)^{\delta}$, where ADTML is average daily traffic on the main line, ADTXS is ADT on the cross street and NXSL is the number of cross street lanes. Table 2 presents the intersection model parameters and descriptive statistics.

Table 1: Road model parameters and descriptive statistics.

ID	Segment Length	# segments	Avg. length	Avg AADT	road type	α	β	φ
1	Short	19536	0.28	5614	all	0.0034	0.7281	1.20
2		3684	0.23	16315	Freeway	0.0022	0.7453	1.82
3		4228	0.13	8714	multi-divided	0.0019	0.8327	0.71
4		19459	0.32	2689	2-lane	0.0013	0.8497	1.17
5		6493	0.37	1225	2-lane low AADT	0.6038*	-0.0106*	0.93
6		6491	0.34	2398	2-lane med AADT	0.0030	0.7228	1.36
7		6478	0.26	4440	2-lane high AADT	0.0000	1.4368	1.22
8	Med	2983	2.59	4785	All	0.0029	0.7433	3.01
9		364	2.36	16166	Freeway	0.0020	0.7583	3.88
10		276	1.98	7963	multi-divided	0.0023	0.7968	5.43
11		2343	2.7	2643	2-lane	0.0013	0.8442	2.86
12	Long	1508	5.1	4185	All	0.0020	0.7904	3.42
13		119	7.23	1574	Freeway	0.0008	0.8555	3.74
14		153	3.65	8324	multi-divided	0.0023	0.7955	7.09
15		1236	5.08	2605	2-lane	0.0014	0.8334	3.24

* model parameter is not statistically significant.

Table 2: Intersection model parameters and descriptive statistics.

Control type	Number of intersections	Avg ADTML	Avg ADTXS	Avg NXSL	Model Form	α	β	γ	δ	φ
Multiphase signal	873	31388	7775	2.804	a	0.067	0.427			1.649
					b	0.047	0.363	0.120		1.727
					c	0.081	0.388		0.224	1.669
Single Phase signal	374	28413	6251	2.5695	a	0.059	0.429			1.330
					b	0.018	0.411	0.164		1.408
					c	0.053	0.419		0.238*	1.340
Thru-stop	3047	14086	789	1.9829	a	0.002	0.684			0.896
					b	0.002	0.515	0.303		1.080
					c	0.002	0.687		-0.144*	0.897

* model parameter is not statistically significant.

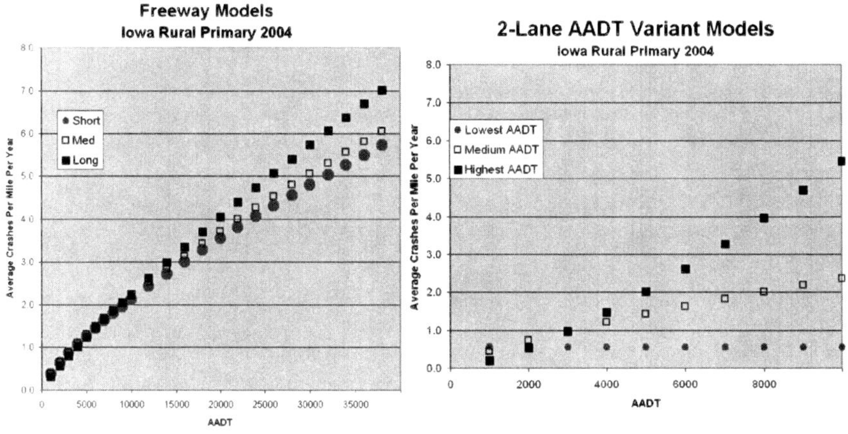

Figure 1: Example road SPFs.

Most of the models fit produced statistically valid results. Exceptions were the low volume 2-lane model and two of the intersection models based on cross street number of lanes as a proxy for cross street ADT (as confidence in the cross street ADT values was low, models were also fit on NXSL as a proxy). Figure 1 illustrates freeway and AADT variant 2-lane models derived from the various levels of segmentation used in this research.

6 Analysis results

To illustrate the effects of segmentation and choice of "comparable data" on the results of the EB procedure, several "high crash" road segments and intersections were selected. These locations were chosen based only on their 2004 crash experience. The purpose was to compare EB estimates for these high crash locations to their five-year crash performance average and to demonstrate the effect of various levels of data aggregation. Recall that data aggregation was performed across two dimensions, segment length (short, medium and long) and similarity of segments (road type, intersection control, AADT class, etc.)

A total of nine road sections, all of the freeway/Interstate class, were selected as "high crash locations." Three each were selected from each of the three road segmentation databases (low, medium and high). Table 3 presents the comparison of EB estimate to five-year average crash frequencies. It can be seen that the EB correction is most accurate when longer segmentation is used. While the shortest segmentation provides the greatest homogeneity, the longer sections values are corrected most closely to their five-year averages.

Three intersections, all of the multi-phase signalized class, were also selected as "high crash locations." Table 4 presents the comparison of EB estimate to five-year average crash frequencies. It can be seen that the EB provides very good adjustments to the single year crash numbers – placing the expected value much closer to the five-year average. (Recall that only one year of data was used to derive the EB corrected estimates.)

Table 3: Road section case studies.

Segmentation	Length	AADT	Crashes in 2004	Model	EB estimate	5yr avg crashes
	0.35	30600	6	3.69	5.63	2.0
	0.46	16300	7	2.87	6.18	5.4
short	0.24	19900	8	1.77	6.22	4.8
	1.01	35444	16	5.79	11.9	10.2
	0.86	38953	23	5.30	15.5	19.8
med	0.65	27948	26	3.11	13.3	15.0
	1.88	22828	25	8.53	20.0	21.6
	0.65	27948	26	3.51	14.4	15.0
long	3.56	17312	35	12.75	30.0	25.4

Table 4: Intersection case studies.

model	ML_AADT	XSTAADT	XSTLANES	Crashes in 2004	EB estimate	φ	5yr average crashes
	22750	3300	2	23	18.4		14.6
a	18700	27200	4	21	16.4	1.649	15.8
	24000	4750	4	20	16.2		12.4
	22750	3300	2	23	18.1		14.6
b	18700	27200	4	21	17.4	1.727	15.8
	24000	4750	4	20	16.1		12.4
	22750	3300	2	23	18.1		14.6
c	18700	27200	4	21	17.0	1.669	15.8
	24000	4750	4	20	16.6		12.4

A more detailed comparison was also conducted across all of the intersections. In this comparison, the standard deviation of the difference between the number of crashes in 2004 and the 5-year average was 2.43. For model a, the standard deviation was 3.95. When the EB formula was used to combine the model with the 2004 observations, the standard deviation was 2.03. In other words, the model by itself provided a poor estimate for the expected number of crashes, but improved the estimates when used with EB and a single year of crash data.

7 Conclusions

This paper demonstrates the effectiveness of EB at improving estimates for the expected number of crashes for road segments and intersections. For road segments, a simple model was applied to fifteen different road segment databases. A sample of nine segments was considered and comparisons made between the 5-year average number of crashes for these segments and the estimates of the expected number of crashes based on a single year of data at that location, a model for crashes at similar locations, and the EB combination of the two. These examples demonstrate how EB improves estimates over use of either a single year of data or the model alone.

These examples demonstrate another feature related how the explanatory power of the model impacts the effectiveness of EB. Table 1 indicates that the term φ is significantly lower for short segments than for medium and long segments. This indicates that, for short segments, there is greater variability about the model estimates than for longer segments. In other words, the model is a better estimator of the expected number of crashes for medium and long segments. The EB formula takes this into consideration when adjusting the estimate for the expected number of crashes. For medium and long segments, the model is more accurate. Because of this, the EB formula places a higher weight on the model, increasing the overall effect of the model on the EB estimate. This is apparent in Table 3 because the EB adjustment for short segments is very small (because φ indicates that the model is not very accurate) and the EB adjustment for medium and long segments is much larger.

For intersections, several different models were developed for three different types of intersections. Table 4 lists the model and EB estimates for 3 example intersections. Even though the differences in φ are small, larger values of φ still correspond to better EB estimates for the 5-year average of the number of observed crashes. A comparison of the single-year, model, and EB estimates for the expected number of crashes for all the intersections with multi-phase signal controllers provides further evidence of the power of EB. EB combined two estimates for the number of crashes at each intersection, one with a root-mean square difference of 2.43 from the average of 5-years of observations and one with a root-mean square difference of 3.95, to produce an EB estimate with root-mean square difference of 2.03. Thus, EB combined two relatively poor estimates for the expected number of crashes at these intersections to produce a significantly improved estimate.

These results demonstrate how EB improves estimates for the expected number of crashes for road segments and at intersections. For the intersections in this study, the use of EB with very simple model resulted in a 20% improvement in estimates for the expected number of crashes at these intersections. Better results would be expected with a more accurate model. The road segment results listed in this paper provide some support for this statement. The improvement in estimates for short segments (where φ was small, indicating more variance unexplained by the model) was less dramatic than for medium and long segments (where φ was larger and there was less unexplained variance).

References

[1] Hauer, E.; Harwood, D.; Council, F.; Griffith, M.; "Estimating Safety by the Empirical Bayes Method: A Tutorial". Transportation Research Record No. 1784, Statistical Methodology: Applications to Design, Data Analysis, and Evaluation. 2002. pp. 126-131.

Section 3
Occupational health

Evaluation of physiological comfort index for workers wearing protective clothing in nuclear or other harsh environments

F. Cumo[1], F. Gugliermetti[1] & G. Guidi[2]
[1]*Department of Fisica Tecnica, Sapienza University of Rome, Italy*
[2]*ENEA, Department of Fusion and Nuclear Technologies, Italy*

Abstract

The assessment of thermal stress and the translation of the stress in terms of physiological strain is complex. There are many indexes evaluating thermal stress but most of them don't take into account physiological variables such as core temperature, heat rate and sweat rate. The need to wear protective clothing in harsh environments, such as for example those affected by nuclear, chemical or biological contamination, may lead to intolerable heat strain, as the clothing limits the workers' ability to lose heat to the environment. A survey on physiological comfort indices showed that PSI (Physiological Strain Index) is the most appreciated one, as individual reactions to it are only based on core temperature and heart rate. Moreover, PSI index can assess in real time both physiological response to heat and heat strain among any combination of climate, clothing and work rate. This index does not consider sweat rate, because of its intrinsic difficulty in performing an on-line measurement: nevertheless this term should be taken into account, especially in the case of short and repeated operations. This work proposes the use of two physiological comfort indices: the first one concerns long-lasting operations and the second concerns short and repeated operations. In order to calculate the value of coefficients in the new physiological comfort index, it is necessary to carry out a measurement campaign on a sufficiently wide statistical population. These measurements should lead to a quantitative evaluation of the importance of the term taking into account the presence of cooling systems in personal protective clothing.
Keywords: physiological comfort index, personal protective equipment, heat stress, heat strain.

WIT Transactions on Biomedicine and Health, Vol 11, © 2007 WIT Press
www.witpress.com, ISSN 1743-3525 (on-line)
doi:10.2495/EHR070111

1 Introduction

The use of personal protective equipment (PPE), when required by hazardous activities, is often opposed by workers because of its lack of comfort, both thermal and physiological. The need to wear protective clothing may lead to intolerable heat strain, as clothing will have a detrimental effect on the workers ability to lose heat to the environment. Even though PPE offer the required protection, in some conditions they may increase the risk of heat strain, that could be a threat to worker's life. When heat stress may cause a risk, this can be assessed directly, by means of physiological measurements, but in many situations it is not practical. Different methods for estimating potential heat stress have been developed and many indices exist, but none of them is widely accepted.

2 Personal protective equipment in nuclear decontamination activities

While in nuclear power plants it is possible to use robots, in nuclear fuel cycle facilities, because of their geometry, this possibility not always occurs. In this case the use of a ventilated-pressurized protective clothing is required to ensure workers against the hazard of radioactive contamination [1].

The clothing is made of impermeable material that protects the whole body (head, hands and feet) and it is equipped with a ventilation system to supply breathable air and to ensure required overpressure. Studies and interventions, performed during the deactivation and decontamination of Hot Cells in ENEA Casaccia Research Centre, showed performance improvements in the protective equipment usage if a direct skin ventilation and an emergency extracting system (ENEA patent, see fig. 1) are used too. Emergency extracting system offers many advantages like: easy employability in limited spaces, simplicity and reliability, ease of removal of the operator to be succoured toward the exit.

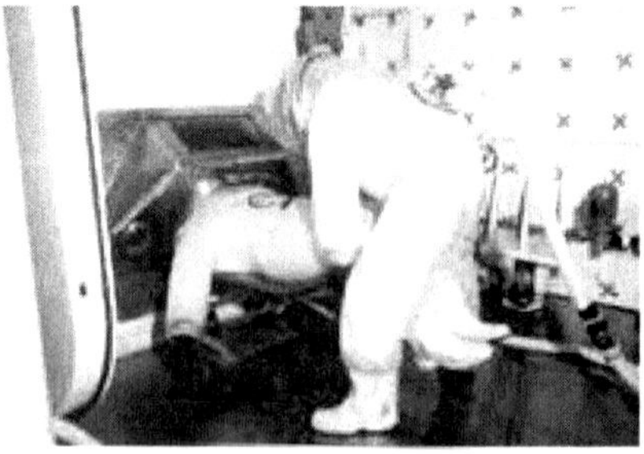

Figure 1: ENEA extracting system.

Direct skin ventilation in ventilated-pressurized protective clothing guarantees a better thermal regulation especially when operations should be performed in hot environments. This system directly ensures cooling of the wearer's skin. The studies, supported by occupational physicians, proved that for the same ventilation rate and the same physical work rate, the acceptability duration may be improved by 50% by means of the body refreshing due to direct skin ventilation, in comparison with the traditional clothing in which the ventilation is fed into the suit, that is only over the underwear [2]. Workers audit carried out in ENEA confirmed the benefit of the ventilated-pressurized clothing especially as regards the increasing in comfort. The acceptability duration is defined as the time at which the wearer, performing a heavy work, has accomplished some physiological limits:

- skin temperature increase $\leq 3°C$
- increase of heart rate $\leq 30\%$
- rectal temperature increase $\leq 2°C$
- body mass loss ≤ 2 kg.

Data collected in ENEA Casaccia Research Centre, over more than 500 interventions, showed that the ventilated-pressurized protective clothing may be successfully used both in hazardous operations developed in nuclear and chemical industry, and in environment with low air contamination levels, due to the following advantages:

- the conspicuous reduction of the wastes volume (with broad advantages for the environment);
- the remarkable decrease of the contamination risk for personnel;
- the operator safety, due to the resistance and reliability of materials and systems.

The usage of a protective clothing places workers at risk because it prevents the loss of heat by convection, radiation and evaporation from the body. When the body temperature rises above about 40°C the mechanisms that usually control body temperature at around 37°C stop working, with potential lethal consequences [3]. If the body cannot lose heat, then even small amounts of heat, generated by doing a physical task, will cause heat strain in less than 30 minutes. Frequently the signs of heat illness, such as nausea, irritability, sluggishness, pallor, lack of sweating, are misunderstood with fatal consequences.

3 Thermal comfort indices

Heat stress is a combination of factors, such as air temperature, air movement, humidity, radiant heat and accomplished work that influence the body heat balance; the physiological responses to heat stress is the heat strain.

Thermal comfort is defined in the ISO 7730 [4] as "that condition of mind that expresses satisfaction with the thermal environment". As a matter of fact thermal comfort is very difficult to define because it is necessary to take into account a range of environmental and personal factors when deciding what will make people feel comfortable.

The assessment of this psychological state may be quantified by means of indices taking into account environmental factors such as:

- air temperature;
- radiant temperature;
- air velocity;
- humidity;

and personal factors such as:

- metabolic heat;
- clothing insulation.

Among the available indices, one of the most widely used index is the PMV (Predicted Mean Vote) and the PPD (Predicted Percentage of Dissatisfied) index. This index predicts the thermal comfort of people working in a given environment. PPD is the predicted percent of dissatisfied people at each PMV. As PMV changes away from zero in either the positive or negative direction, PPD increases.

The ISO 7243 [5] provides a simple method and uses the Wet Bulb Globe Temperature (WBGT) index to assess hot environments. This index is obtained from three parameters: black globe temperature (T_g) which reflects the solar radiation, wet bulb temperature (T_w) and dry bulb temperature (T_a). This index is calculated as follows:

$$WBGT = 0.7T_w + 0.2T_g + 0.1T_a \quad (1)$$

The WBGT index was found to be limited in evaluating heat stress, due to the inconvenience of measuring T_g. Besides the correlation of this index to physiological responses was only partially tested.

Other indices exist, such as for example HSI (Heat Stress Index) and ESI (Environmental Stress Index) index, proposed by Moran et al [6], but none of them takes into account physiological parameters.

While indices of heat stress have become widely used in occupational settings, attempts at developing indices of heat strain have been less successful. The increased needs for workers to wear heavy, impermeable clothing while working in hot environments, has the potential to increase heat related injuries.

The high number of heat stress indices developed over the years, the lack of broad acceptance of any single index reinforce the problems of managing heat stress, especially in occupational setting. The problem of clothing, and personal protective equipment in particular, is another item, in addition to the above mentioned ones. Most indices are used to predict whether continuous work is possible or some sort of work/rest cycle is required under particular conditions.

4 Physiological comfort indices

In order to monitor heat strain, physiological variables must be taken into account. Physiological comfort indices try to quantify thermal environment comfort with regard to the physiological reactions to heat exposure. Many attempts have been carried out in order to combine environmental parameters with the physiological ones to develop a single index [7]. Currently there are many indices but none of them is widely accepted. The main reason lies in the greatest complexity and plurality of interactions among the main factors to take into account when defining the index.

A simple, easily calculated physiological strain index for use in hot environments, that provides a rapid and accurate assessment of the heat strain, could reduce the risk of heat exposure. Moran et al. [8] developed a Physiological heat Strain Index (PSI) based upon the summation, with equal weight factors, of individual strains for core temperature (T_c) and heart rate (f_c) as follows:

$$PSI = 5\frac{(T_{cf} - T_{c0})}{39.5 - T_{c0}} + 5\frac{(f_{cf} - f_{c0})}{180 - f_{c0}} \quad (2)$$

where T_{cf} and f_{cf} are simultaneous measurements taken at any time during the exposure and T_{c0} and f_{c0} are the initial measurements. The index represent the combined strains of the termoregulatory and cardiovascular systems. Each strain system was scaled between 0 and 5. The PSI index places the heat strain on a scale of 0 through 10. It can be applied at any time, including rest or recovery periods, whenever T_c and f_c are measured.

5 Proposal for the definition of a new physiological comfort index

A survey on physiological comfort indices has been carried out. It showed that PSI (Physiological Strain Index) is the most appreciate one. It offers advantages such as the following ones:

- it gives on line values, for a real time evaluation of physiological response to heat. It can be calculated while the subject is exposed to heat stress and it is not necessary to wait till the end of the exposure to analyze the heat strain; moreover it allows to take action quickly, before physiological parameters reach dangerous values for the operator's health;
- it can also be calculate in rest situations, when the values of core temperature and heart rate are recorded;
- it is able to evaluate heat strain under different combinations of work rate, environmental conditions and clothing.

The PSI index does not contain sweat rate intentionally, because of its inherent on-line measurement difficulty even if, as everybody knows, it is a parameter that should be taken into account in order to have a whole evaluation.
For these reasons it is possible to alter the Moran et al. definition of PSI index in order to introduce some improvements:

- in PSI index, core temperature and heart rate have equal weights; it could be possible to modify the weight of the two parameters if experimental proofs justify a different influence of the above mentioned parameters to physiological comfort;
- PSI index has been obtained for healthy young men; for this reason 3°C and 120 beats/min were the maximal rise for core temperature and heart rate respectively from normothermia to hyperthermia during exposure to heat stress. It is generally known that heat stress tolerability for middle-aged men and women is less than for those younger; to apply PSI to women and different age groups, corrective coefficients, taking into account the age and the sex of individuals, should be brought in;
- insert a term linked to sweat rate;
- put in a corrective term, reducing the index value when there is an appropriate skin ventilation system in the personal protective equipment, worn by the operator.

The term referred to sweat rate is easily measurable, in case of short-lasting and repeated operations, by means of the difference between the weight of the subject before and after the operation. This term, especially when short-lasting and repeated operations should be performed in harsh environment, should be taken into account.

Two indices are proposed, to employ depending on the intervention length, for operators wearing personal protective equipment:

1) index for long-lasting operations;
2) index for short-lasting operations.

On first approximation an intervention is considered long-lasting when its length is greater than 40 minutes.

In case of long-lasting operations the authors propose an index very similar to PSI including, as far as concerns the physiological parameters, only the two terms: core temperature and heart rate.

As regards the core temperature measurement, it is manifest that a system based upon the on-line measurement of the rectal temperature is rather awkward for operators performing long-lasting operations and still are up for numerous and also hard movements. Therefore it is proposed, in case of long-lasting operations, the use of an alternative core temperature measurement method, based on the aural temperature. The walls of the auditory meatus, immediately adjacent to the tympanum, are vascularized by the external carotid artery and their temperature is affected both by the arterial blood temperature at the heart and by the cutaneous blood flow around the ear and adjacent parts of the head. A temperature gradient is thus observed between the tympanum and the external orifice of the auditory meatus. Insulating the ear adequately from the external climate may reduce this gradient [9]. Literature data highlight that this method shows greater errors than the one based on rectal temperature measurement; nevertheless these errors, which are affected by the external climate, in the case of operators wearing ventilated full suit, are undoubtedly smaller in comparison with the case of operators wearing standard clothing and working outdoor.

It is suggested to carry out preliminarily a comparative study on the operators which will be involved in the operational campaign, between the rectal temperature and the aural temperature, in order to establish the correlation between them. Just after that it could be possible to make use of the following formula containing the rectal temperature as a measure for core temperature. This formula includes a third term taking into account a possible presence of cooling equipment in the personal protective equipment under consideration (for example direct skin ventilation):

$$PCI = a\frac{(T_{Ct} - T_{C0})}{39.5 - T_{C0}} + b\frac{(HR_t - HR_0)}{180 - HR_0} - rC \tag{3}$$

where:
PCI is the physiological comfort index;
a is a coefficient;
T_{Ct} is the core temperature during the intervention;
T_{C0} is the core temperature at the beginning;
b is a coefficient;
HR_t is the heart rate at the end of the intervention;
HR_0 is the heart rate at the beginning;
r is a coefficient;
C is the term taking into account the presence of cooling equipment in the personal protective equipment.

For short-lasting and repeated operations two terms should be added compared to PSI index:

- the first one pertains to sweat rate;
- the second one takes into account the presence of a cooling system in the personal protective equipment.

The numerator of the term concerning the sweat rate contains the sweat rate, obtained from the difference between the worker body mass before and after the operation, adjusted for water intake and urine output. The denominator contains the numeric value 1.25 is referred to the limit for sweat rate, as indicated by ISO 7933 [10] for acclimatized subjects (1.25 l/h):

$$PCI = a\frac{(T_{Ct} - T_{C0})}{39.5 - T_{C0}} + b\frac{(HR_t - HR_0)}{180 - HR_0} + c\frac{M}{1.25 * t} - rC \qquad (4)$$

where:
PCI is the physiological comfort index;
a is a coefficient;
T_{Ct} is the core temperature during the intervention;
T_{C0} is the core temperature at the beginning;
b is a coefficient;
HR_t is the heart rate at the end of the intervention;
HR_0 is the heart rate at the beginning;
c is a coefficient;
M is the sweat rate, equal to the difference between the worker body mass before and after the operation;
t is the duration of the operation;
r is a coefficient;
C is the term taking into account the presence of a cooling equipment in the personal protective equipment.

In order to calculate the numeric value of a, b, c coefficients pertaining to the three physiological parameters (core temperature, heart rate and sweat rate), an ad hoc measurement campaign will be necessary on an enough wide statistical population, because of variability of individual physiological reactions.

In the case of workers wearing personal protective equipment the thermal load is most of all of metabolic type, rather than environmental. Workers wearing ventilated-pressurized protective clothing experienced the presence of sweating inside the suit at the end of the operation. The sweating quantity surely has to be correlated to physiological strain. The quantification of the negative corrective term, linked to the cooling system, if it exists in the protective equipment, should be experimentally obtained, evaluating the trend of the three physiological parameters in the presence and in the absence of the system itself.

6 Conclusions

The WBGT index is essentially a first stage assessment method: it can be used to evaluate the heat stress only on first approximation. Furthermore WBGT index is limited in evaluating heat stress due to the inconvenience of measuring T_g (the black globe temperature) and it is not well-suited in measuring the body reactions to heat, particularly when workers wear impermeable personal protective equipment [11]. The ESI index does not consider any physiological parameter revealing body reactions.

The PSI index takes into account physiological parameters such as core temperature and heart rate, but it does not consider the body mass loss. This index has been validated on young and healthy men, performing work outdoor and wearing different kind of clothing.

This work proposes to make use of two new indices, to apply depending on the heat exposure duration and trying to overcome limits of PSI index. Both new indices contain a term reckoning with the possible presence of cooling systems inside the protective equipment, capable of improving operators' physiological comfort. It could be convenient to carry out experimental surveys aiming, first of all, at a quantitative assessment of this contribution. These surveys should also lead up to the determination of a, b, c and r coefficients when workers wear protective equipment in harsh environments. Only by means of these experimental surveys it could be possible to attain a correct definition of a physiological comfort index: it is an important item because it allows to determine the maximum employment time for the protective equipment as well as the duration of work-rest cycles.

Acknowledgement

Authors wish to thank ISPESL (National Institute for Occupational Safety and Prevention) for supporting the study.

References

[1] Caporossi G., Cumo F. & Guidi G., Intervento diretto dell'uomo in ambienti contaminati: esperienza in un impianto del ciclo del combustibile nucleare. *Atti del Convegno Nazionale di Radioprotezione "Sanità e Ambiente: ricerca e radioprotezione operativa", Verona, 16-18 settembre 2004.*

[2] Bruhl G., Bisceglie G.P., Caporossi G. & Marangio G., Progress made in the design and the use of ventilated-pressurized protective clothing against contamination. *Proc. of the International Conference on Harmonization in radiation protection: from theory to practical applications, Taormina, 11th- 13th October 1993.*

[3] Crockford G.W., Protective clothing and heat stress: introduction. *The Annals of Occupational Hygiene,* **43(5)**, pp. 287-288, 1999.

[4] ISO 7730, Moderate thermal environments – determination of the PMV and PPD indices and specification of the conditions for thermal comfort, ISO, Geneva 1994.

[5] ISO 7243, Hot environments – estimation of the heat stress on working man, based on the WBGT index, ISO, Geneva 1989.

[6] Moran D.S., Pandolf K.B., Shapiro Y., Heled Y., Shani Y., Matthew W.T., & Gonzales R.R., An environmental stress index (ESI) as a substitute for the wet bulb globe temperature (WBGT). *Journal of Thermal Biology*, **26,** pp. 427-431, 2001.

[7] Cumo F. & Guidi G., Indici di comfort fisiologici utilizzati per valutare lo stress subito da lavoratori che indossano dispositivi di protezione integrali. *Atti del 60° Congresso Nazionale ATI "Energia e ambiente: valori condivisi", Roma, 13-15 settembre 2005.*

[8] Moran D.S., Shitzer A. & Pandolf K.B., A physiological strain index (PSI) to evaluate heat stress. *American Journal of Physiology* **274(44)**, R129-R134, 1998.

[9] ISO 9886, Evaluation of thermal strain by physiological measurements, ISO, Geneva 1992.

[10] ISO 7933, Hot environments – analytical determination and interpretation of thermal stress using calculation of required sweat rate, ISO, Geneva, 1989.

[11] Hanson, M.A., Development of a Draft British Standard: the Assessment of Heat Strain for Workers Wearing Personal Protective Equipment. *The Annals of Occupational Hygiene,* **43(5)**, pp. 309-319, 1999.

Environmental health risk from past uranium mining and milling activities

F. P. Carvalho
Instituto Tecnológico e Nuclear, Departamento de Protecção Radiológica e Segurança Nuclear, Portugal

Abstract

In the last few years several European countries undertook closure and environmental remediation of old uranium mining sites. This is the case for Portugal. Due to concerns about public health, environmental radioactivity was recently investigated in a number of counties in the Centre-North of Portugal where the extraction and chemical treatment of uranium ore was carried out, as well as in reference areas. The results of this environmental research and of an assessment of the health condition of local populations allowed the conclusion that some exposure to radioactivity from uranium mining waste occurs in these areas. The reduction of such exposure should be achieved through environmental remediation measures. However, as radio nuclides in uranium mining and milling waste are very long lived and their potential to cause health hazards will last for centuries, remediation measures should be effective for generations. To achieve this goal adequate radioactivity monitoring around sites is needed and institutional custody of waste repository sites should be ensured.
Keywords: uranium mining, radioactive waste, ionizing radiation effects, public health, environmental remediation.

1 Introduction

Mining of radioactive ores in European countries took place during most of the last century. With the opening of very large uranium mines in Australia, Canada and Africa, uranium mining activities were displaced to these regions and former radium-uranium European producing countries closed their mines and radioactive ore treatment plants by the turn of the century. Since then, these countries started environmental remediation of former uranium mining and

www.witpress.com, ISSN 1743-3525 (on-line)
doi:10.2495/EHR070121

milling facilities. This occurred in France, East Germany, Spain, and in Portugal as well [1]. Growing environmental concerns and recommendations developed by international organisms for enhanced measures in the field of radiological protection of workers and members of the public, such as the Basic Safety Standards developed by the International Atomic Energy Agency [2] and the Basic Safety Standards approved by the European Union [3], fostered environmental remediation in former uranium mining areas and provided a technical framework for remediation goals.

In the beginning of uranium mining activity there was no awareness of ionizing radiation risks and environmental protection measures were less strict than they are today. In the present, the legacy of large uranium mining and milling waste deposits raises concerns about the risk of exposure of man through environmental pathways. Today, most of former uranium producing countries must deal with this legacy. These mining and milling wastes contain high concentrations of long lived radio nuclides, such as radium (^{226}Ra) with a half-life of 1600 years. Therefore, on one hand, environmental remediation measures shall be effective for long time in preventing the environmental contamination and exposure of populations to radioactivity. On the other hand, with the rising price of uranium, some countries may re start uranium mining and, thus, lessons from previous time must be taken into account in future activities.

This paper gives an account of the radium and uranium mining industry in Portugal, of waste generated and environmental radioactivity enhancement in old mining areas as well as of exposure of populations. Lessons to be retained are discussed.

2 Uranium mining industry in Portugal

Radioactive ores were exploited in Portugal during most of the last century. In total 61 mines mostly located in the uraniferous region at centre-North of the country (Fig. 1), were exploited as open pits or underground mines or in a combination of both methods.

For radium production the ores were chemically treated in the Uranium Salts Factory (1909-1926) located in Barracão, near Guarda. Later, for uranium production, ores from small mines were sent to one of the main facilities for uranium extraction. The largest mill and chemical treatment plant operated (1951-2001) at the Urgeiriça mine, in Canas de Senhorim, near the city of Viseu (Fig 1). These facilities ceased activity in 2001 and are now in the decommissioning process.

During the decades of radium-uranium mining, 50 – 100 grams of radium and 4370 tons of uranium oxide (U_3O_8) were produced. This activity generated solid wastes amounting to about 13 million tons including low radioactivity barren rocks, sands from extracted ores, and sludge from acid mine water treatment. From this total, near 3 million tons are located in the facilities of Urgeiriça mine, in low grade ore heaps (not extracted), milling tailings, and sludge ponds. Other waste heaps are deposited near other uranium mines in the region, such as Cunha Baixa, Quinta do Bispo and Bica [4].

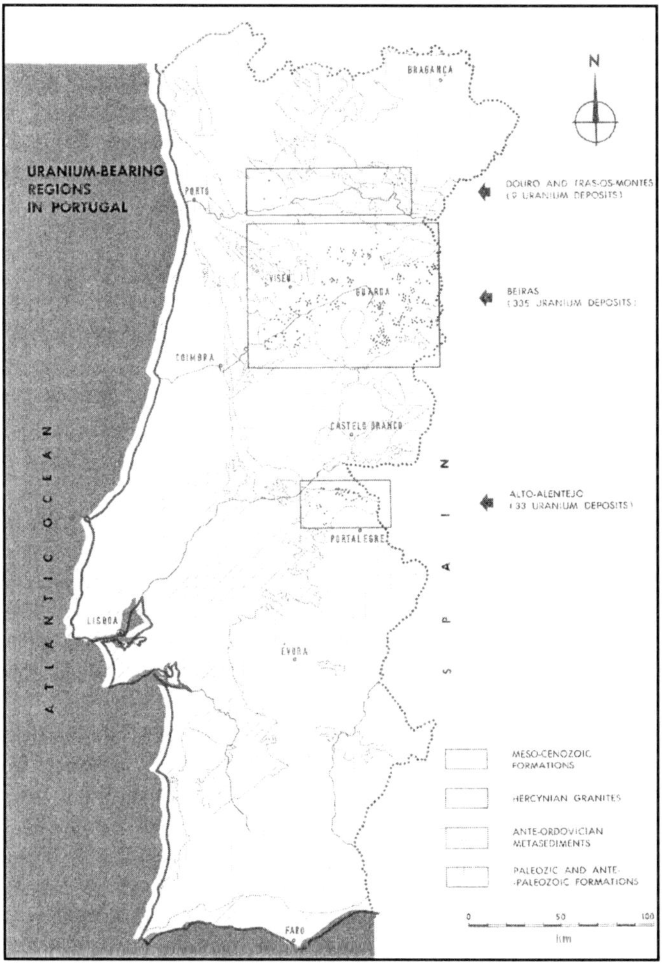

Figure 1: Location of the main uranium deposits in Portugal in a historic map (Source: JEN, 1969).

At the Urgeiriça mine site, liquid effluents from ore processing, surface runoff and drainage from the mill tailings have been released into a creek, Ribeira da Pantanha, flowing into the Mondego River, a major hydrographic basin in the region, causing some dispersal of radio nuclides in the environment [5]. During decades of mining activity, the U mining company has controlled the area and restricted the access to the waste tailings, thus minimizing the spread of contaminated materials in the region. Sulfuric acid was used in this underground mine for *in situ* uranium extraction. This procedure generated acid waters that infiltrate into groundwater.

Human activities may have contributed to enhance environmental radioactivity levels in the surrounding areas, for example through dispersal of materials recuperated from mining waste, such as sands and gravel used in improving rural roads and in construction. Further contributions might have come from wind erosion and radon emanation from tailings. This enhancement of environmental radioactivity levels may have caused exposure of populations to ionizing radiation above the natural background levels.

3 Assessment of environmental radioactivity

An assessment of environmental radioactivity was carried out in the county of Canas de Senhorim, Urgeiriça mine (Zone A), where U mining and milling wastes are accumulated in larger amounts than elsewhere. This assessment was extended to other counties with old uranium mines (Zone B) and also to counties with no past uranium mining (Zone C) in order to use the last ones as a reference area. All are located in the same geologic region.

The ambient radiation dose measured in Canas de Senhorim, outside the mining areas, averaged 2.5 mSv a^{-1}. Within the statistical uncertainty, this value compares to doses determined in counties with no uranium mining activities and no residues (Table 1). However, measurements made in the county of Canas de Senhorim but inside areas affected by the uranium mining activities, showed elevated radiation doses. These doses may reach for instance 41.2 mSv a^{-1} at the ore discharge in the milling facility.

It is interesting to observe the differences in radiation doses determined on two tailings, "Barragem Velha" and "Barragem Nova", existing in the area. While on "Barragem Velha" (dumpsite for extracted ore) the ambient dose amounts to 18.6 mSv a^{-1}, on "Barragem Nova" (dumpsite for sludge from mine water treatment) the dose is much lower, 3.4 mSv a^{-1} (Table 1). The reason for the difference was clarified through spectrometric analysis of waste materials and relates to the origin of waste. Milling waste (deposited in "Barragem Velha") corresponds to sandy materials rejected after uranium extraction and contains low concentrations of uranium and high concentrations of uranium descendants, such as ^{230}Th, ^{226}Ra, ^{210}Pb and ^{210}Po. Sludge from acid mine water treatment (accumulated in "Barragem Nova") has a different composition and displays uranium activity concentrations much higher than those of U descendants delivering lower gamma dose rate (Table 2).

As tailings are exposed to weathering, surface runoff may transport radio nuclides in the particulate phase, as well as rainwater seepage may transport dissolved radio nuclides into the surface water streams and sub-surface water reservoirs. Concentrations measured in surface drainage (BV1) and water percolated through the tailings (BV2) collected at "Barragem Velha" were very high for dissolved uranium and confirmed the role of these transport pathways. Acid water from the underground mine of Urgeiriça displays also very high radionuclide concentrations that may exceed concentrations in uncontaminated surface waters of Ribeira da Pantanha by three orders of magnitude (Table 2) [5, 6].

Analysis of radionuclides in agriculture soils has shown enhanced concentrations in soils in the vicinity of mining and milling areas. This was the case in the county of Canas de Senhorim, for instance. Nevertheless, apart the area of mining facilities soils do have naturally-occurring radionuclide concentrations comparable to soils in reference counties.

Table 1: Environmental annual dose equivalent, in mSv [6].

Zone	Site	Arithmetic mean ($mSv\ a^{-1}$)	Geometric mean ($mSv\ a^{-1}$)
A	Canas de Senhorim (a) outside mining concession	2.5 ± 0.8	2.4 ± 0.1
	Tailing Barragem Velha (b)	18.6 ± 27.6	8.8 ± 1.8
	Tailing Barragem Nova (b)	3.4 ± 1.4	3.2 ± 0.3
	Ore discharge at mill station (b)	41.2 ± 27.9	32.0 ± 11.0
B	Moreira de Rei	2.2 ± 0.4	2.2 ± 0.1
	Rio de Mel	2.3 ± 0.5	2.3 ± 0.1
C	Sátão	1.3 ± 0.3	1.23 ± 0.04

(a) Without the mining areas; (b) Mining areas and contiguous land.

The results indicate that dispersion of solid radioactive wastes from Urgeiriça mining facilities did occur into adjacent soils and into river basins in the region to some extent. Enhanced radioactivity levels were measured also in water from wells in this area and in other old mining areas. Although generally not used as drinking water supply anymore, wells still are currently used as irrigation water source. Measurements of radon and aerosols in surface air have shown enhanced concentrations also of radio nuclides in the atmosphere of the region.

Altogether these enhanced concentrations of uranium daughters in the environment increased the exposure of local inhabitants to ionizing radiation. It was concluded that the urgent issues are to confine residues, preventing further waste dispersal in the environment, and to protect the water lines from discharges of contaminated leaching and surface runoff from tailings. Otherwise radioactivity will spread further and human exposure to ionizing radiation may increase.

4 Effects on population health

The effects of exposure to environmental radioactivity from past uranium mining activities on populations' health were evaluated in two ways. One, through statistical tests on differences of biological parameters measured in the population of Canas de Senhorim (A) and in the populations used as a comparison term (B+C). The other, through looking at indicators of internal accumulation of radio nuclides and genetic damage induced in chromosomes by radiation.

Table 2: Concentration of alpha emitting radio nuclides (Bq kg^{-1} ± 1σ) in samples from mining and milling tailings at the Urgeiriça mine [5].

	^{238}U	^{230}Th	^{226}Ra	^{210}Po
Uranium tailings				
BV- Barragem Velha	2530± 94	10337 ± 598	24717 ± 2039	20354±681
BN- Barragem Nova	41598 ±1228	13390 ± 613	1690 ±150	1176±43
MS- Milling station	38316 ± 1154	30115 ± 1123	15569 ± 707	30824±1147
Acid mine water (Urgeiriça mine)				
Filtered water (-20 m)	2.17±0.07	0.015±0.003	1.48±0.06	0.146±0.004
Suspended matter (-20 m)	(35.1±1.7)x10^3	(1.8±0.1)x10^3	(12.1±0.5)x10^3	(52.5±2.8)x10^3
Runoff from tailings				
BV1- Surface runoff (Dissolved)	13.2±0.6	1.17±0.08	0.672±0.06	0.69±0.03
BV2– Percolation water (Dissolved)	35.7±1.1	1.06±0.06	1.84±0.03	0.70±0.04

Analyses of bio-medical parameters in populations confirmed that

- population A displays results compatible with a reduced performance of several biological functions in comparison with B+C populations,
- this reduction in performance was more clearly observed in the male reproductive health, thyroid function and blood cell counts,
- concentrations of lead, copper, and zinc in blood serum were also higher in A,
- although less significant, results suggest also a reduction of the woman's reproductive health and of the kidney function in A.

Notwithstanding, the observation method used in this study does not allow to identify the causes for the health differences measured in these population groups. However, the long term exposure of A population to radio nuclides and heavy metals from uranium mining is the most plausible cause for the differences measured [6].

Additional studies were carried out to assess the exposure of populations to radio nuclides. These were performed through analysis of radio nuclides in human hair and analysis of chromosome aberration in lymphocytes from peripheral blood. Analyses of ^{210}Po and ^{210}Pb in human hair have shown that the population living near the mining and milling tailings eliminates more ^{210}Po in the hair than reference groups [7]. This implies that the body burden of this population group in ^{210}Po parent radio nuclides, i.e., ^{226}Ra and ^{210}Pb, is higher than in the reference population. Furthermore, the genetic analyses indicated that the exposed population may have slightly higher chromosome aberrations that non exposed groups, and do have more efficient repair mechanisms for induced genetic lesions than the reference group which implies a previous exposure to ionizing radiation [6].

This investigation on exposure and effects on humans confirmed that environmental radioactivity and toxic metals from uranium mining waste, although relatively confined in space, have exposed local populations through environmental transfer pathways. These findings underscored the need to carry out environmental remediation and to monitor the environmental radioactivity and food chain transfer of radio nuclides in these areas.

5 Environmental remediation

Environmental remediation of the old mining areas was decided by the Government [8]. Remediation plans foresee the disposal of solid waste in the main open pits of each mining area, five in total. The tailings of Urgeiriça will be reshaped and capped in the same place where they have been located for decades, after cleaning the area of the chemical treatment plant and adding these residues to the dump site. Capping the waste dump will be performed with geo-textile membrane and soil from the region. The underground mine will be flooded and the acid water monitored as well as the leaching from the tailings.

The closure of waste disposal sites requires radioactivity surveillance for some time after completion of the remediation intervention. This surveillance should assess the exposure of populations through ingestion of local agriculture products, water, and aerosols inhalation. This surveillance should be carried out for compliance also with Euratom treaty Art. 35.

6 Future radiological risks and stewardship of sites

Environmental remediation is expected to immediately reduce ambient radiation doses. Furthermore, capping must also reduce radon emanation from tailings into the atmosphere, and thus will contribute to abate irradiation of lungs through inhalation. Nevertheless, the weathering of waste dumps will continue through decades and centuries and, thus, maintenance of the sites must be foreseen in order to prevent removal (erosion, intrusion, etc.) of capping materials. Water may flow through the waste and generate radioactive leaching that eventually could reach groundwater. These risks require a periodic monitoring of radioactivity in the environment and corrective measures as needed.

Stewardship of remediated sites is needed but costs may vary according to the engineered solutions. Solutions based on active treatment of effluents and sophisticated maintenance will be costly and subject to undue interruption in the future and, therefore, seem too much contingent to last for generations. May be a better choice would be the adoption of natural remediation processes, requiring minimal maintenance.

Past uranium mining activities were justified and profitable. In the present, the mining and milling waste accumulated desirably should be out of the biosphere in order to prevent radiological exposure of man. This has to be achieved in old uranium mining areas and requires environmental remediation and radiological surveillance for the next decades to ensure that waste disposal methods are protecting the public health in an effective manner.

References

[1] M. Hagen, A.T. Jakubick (2006). Returning the WISMUT legacy into productive use. *In*: Uranium in the Environment: Mining Impacts and Consequences, pp 11-26. B.J. Merkel and A. Hasche-Berger (Ed.). Springer-Verlag, Berlin Heidelberg.

[2] International Basic Safety Standards for Protection against Ionizing Radiation and for the Safety of Radiation Sources. Safety Series N° 115. International atomic Energy Agency, Vienna, 1996.

[3] European Union Directive 96/29/EURATOM.

[4] F.P.Carvalho, M.J. Madruga, M.C. Reis, J.G. Alves, J.M. Oliveira, J. Gouveia, L. Silva (2005). Radioactive survey in former uranium mining areas in Portugal. Proceed. of an *International Workshop on Environmental Contamination from Uranium Production Facilities and Remediation Measures*, held in Lisbon 11-13 Feb 2004, pp.29-40. International Atomic Energy Agency, Vienna.

[5] F.P.Carvalho, J.M.Oliveira, M.J.Madruga, I.Lopes, A.Libanio, L.Machado (2005). Contamination of hydrographical basins in uranium mining areas of Portugal. *In*: Uranium in the Environment: Mining Impacts and Consequences, pp 691-702. B.J. Merkel and A. Hasche-Berger Ed. Springer-Verlag, Berlin Heidelberg.

[6] J.M. Falcão, F.P. Carvalho, M.M. Leite, M. Alarcão, E.Cordeiro, J. Ribeiro, et al. (2005). MinUrar-Minas de Uranio e seus Resíduos.Efeitos na Saúde da População. Relatório Científico I (Julho de 2005). Publ. INSA, INETI, ITN.(available from www.itn.pt)

[7] F. P. Carvalho and J. M. Oliveira (2006). Natural radioisotopes ^{210}Po and ^{210}Pb in human hair as an indicator of exposure. In: *Metal Ions in Biology and Medicine, Vol 9,* pp.570-576. M Alpoim and P. Collery Ed., J. Libbey Eurotext Publishers, Paris.

[8] Santiago Baptista A. (2005). The programme for remediation of contaminated sites: its regulation and follow-up in Portugal. Proceed. of an *International Workshop on Environmental Contamination from Uranium Production Facilities and Remediation Measures*, held in Lisbon 11-13 Feb 2004, pp.223-232. International Atomic Energy Agency, Vienna.

The role of measurement accuracy on the heat stress assessment according to ISO 7933: 2004

F. R. d'Ambrosio Alfano[1], B. I. Palella[2] & G. Riccio[2]
[1]*DIMEC, Dipartimento di Ingegneria Meccanica, Università di Salerno, Italy*
[2]*DETEC, Dipartimento di Energetica, Termofluidodinamica Applicata e Condizionamenti Ambientali, Università di Napoli Federico II, Italy*

Abstract

The thermo-hygrometric risk analysis, regulated by several International Standards, is one of the more relevant facets of workplace assessment. Based on the predicted heat strain (PHS) model, the last version of ISO Standard 7933 devoted to the hot stress evaluation requires the measure of four physical (air temperature, mean radiant temperature, humidity and air velocity) and two subjective (metabolic rate and thermal clothing insulation) parameters. As far as the measurement of microclimatic parameters is concerned, ISO 7726 Standard suggests minimum and maximum accuracy values. On the other hand, for subjective measurements the situation does not appear so clear since the metabolic rate accuracy requirements are strictly related to the calculation method, whereas any accuracy is actually suggested for the clothing insulation evaluation. In order to evaluate the effect of the measurement accuracy on the reliability of the hot stress assessment, this work reports a sensitivity analysis of the PHS model to its independent variables. The results obtained clearly show that the mean radiant temperature measurement appears a tricky matter since only an error within the accuracy range can result in a very strong overestimation (up to 5 hours) of allowable exposure times.
Keywords: heat stress assessment, accuracy, predicted heat strain.

1 Introduction

In the last sixty years several efforts have been devoted by the scientific community to the formulation of a reliable index/method for the heat stress

WIT Transactions on Biomedicine and Health, Vol 11, © 2007 WIT Press
www.witpress.com, ISSN 1743-3525 (on-line)
doi:10.2495/EHR070131

assessment [1, 2]. The different ways of treating the matter result in an impressing number of indices (often empirical) characterised by a balanced compromise among the reliability of the assessment, a user-friendly calculation and a reduced number of measurements. In spite of this apparent confusion, the ISO layout for hot extreme environments [3] is very clear: for a rough preliminary assessment the calculation of the WBGT index [4], whereas, for an in-depth analysis of the working situation, the Predicted Heat Strain (PHS) approach [5], are required. Based on the heat balance equation of the human body [6, 7], PHS method requires the measure of four physical (air temperature, mean radiant temperature, humidity and air velocity) and two subjective (metabolic rate and thermal clothing insulation) variables in order to evaluate maximum allowable exposure time compatible with a limit rectal temperature of 38°C and a maximum water loss of 5% of the overall subject weight [5].

Since the thermal response of the subject predicted by PHS model is strictly related to the six variables quoted above, both accuracy and a right procedure for measuring the whole of the variables involved in the assessment appear a crucial need: as a matter of fact one or more errors could result in a wrong estimation of the maximum allowable exposure time.

On this point of view we need to underline that:

- ISO 7726 Standard [8] suggests the minimum characteristics (required and desirable) of instruments for measuring the four physical parameters;
- ISO 8996 Standard [9] specifies methods for estimating metabolic rate and their accuracy on the base of four different measurement levels (screening, observation, analysis and expertise), suggesting as far as possible, the most thorough method.
- ISO/DIS 9920 Standard [10] deals with methods for estimating thermal characteristics of clothing ensemble, also taking into account the pumping effect due to body movements [11] but it does not suggest their accuracy.

The need of a right heat stress assessment provided some crucial answers:

- Minimum and maximum accuracy levels required by Standards actually in force are enough for a reliable assessment of the working situation?
- In case suggested accuracy levels should not be enough, what kind of strategy is required?
- Which variables play a more significant role in the assessment phase? Microclimatic ones? Subjective ones or both?

In order to thoroughly answer these questions a valid investigation tool is undoubtedly the sensitivity analysis of PHS model to its independent variables. On one hand this approach allows to establish how the measurement errors affect the heat stress assessments; on the other one it could suggest more or less restrictive accuracy requirements with the consequent choice of more adequate measurements devices or methods.

2 Methods

As the mathematical function binding subjective and microclimatic variables to the physiological response of the subject to the thermal environment according to the PHS model is not handy to treat [5,11], the sensitivity analysis has been carried out by means of a special software designed according to ISO 7933 [11]. More in particular, this software is able to return:

a) The final values of the rectal temperature and the water loss after eight hours of continuous work starting from a full data set of two subjective and four microclimatic parameters;

b) Temperature-humidity limit curves allowing 8 hours of continuous work starting from a data set of two subjective and two microclimatic (mean radiant temperature and air velocity).

Two levels of subjective variables have been investigated: concerning the metabolic rate (M) 1,7 and 2,8 met corresponding to a light and a moderate activity [9], whereas, concerning the clothing insulation (I_{cl}) 0,60 and 1,0 clo, typical values of summer and winter clothes [10]. As far as the microclimatic parameters are concerned, table 1 summarizes the investigated ranges of air temperature, mean radiant temperature, air velocity and humidity.

Table 1: Microclimatic variables ranges investigated.

Microclimatic variable	Symbol	Range
Air velocity	v_a	0,20 m/s
Mean radiant temperature	t_r	15÷45°C
Air temperature	t_a	15÷45°C
Humidity ratio	RH	0÷100%

Table 2 briefly summarises the whole of the non-measurable parameters (i.e. weight, height, posture, acclimatization status, drinking possibility and so on), required by PHS for the hot stress assessment [5].

Table 2: Non-measurable parameter values required by PHS method [5].

Parameter	Value
Weight	75 kg
Height	1,70 m
Posture	Standing
Clothing vapour permeability	0,38
Acclimatization status	Not acclimatised
Freely drinking possibility	Yes

The sensitivity analysis reported here, by varying each variable in the range of desired and required accuracy required by ISO 7726 Standard [8] for typical hot stress situation (S class), has been carried out. Concerning clothing insulation an accuracy of ±10% has been used, since any indication is actually required by ISO/DIS 9920 [10]. About the metabolic rate accuracy ISO 8996 reports typical precision values in the range 5÷20% depending on the method used for the evaluation of the metabolic rate (i.e. tables, heart rate measurement, oxygen consumption measurement, double labelled water method, direct calorimetry) [9]. We made use of a value ±10% corresponding to the typical accuracy of metabolic rate assessed by means of the heart frequency values. A summary of investigation is reported in table 3.

Table 3: Summary of accuracy values used in this investigation.

Variable	Required Accuracy	Desired Accuracy
t_a	±0,50°C	±0,25°C
t_r	±5,00°C	
v_a	$\pm(0{,}1 + 0{,}05\ v_a)$	$\pm(0{,}05 + 0{,}05\ v_a)$
p_a	±0,15 kPa	
M	±10%	
I_{cl}		

The calculation phase has been organized in three different steps:

1) Starting from nominal values of each variable, temperature-humidity curves (called nominal limit curves) corresponding to 8 hours of continuous work have been preliminarily obtained. By this way safe working conditions have been depicted on special psychometrics charts (fig. 1 and fig. 2).
2) In the second phase each variable (subjective or physical) has been "disturbed" of an amount equal to its accuracy (required and desired according to tab. 3) in order to highlight the nominal limit curve shifting and the onset of uncertain regions.
3) On the over nominal limit curve the maximum allowable exposure times have been finally calculated taking into account the measurement errors: by this way the accuracy effect in terms of the corresponding reduction of the allowable exposure times has been expressed (fig. 3).

3 Results and discussion

Figure 1 shows the effect on accuracy of subjective parameters on the nominal limit curves under typical summer/winter clothing situations and for two metabolic rate levels. Fig 1A clearly highlights an even reduced error on the metabolic rate assessment, which strongly affects the safety regions amplitude. As a matter of fact, for 1,7 met (continuous curves in fig. 1), the variation of the metabolic rate within its accuracy (±10%) results in a shift of the nominal limit curve corresponding to an uncertainty region of about 2,6÷2,9°C at 0,6 clo (3,1÷3,6 at 1,0 clo) depending on the humidity levels. It is noteworthy to point out that, according to our early findings [12], the discontinuity of limit curves (more evident at lower metabolic rate) is mainly due to the different protection criterion required for the assessment phase. More in particular at lower temperature and high humidity values the sweating efficiency is so low that the subject is not able to get over the heat accumulation reaching a core temperature of 38°C, whereas, at lower humidity levels and higher temperatures, the sweating mechanism is so efficient that after 8h of continuous work maximum water loss is reached. An amplified behaviour for I_{cl}=1,0 clo has been obtained with a general increasing trend of uncertainty regions especially at a higher metabolic rate (dashed curves). According to fig. 1B, the clothing insulation accuracy effect appears undoubtedly milder (3,0°C of uncertainty at 2,8 met and 1,0 clo) while a simultaneous error on both subjective variables (fig. 1C) results in an almost randomness of the thermal environment assessment since the width of uncertainty regions reaches 7,0°C.

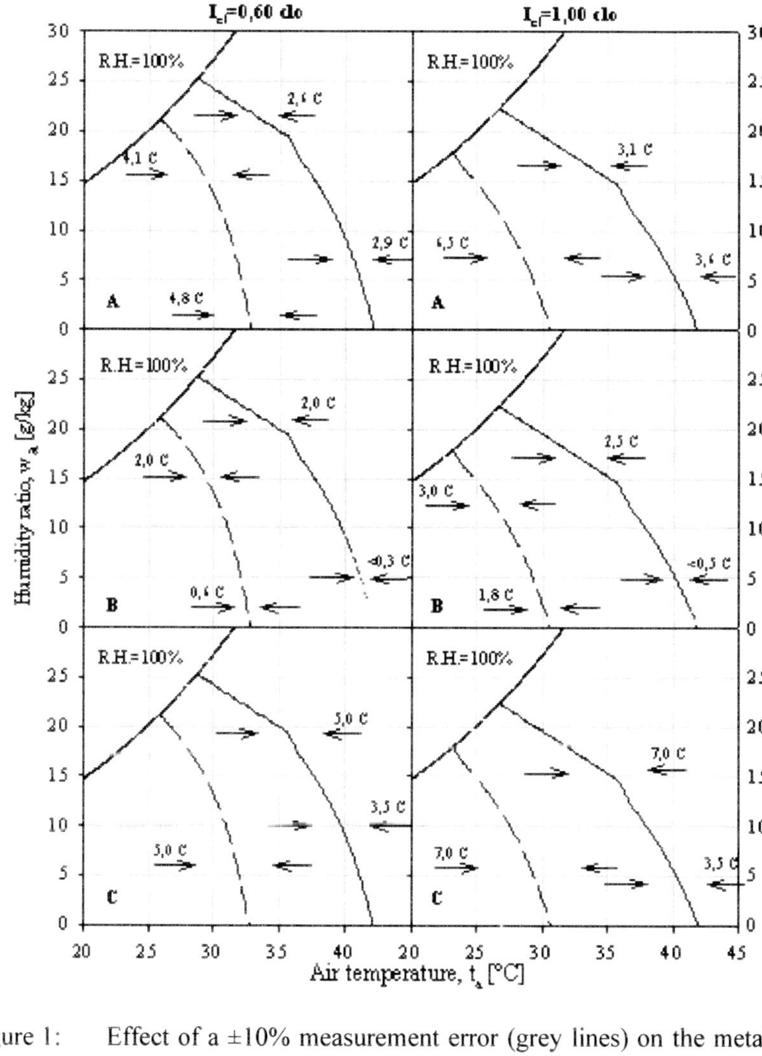

Figure 1: Effect of a ±10% measurement error (grey lines) on the metabolic rate (A), the clothing insulation (B) and both metabolic rate and clothing insulation (C) on the nominal exposition limit curves (black lines) corresponding to 8 hours of continuous work. Metabolic rate: 1,7 met (continuous curves), 2,8 met (dashed curves); absolute air velocity, v_a = 0,20 m/s, ($t_a = t_r$).

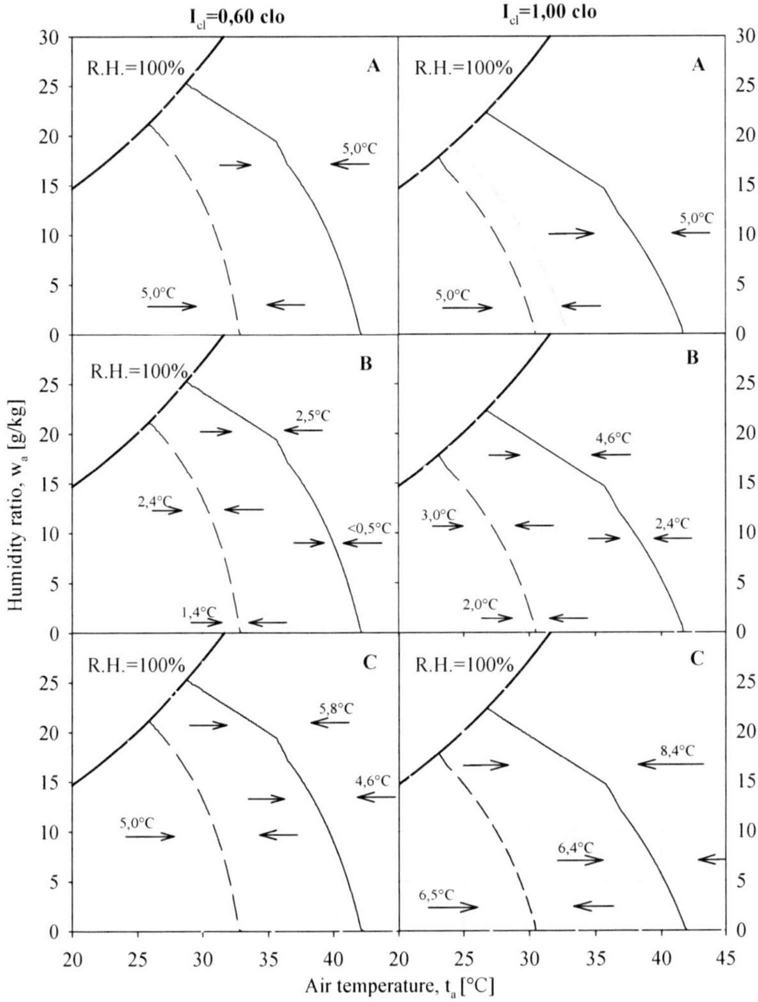

Figure 2: Effect of the measurement accuracy of the mean radiant temperature (A), the air velocity (B) and the whole of physical parameters (C) on the nominal limit curves (black lines) corresponding to 8 hours of continuous work according to ISO 7933. Metabolic rate: 1,7 met (continuous curves), 2,8 met (dashed curves); absolute air velocity, v_a = 0,20 m/s, ($t_a = t_r$). Grey curves refer to the required accuracy values suggested by ISO 7726 Standard.

A similar investigation has been carried out on the effect of required accuracy of physical parameters, as shown in fig. 2.

Fig. 2A clearly shows up a strong effect of the mean radiant temperature on the thermal stress assessment [13]: in fact, a t_r error within the required accuracy results in an uncertainty area width of about 5,0°C (for both M and I_{cl} investigated values). On the contrary hand, the air velocity (fig. 2C) exhibits a slighter sensitivity with smaller areas (in the 0,3÷3,0°C depending on the metabolic rate and the clothing insulation).

According to fig. 2C, where the whole of the microclimatic variables have been taken into account, a reliable assessment of working conditions appears almost a hard matter since the presence of measurement errors result in uncertain areas wider than 8,0°C with unexpected effects on the health care of workers. A similar investigation on the desired accuracy levels has been carried out (only for t_a and v_a according to tab. 3), showing only a milder effect.

In order to lead to the formulation of a relative scale of sensitivity to errors on the hot stress assessment carried out according to PHS method, in figure 3 the variations of allowable exposure times (ΔD_{lim}) obtained by "disturbing" over nominal limit curves each parameter of an amount equal to its required or desired accuracy, has been reported. This kind of analysis should be generally described by means of a special 3-d plot (temperature-humidity-exposure time). In order to avoid a complex representation, two combined plots have been used: in the lower box for the desired metabolic rate activity the nominal microclimatic conditions (evaluated in the absence of errors) allowing 8 hours of continuous work have been depicted; following the arrow, the corresponding reduction of the exposure time (with respect to 8h) calculated taking into account errors on each parameter on the upper plots has to be read.

Obtained results lead to highlight several interesting features:

1) For moderate metabolic activities (M=1,7 met) a dual behaviour depending on the working place humidity has been found:
   - under hot and dry condition (i.e. RH<50%) the variation of allowable exposure times does not appear very significant (only metabolic rate and the mean radiant temperature, according to previous results on the thermal comfort assessment [13], exhibit a reduction of the allowable exposure times of almost 60 min and 90 min, respectively) with the following relative sensitivity scale:

$$t_{a,des} \cong t_{a,req} < I_{cl} \cong v_{a,des} \cong p_a < v_{a,req} < M < t_r$$

   - under hot and humid conditions (i.e. RH>50%) a dramatic decreasing of allowable exposure times has been observed (more than 5h) with the following sensitivity scale:

$$t_{a,des} < t_{a,req} < I_{cl} < v_{a,des} < M \cong p_a < v_{a,req} < t_r$$

2) For higher metabolic rates (M=2,8 met) above quoted phenomena begin to disappear with a more homogeneous behaviour. As a matter of fact the sensitivities to the air temperature, the air velocity (within the desirable accuracy range), humidity and the clothing insulation appear almost negligible (the allowable exposure time reduction has always been in the range 20÷60 min) on the whole limit curve, while only for highest humidity values (RH>70%) an "on-off" behaviour similar to that observed at lower metabolic rate has been detected.

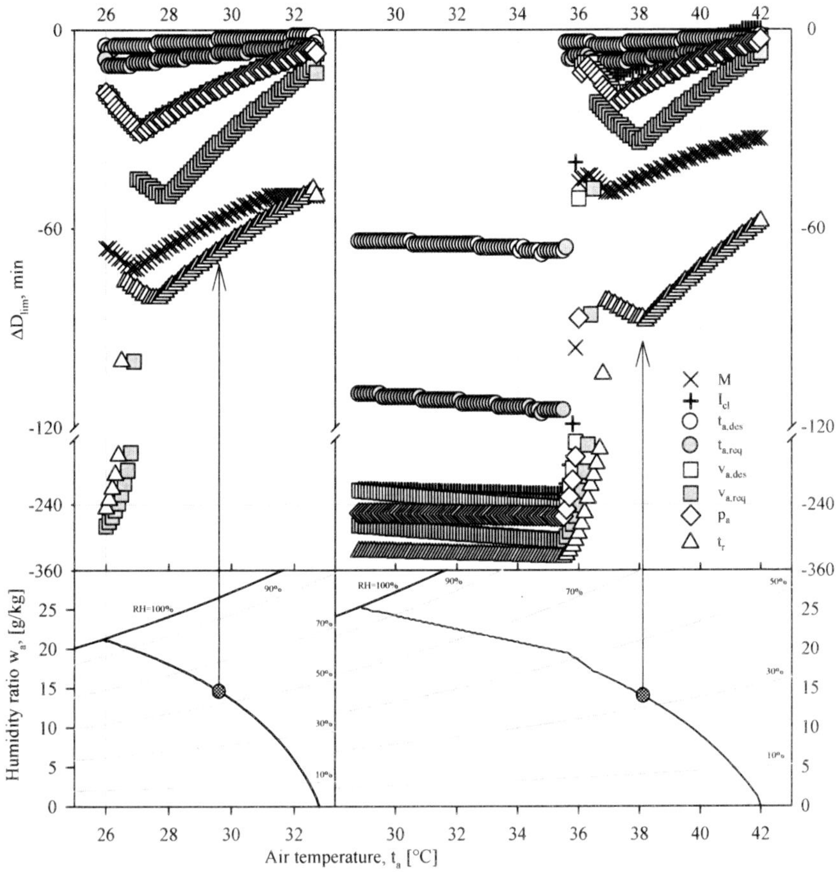

Figure 3: Sensitivity of the PHS model to the measurement errors. Nominal values of independent variables: M=1,70 met (right side), M=2,80 met (left sides), I_{cl}=0,60 clo, v_a=0,20 m/s. On the upper side the reduction of exposition times ΔD_{lim} with respect to microclimatic states corresponding to 8 h of continuous work (reported on the lower side) have been reported.

In these cases errors due to the mean radiant temperature and the air velocity (within the required accuracy range) lead to an overestimation of allowable exposure times more than 4h. Finally, the sensitivity scale obtained in such conditions was:

$$t_{a,des} \cong I_{cl} \cong v_{a,des} \cong t_{a,req} \cong p_a < M < v_{a,req} < t_r$$

Observed phenomena could be explained taking into account the different efficiency of thermoregulations mechanisms, by changing microclimatic conditions, on which the PHS model is based [7]. According to this hypothesis, under hot dry microclimatic conditions (where the maximum exposure time is related to the attainment of the maximum water loss), lower humidity values result in a highest efficiency of sweating, therefore a little perturbation of any parameter is easily counterbalanced by the human body. On the contrary hand, under hot humid situations (where the maximum exposure time is related to the attainment of the maximum rectal temperature), the lowest sweating efficiency combined with a lowest evaporative driving force avoids an effective removal of the heat accumulation so much that even a little variation of the parameters results in a dramatic reduction of exposure times. In other words, the PHS models appear more sensitive to the whole of the microclimatic situations where the behavioural thermoregulation mechanism efficiency is poor.

4 Conclusions

This paper has been devoted to the measurement error effect of subjective and microclimatic parameters involved in the hot stress assessment carried out according to ISO 7933 Standard. The data elaborations by means of special software designed in accordance with thermal environment Standards actually under force has been carried out.

Obtained results highlight a behaviour strictly related to the efficiency of thermoregulation mechanisms regulating the heat accumulation removal. In particular, at lower metabolic rate, in the whole of situations characterised by a reduced efficiency of sweating mechanism, the obtained sensitivity scale has clearly shown the crucial role of mean radiant temperature measurement whose errors can lead to an underestimation of maximum allowable exposure time of more than 5 hours. A strong effect of the air velocity errors and a milder influence of metabolic rate and clothing insulation have been also detected.

Under higher metabolic rates (high sweat production) or drier microclimatic situations (high sweating efficiency) the effects of measurement errors seems to be milder, although the sensitivity to the mean radiant temperature still appears a crucial matter.

Finally, the strong uncertainty of the hot stress assessment related to the mean radiant temperature measurement would make either an increase of accuracy required by ISO 7726 for Class S devices or turning to more careful measurement techniques (i.e. indirect methods as the plane radiant temperature methods) necessary. Similar interventions to the air velocity and the humidity accuracies, which often affect the "subject-environment" heat transfer should be hoped. Concerning subjective parameters more thorough method should be devoted only for higher metabolic rates or clothing insulation values.

Acknowledgements

This work was funded by the Italian MURST (Italian Ministry for University and Scientific-Technological Research) in the area of the PRIN COFIN 2005 Project entitled "Studio termofluidodinamico di componenti di facciata adattativi per il comfort ed il risparmio energetico".

References

[1] Lee, D.H.K., Seventy-five years of searching for a heat index. *Environmental Research* 22, pp. 331-356, 1980.

[2] d'Ambrosio Alfano, F.R. Palella, B.I., Riccio, G., Manuscript under preparation.

[3] ISO, 2004. Ergonomics of the thermal environment - Risk assessment strategy for the prevention of stress or discomfort in thermal working conditions – ISO Standard 15265 – Geneva: International Standardization Organization.

[4] ISO, 1989. Hot environments - Estimation of the heat stress on working man, based on WBGT-index (wet bulb globe temperature) – ISO Standard 7243. Geneva: International Standardization Organization.

[5] ISO, 2004. Ergonomics of the thermal environment – Analytical determination and interpretation of heat stress using calculation of the predicted heat strain. ISO Standard 7933. Geneva: International Standardization Organization.

[6] Fanger, P.O., Thermal Comfort. McGraw-Hill, New York, 1970.

[7] Malchaire, J.B., Piette, A., Kampmann, B., Menhert, P., Gebhardt, H., Havenith, G., Den Hartog, E., Holmer, I., Parsons, K., Alfano, G., Griefahn, B., Development and Validation of the Predicted Heat Strain Model. *Annals of Occupational Hygiene*, **45(2)**, pp. 123–135, 2001.

[8] ISO, 1985. Thermal environments - Instruments and methods for measuring physical quantities. Geneva: International Standardization Organization.

[9] ISO, 2004. Ergonomics of the thermal environment - Determination of metabolic rate - ISO Standard 8996. Geneva: International Standardization Organization.

[10] ISO, 2004. Ergonomics of the thermal environment – Estimation of the thermal insulation and evaporative resistance of a clothing ensemble – ISO/DIS 9920. Geneva: International Standardization Organization.

[11] d'Ambrosio Alfano, F.R., Palella, B.I., Riccio, G., TEE (Thermal Environment Assessment): a friendly tool for thermal environment evaluation. *Proc. Of. 11th International Conferences on Environmental Ergonomics*, Eds. Ingvar Holmér, Kalev Kuklane and Chuansi Gao, pp.503-506, 2005.

[12] d'Ambrosio Alfano, F.R., Palella, B.I., Riccio, G., Criteria for assessment of hot environments: WBGT index and PHS (predicted heat strain). *Medicina del Lavoro,* **95(4)**, pp. 255-280, 2004.

[13] d'Ambrosio Alfano, F.R., Dell'Isola, M., Palella, B.I., Riccio, G., Russi, A., La misura della Temperatura Radiante. *Atti del 61° Congresso Nazionale ATI*, Eds. Morlacchi Editore: Perugia (Italy), pp. 285-290, 2006 (in Italian).

Section 4
Water quality issues

Evaluating safety of drinking water using animal cell bioassays

G. K. Luk
Department of Civil Engineering, Ryerson University, Toronto, Ontario, Canada

Abstract

Disinfection byproducts (DBPs) such as trihalomethanes (THMs), haloacetic acids (HAAs), 3-chloro-4-(dichloromethyl)-5-hydroxyl-2(5H)-furanone (MX) and other hazardous compounds are produced by chlorination of raw water in the water treatment plants. Most chlorinated by-products are formed by the interaction of chlorine and natural organic matter (NOM) such as fulvic and humic acids, which are present in most surface waters. Many of these by-products are suspected to be mutagenic or carcinogenic in nature. The objective of the paper is to demonstrate the effectiveness of bioassay-directed research in evaluating the safety of chlorinated drinking water, and to investigate the effect of pH on the genotoxicity of chlorinated sample water.
Keywords: disinfection byproducts, chlorination, drinking water, bioassays.

1 Introduction

Although water disinfection has been quite successful in eliminating many acute waterborne diseases in the developed world, many potential health hazards related to disinfection by-products (DBPs) have been reported [1, 2]. Epidemiological studies demonstrate that many potential health risks such as cancers of the stomach, pancreas, kidney, bladder, and rectum, as well as Hodgkin's and non-Hodgkin's lymphoma have been linked to exposure to DBPs [3]. DBPs such as trihalomethanes (THMs), haloacetic acids (HAAs), 3-chloro-4-(dichloromethyl)-5-hydroxyl-2(5H)-furanone (MX) and other hazardous compounds are produced by chlorination and other disinfection methods of raw water in the water treatment plants. Most chlorinated by-products are formed by the interaction of chlorine and natural organic matter

WIT Transactions on Biomedicine and Health, Vol 11, © 2007 WIT Press
www.witpress.com, ISSN 1743-3525 (on-line)
doi:10.2495/EHR070141

(NOM) such as fulvic and humic acids, which are present in most surface waters [4]. The problem is intensified with the presence of bromine which can be found in most natural waters. Many of these by-products are suspected to be mutagenic or carcinogenic in nature [5, 6].

The purpose of this study is to demonstrate the effectiveness of bioassay-based research for the investigation of genotoxic potential of chlorinated water. Past studies on bioassay-directed research has confirmed many advantages over traditional clinical studies involving lab animals, resulting in tremendous saving in time and cost. For instance, it has been found through bioassays that the mutagenicity of chlorinated water is dependent on pH and temperature [7–10], albeit the nature of dependency over a wide range of pH has not been studied in detail. The objective of this paper is to evaluate the genotoxicity of total organic halides (TOXs) produced by the reaction of chlorine and NOM, in the form of humic acid, under different raw water pH conditions. As a measure of genotoxicity, the *in vitro* bioassay test measuring chromosomal aberrations using Chinese hamster lung (CHL/IU) cells was carried out, and was used as an index to examine the change of activity inducing chromosomal aberrations after chlorination of water samples containing humic acid.

2 Health effects and regulations of DBPs

Since the discovery of chlorinating byproducts in drinking water in 1974, numerous toxicological studies have been conducted. These studies have shown several disinfection byproducts, such as bromate, certain trihalomethanes (THMs) and haloacetic acids (HAAs), to be carcinogenic in laboratory animals. Other disinfection byproducts including chlorite, certain THMs and HAAs have also been shown to cause adverse reproductive or developmental effects in laboratory animals. However, there is considerable uncertainty involved the results of high-dose, toxicological studies of some byproducts occurring in disinfected drinking water to estimate the risk to humans from chronic exposure to low doses of these and other byproducts.

In the area of epidemiology, a number of studies have been completed investigating the relationship between exposure to chlorinated surface water and cancer. Even though the results are not complete, the US-EPA [11] established that based on available evidence, there is a causal link between exposure to chlorinated surface water and cancer, and that these studies have suggested an association, albeit small, between bladder, rectal, and colon cancer and exposure to chlorinated surface water. In conclusion, the US-EPA believes the weight-of-evidence presented by the available epidemiological studies on chlorinated drinking water and toxicological studies on individual disinfection byproducts supports a potential hazard concern and warrant regulatory action. In January 2006, the U.S. EPA published the Stage 2 Disinfectants/Disinfection Byproducts Rule [12] that requires public water systems to use treatment methods to reduce the formation of disinfection byproducts and to meet the following standards, among others: total trihalomethanes (TTHM) (measured as the sum concentration of chloroform, bromoform, bromodichloromethane, and dibromochloromethane) at 80 parts per billion (ppb), five haloacetic acids (HAA5) (measured as the sum concentration of monochloroacetic, dichloroacetic, trichloroacetic, monobromoacetic, and dibromoacetic acids) at 60 ppb, bromate at 10 ppb, and chlorite at 1.0 parts per million (ppm). The standards for TTHM, HAA5, and bromate are annual averages. For chlorite, the standard is an average of a three samples taken at least monthly.

3 In vitro chromosome aberration assays

The past century has been witness to enormous advances in the study of genetic toxicity, which focuses on the processes of mutagenesis, including the induction of DNA damage, gene mutation and chromosome aberration, at the cell level. These genotoxic effects are considered important precursors to the development of adverse health effects such as cancer. As important primary screening tools for the assessment of genetic hazard, genetic toxicity test systems are categorised by the end points that they measure, such as gene mutation, chromosome damage or DNA damage [13]. The strong association between these end points and known mechanisms of oncogeny activation or loss of tumour suppressor gene function places great importance on genotoxicity testing to evaluate the mutagenic and carcinogenic potential of consumer and industrial products, pharmaceutical and agricultural agents, and environmental samples.

The chromosome aberration assay provides a technique for evaluation of damage to chromosomes through direct visualization of the damage caused by the test article under investigation. The purpose of this test is to identify agents that cause chromosome aberrations in cultured mammalian cells, as well as to screen populations for chromosome anomalies arising as a result of environmental agents. More specifically, Putman *et al* [13] stated that the aim of the *in vitro* cytogenetics assay is to evaluate the clastogenic or chromosome breakage potential of a test contaminant and its metabolites based upon their ability to induce chromosome aberrations in a culture. The use of cell cultures as a test system has been demonstrated to be an effective method of detection of chemical clastogens and the induction of chromosome breakage *in vitro* is an indication that the test article is potentially genotoxic [14]. The chromosomal aberration assay is vital because there is strong evidence to suggest that chromosome mutations and related events cause alterations in the oncogenes and tumour suppressor genes of somatic cells and are involved in cancer induction in humans and animals [15].

3.1 Chromosomal aberrations

Two types of chromosomal abnormalities can be detected using the *in vitro* chromosome aberration assay: structural chromosome aberrations and numerical chromosome aberrations. Structural aberrations include deviations such as breaks and rearrangements and can result in a discontinuity in the chromosomal DNA. These discontinuities may be repaired, rejoined inappropriately, or left unrejoined, causing a break or a deletion in the chromosome [13]. Structural aberrations may be of two types, chromosome or chromatid. Chromosome-type aberrations are expressed as a breakage or a breakage and reunion of both chromatids at an identical site. The majority of chemical mutagen induced aberrations are chromatid type, in which structural chromosome damage is expressed as breakage of single chromatids or breakage and reunion between chromatids [16], as shown in fig. 1.

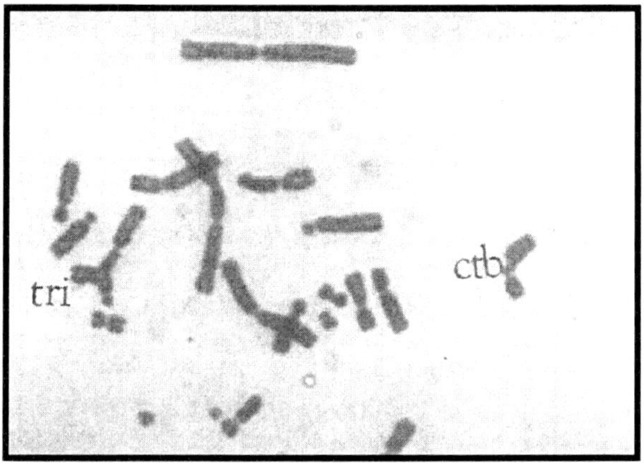

Figure 1: Chromatid type structural aberrations in Chinese hamster ovary (CHO) chromosomes; chromatid break (ctb) and triradial chromatid rearrangement (tri).

For the most part, structural aberrations are lethal to the cell or to the daughter cells in the first few cell cycles after their appearance. However, these structural deviations may also serve as an indicator of the occurrence of transmittable aberrations, such as balanced translocations, duplications, inversions or small deletions, and may play a role in tumor initiation and progression in somatic cells [15].

On the other hand, numerical aberrations are variations in the number of chromosomes in the nucleus from the normal number characteristic of the cell. Studies have generally found that numerical chromosome aberrations are not due to the direct interaction of an environmental agent with the chromosomal DNA [13]. Although numerical aberrations do not seem to play a key role in the initiation of tumours and the physiological and genotoxic impacts of polyploidy and endoreduplication are less than clear, they may be indicative of the evolution of karyotypic instability within a population of tumour cells. The *in vitro* cytogenetics assay was not designed to measure numerical aberrations and is not routinely used for that purpose.

3.2 Cell selection

The chromosome aberration test system can be run using either established cell lines or primary cell cultures. The cell lines routinely used in this assay are

Chinese hamster ovary (CHO) cells and Chinese hamster lung (CHL) cells grown in mono-layer cultures, as shown in fig. 2. There are a number of advantages to using established cell lines from frozen stocks. Cell lines are genetically more homogeneous than primary cell cultures and thus tend to show less inter-experimental variability within the cell types [13]. Secondly, the established Chinese hamster cell lines are advantageous for use in the *in vitro* cytogenetics assay because they are easily cultured in standard media, have a small number of large chromosomes each with a more or less distinctive morphology, and have a relatively short cell cycle [17]. On the other hand, primary cell cultures, such as human peripheral blood lymphocytes (HPBL), show some variability among donors in their response and sensitivity to test articles compared to established cell lines [18], but the relevance of these systems to human exposure to test articles cannot be overlooked.

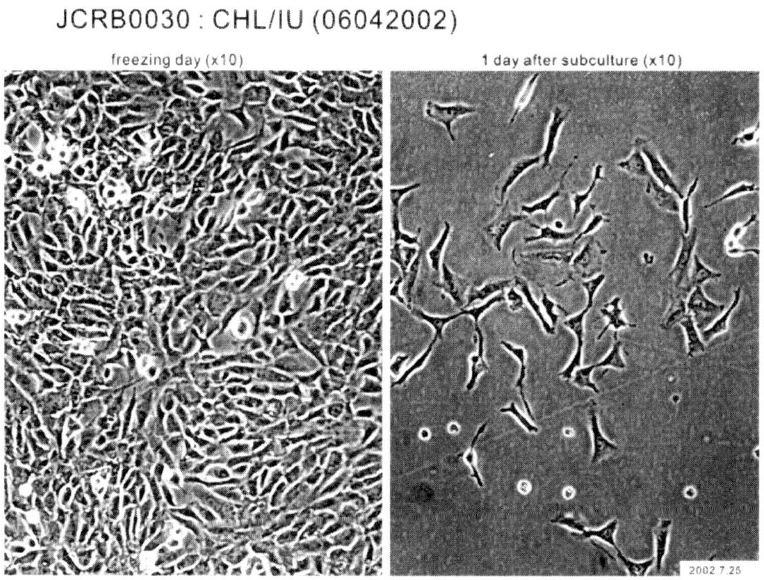

Figure 2: Cultured CHL metaphase with 100x magnification.

During cell culturing, treatment and preparation of samples for mounting, there is extensive chromosome rearrangement and it is an inherent property of most established cell lines that the chromosome number varies around a modal value [18]. As such, it is necessary to establish criteria for defining analyzable cells; current criteria are that cells with the modal chromosome number ± 2 chromosomes are acceptable for microscopic analysis [13]. For CHL cells, which have a modal chromosome number of 25, all cells with chromosome numbers ranging from 23 to 27 are considered as acceptable samples for the reading. This criterion has been adopted for the present study.

Prior to the start of the assay, frozen stocks should be established and cells checked for contamination by parasitic, pathogenic microorganisms, such as mycoplasma [19]. Since the objective of the chromosome aberration assay is to determine whether test chemicals induce aberrations in a culture, environmental factors, such as pH, cytotoxicity and osmolality, must be carefully monitored and adjusted to physiological levels if necessary, as extremes of these factors can cause chromosome aberrations [13]. As there are natural background levels of mutation, a negative control test is also required to assess the relative increases in the measured end-point, in this case structural or numerical aberrations. It is necessary to determine how many aberrations occur in the control (untreated or solvent control) sample, and subtract that base number from all of the test samples.

4 Experimental design

The chromosome aberration assay was conducted in two stages: the preliminary toxicity assay and the chromosome aberration assay. The preliminary toxicity assay served as a dose range-finding assay for the definitive portion of the study. There are a number of protocols in place for determining which exposure concentrations should be tested in order to ensure that concentrations cover the range from the maximum to little or no toxicity (e.g. >50% reduction in cell growth or confluency) [13, 16]. In cases where the contaminant in question is wide-spread in the environment, either from long-time human use or disposal practices, it may be possible to use a dose range that reflects the concentrations of the chemical found in natural systems. This was the method used in this study, in which both chlorination level and concentration of humic acid were pre-determined to reflect worst-case values in real life. In the chromosome aberration assay, the clastogenic potential of the contaminant is evaluated microscopically. After cells are exposed to the test substance for 24 h, they are treated with a metaphase-arresting substance, harvested, stained and examined microscopically. As shown in fig. 3, the cells are first inspected with a magnification of 400x for identification, and further magnified with a minimum magnification of 1000x for the presence of both numerical and structural aberrations.

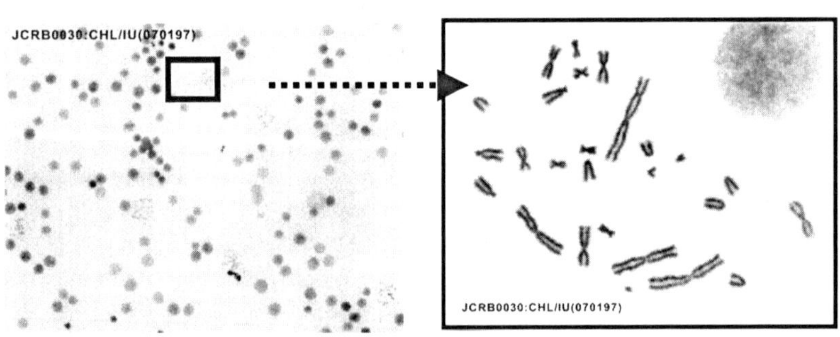

Figure 3: Views of slide at 400x (left) and 1000x (right) magnification.

The chromosomal aberration test was carried out on a Chinese hamster lung (CHL/IU) cell-line supplied by Dainihon Pharmaceutical Co. Ltd., and cultured at 37°C in a 5% CO_2 incubator. The cells are kept in 50 mL disposable ventible culture bottles with 10-11 mL of Eagle's MEM medium supplemented with 10% fetal bovine serum. Mutagenesis assays were performed in duplicates, and 100 metaphase cells were analysed for structural aberration from each duplicate. To assess the activity-inducing chromosomal aberrations in the cells, a 1-mL study sample was added to a 1-day-old CHL culture containing 1 mL of cell mixture and 5 mL of MEM media, and incubated for 24 hours. Bacteria in the samples were eliminated prior to addition with a sterile syringe-driven 0.22 μm filter unit (Millex®-FG SLFG 025 LS). Chromosome preparations were fixed on microscopic slides with a fixation solution made of a 3:1 v/v methanol and glacial acetic acid (with >96% purity), and stained with a 1.5% Giemsa solution prepared with a phosphate buffer at pH 6.8. Bioassays were carried out for samples at a pH of 5, 7, and 9 respectively, and covering a chlorine concentration range of 0 to 1500 mg Cl/L.

5 Results and discussion

The experimental results are summarized in fig. 4. It was observed that chromosomal aberrations increase almost linearly with increasing chlorine concentration. It can also be observed that the amount of TOCl decreased by 70% when pH was increased from 5 to 9, at a chlorination level of {HOCl} = 1,500 mg Cl_2/L. In spite of this, there did not seem to be any noticeable difference in the activity inducing chromosomal aberrations with pH change.

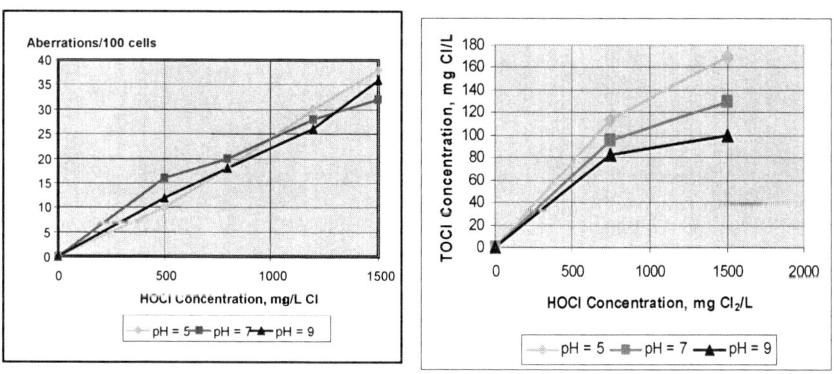

Figure 4: Bioassay (left) and analytical results.

When a reasonable margin of error for the chromosomal aberration test (+/- 10%) was considered, the bioassay data taken from samples with three different pHs falls practically on the same linear trend, and the best-fit linear regression equation is given by:

$$N = 0.0236 \{HOCl\} \quad (R^2 = 0.9779) \tag{1}$$

where N is the number of activity inducing chromosomal aberrations per 100 cells, and {HOCl} is the concentration of HOCl in mg Cl_2/L. To investigate the reasons behind this peculiar observation, it is necessary to evaluate the aberration initiation strength, defined as the number of chromosomal aberrations per mg Cl/L of TOCl, and given by the following equation:

$$A_{TOCl} = \frac{N}{\{TOCl\}} \bullet DF \tag{2}$$

where N is the number of chromosomal aberrations per 100 cells, {TOCl} is the concentration of TOCl in mg Cl/L, and DF is the dilution factor for the sample during the bioassay experiments. According to the standard chromosomal aberration test procedure, a 1-mL sample is added to 1 mL of cell mixture submerged in 5 mL of MEM cell growth medium, giving a total volume of 7 mL. Therefore, the dilution factor of the sample is 7 for all tests. When the A_{TOCl} values were evaluated and averaged for each pH, as shown in table 1, it can be observed that the aberration initiation strength increased by 49.6%, from 1.25 to 1.87 aberrations per mg Cl/L, when the pH was changed from 5 to 9. Therefore, it can be concluded that while the amount of TOCl decreases when pH is increased, the aberration initiation strength increases, thus creating a "compensation effect" which results in no discernable difference in genotoxicity with pH.

Table 1: Aberration per unit TOCl at different pH values.

pH	**Chlorination (mg Cl_2/L)**	**Aberrations per 100 cells**	**TOCl (mg Cl/L)**	**A_{TOCl} (per mg Cl/L)**
5.0	500	10	76	0.132
	800	18	118	0.153
	1200	30	147	0.204
	1500	38	170	0.224
				Avg. = 1.25
7.0	250	5	53	0.094
	500	8	62	0.129
	750	10	92	0.108
	1000	11	95	0.116
	1250	15	151	0.099
	1500	16	140	0.115
				Avg. = 1.54
9.0	500	12	55	0.218
	800	18	84	0.214
	1200	26	95	0.274
	1500	36	100	0.360
				Avg. = 1.87

It should be noted that although the *in vitro* chromosome aberration assay is an important tool for screening potential mutagens and carcinogens, it does not give a perfect correlation between the results and carcinogenicity. It has been documented that a test chemical for which there is a negative result, indicating that the test chemical does not induce aberrations, may still be a carcinogen, since carcinogens may act through mechanisms other than direct DNA damage [15, 16]. Despite these potential limitations, the chromosome aberration assay provides two distinct advantages. First, the test is very useful for comparisons of chemicals in the same class and provides a direct measure of their relative toxicity. Secondly, the test is not financially prohibitive and is feasible even for smaller laboratories. The test does not require the use of laboratory animals or the space to house and care for them; there are fewer requirements for additional staff (animal care technicians, etc.) and/or training, and equipment.

6 Conclusions

Based on the results from in this study, it is concluded that while genotoxicity increases with increasing chlorination, the effect of pH on genotoxicity is not significant owing to the compensation effect of the aberration initiation strength. The study also demonstrated that *in vitro* chromosome aberration assay provides an excellent opportunity to quickly and efficiently test a large number of potential genotoxins, under a wide range of conditions. This in turn allows for the prioritization of further research through laboratory or clinical trials.

References

[1] Richardson, S.D., Drinking water disinfection by-products. *Encyclopedia of Environmental Analysis and Remediation*, ed. R.A. Meyers, John Wiley & Sons, pp. 1398-1421, 1988.

[2] Bull, R.J. Drinking water disinfection. *Environmental toxicants: human exposures and their health effects,* ed. M. Lippmann, John Wiley & Sons, pp. 267-317, 2000.

[3] Nieuwenhuijsen, M.J., Toledano, M.B., & Elliott P., Uptake of chlorination disinfection by-products: a review and a discussion of its implications for exposure assessment in epidemiological studies. *J. Expos. Analy. Environ. Epidem.*, **10**, pp. 586-599, 2000.

[4] Weinberg, H.S., Krasner, S.W., Richardson, S.D. & Thurston, A.D. Jr. *The Occurrence of Disinfection By-products (DBPs) of Health Concern in Drinking Water: Results of a Nationwide DBP Occurrence Study*, National Exposure Research Laboratory, US Environmental Protection Agency, 2002.

[5] Wilcox, P. & Williamson, S., Mutagenic activity of concentrated drinking water samples. *Environ. Health Perspect.*, **69**, pp. 141-149, 1986.

[6] Plewa, M.J., Wagner, E.D., Jazwierska, P., Richarson, S.D., Chen, P.H. & McKague, A.B., Halonitromethane drinking water disinfection by-products: chemical characterization and mammalian cell cytotoxicity and genotoxicity. *Env. Sc. & Tech.*, **38**, pp. 62-68, 2004.

[7] Meier, J.R., Lingg, R.D. & Bull, R.J., Formation of mutagens following chlorination of humic acid: a model for mutagen formation during water treatment. *Mutat. Res.*, **118**, pp. 15-41, 1983.
[8] Fukui, S., Yoshimura, Y., Ogawa, S. & Hanazaki, Y., Formation of non-volatile potent mutagens in domestic sewage by chlorination. *Chemosphere*, **21(6)**, pp. 705-716, 1990.
[9] Itoh, S., Murakami, H. & Sumitomo, H., Activities inducing chromosomal aberrations of waters treated with disinfectants and the stability of them. *Proc. IWSA Specialized Conference on Advanced Treatment and Integrated Water Systems Management into the 21st Century*, Osaka, Japan, Vol. 1:134-139, 1995.
[10] Kamaguchi, H., Behaviour of disinfection by-products by pH adjustment of drinking water", *J. Water Waste*, **38(12)**, pp. 20-26, 1996 (in Japanese).
[11] National Research Council. *Drinking Water and Health: Disinfectants and Disinfectant By-Products*, Vol. 7, National Academy Press, Washington D.C., 1987.
[12] U.S. Environmental Protection Agency. Stage 2 Disinfectants and Disinfection By-Products Rule, Vol. 71, No. 2, Ref. 71FR388, 2006. www.epa.gov/safewater/disinfection/stage2/
[13] Putman, D.L., Gudi, R., Wagner III, V.O., San, R.H.C. & Jacobson-Kram, D., Genetic toxicology. *Toxicology Testing Handbook: Principles, Applications, and Data Interpretation*, eds. D. Jacobson-Kram & K.A. Keller. Marcel Dekker, Inc.: New York, pp. 127-194, 2001.
[14] Preston, R.J., Au, W., Bender, M.A., Brewen, J.G., Carrano, A.V., Heddle, J.A., McFee, A.F., Wolff, S. & Wassom, J.S., Mammalian in vivo and in vitro cytogenetic assays: a report of the U.S. EPA's Gene-Tox program. *Mutation Research*, **87**, pp. 143, 1981.
[15] Tlsty, T.D., Briot, A., Gualberto, A., Hall, I., Hess, S., Hixon, M., Kuppuswamy, D., Romanov, S., Sage, M. & White, A., Genomic instability and cancer. *Mutation Research*, **337:1**, 1995.
[16] OECD, In vitro mammalian chromosome aberration test. *Guideline for the Testing of Chemicals*, OECD Press, **473**, 1997.
[17] Ishidate, M., Harnois, M.C. & Sofuni, T., A comparative analysis of data on the clastogenicity of 951 chemical substances tested in mammalian cultures. *Mutation Research*, **195**, pp. 151, 1988.
[18] Kirkland, D., Chromosomal aberration tests in vitro: problems with protocol design and interpretation of results. *Mutagenesis*, **7**, pp. 95, 1992.
[19] International Conference on Harmonisation (ICH), Technical requirements for registration of pharmaceuticals for human use. *Genotoxicity: A Standard Battery for Genotoxicity Testing of Pharmaceuticals*, 1997.

Health risk related to radon in a thermal spa utilizing waters from Guarani aquifer

D. M. Bonotto & T. O. Santos
Departamento de Petrologia e Metalogenia,
Instituto de Geociências e Ciências Exatas-UNESP, Rio Claro, Brazil

Abstract

This investigation was carried out within the Paraná sedimentary basin, Brazil, involved the sampling of groundwater and air, and was realized with the purpose of evaluating the radioactivity, due to radon gas, in a thermal spa utilizing the waters from Guarani (Botucatu-Pirambóia) aquifer. The results reported here provide additional information relative to that of previous studies focusing on the presence of radionuclides in the aquifer, which have mainly characterized those belonging to uranium and thorium series decay, such as the uranium isotopes (^{238}U and ^{234}U), radium isotopes (^{226}Ra and ^{228}Ra), radon daughters (^{214}Bi and ^{214}Pb) and radon (^{222}Rn) itself. The results obtained were compared with the maximum permissible concentration limits in air and drinking water defined by international standards, such as the guidelines for drinking water quality established by the World Health Organization. The possible processes responsible for the presence of radon in the aquifer were also considered in order to evaluate the data obtained.
Keywords: radon, air, groundwater, Guarani aquifer, thermal spa.

1 Introduction

Radon (^{222}Rn, half-life 3.84 days) is a naturally occurring volatile noble gas formed from the normal radioactive decay series of ^{238}U, according to the following decay sequence: ^{238}U (4.49 Ga, α) $\rightarrow$ ^{234}Th (24.1 d, β^-) $\rightarrow$ ^{234}Pa (1.18 min, β^-) $\rightarrow$ ^{234}U (0.248 Ma, α) $\rightarrow$ ^{230}Th (75.2 Ka, α) $\rightarrow$ ^{226}Ra (1622 a, α) $\rightarrow$ ^{222}Rn (3.83 d, α) $\rightarrow$ ^{218}Po (3.05 min, α) $\rightarrow$ … It is a colorless, odorless, tasteless, chemically inert and radioactive gas produced continuously in rocks and soils through α-decay of ^{226}Ra, with some atoms escaping to the surrounding fluid

WIT Transactions on Biomedicine and Health, Vol 11, © 2007 WIT Press
www.witpress.com, ISSN 1743-3525 (on-line)
doi:10.2495/EHR070151

phase, such as groundwater and air. It is subjected to recoil at "birth", with the emanated fraction relatively to that produced in the solid phase being dependent on factors such as total surface area of solids and concentration/distribution of ^{238}U (^{226}Ra) in the minerals [1]. On the other hand, ^{222}Rn also generates several daughters (heavy metals) through a sequence decay that finishes with lead, i.e. ^{222}Rn (3.84 d, α) $\rightarrow$ ^{218}Po (3.05 min, α) $\rightarrow$ ^{214}Pb (26.8 min, β^-) $\rightarrow$ ^{214}Bi (19.7 min, β^-) $\rightarrow$ ^{214}Po (0.16 ms, α) $\rightarrow$ ^{210}Pb (22.3 a, β^-) $\rightarrow$ ^{210}Bi (5 d, β^-) $\rightarrow$ ^{210}Po (138.4 d, α) $\rightarrow$ ^{206}Pb.

High ^{222}Rn concentrations occur in groundwater in many areas where wells are used for domestic water supply and thermal spas, including small rural water supplies [2,3]. Exposure to radon and its progeny is believed to be associated with increased risks of several kinds of cancer [4]. When radon or its progeny are inhaled, lung cancer accounts for most of the total incremental cancer risk, while ingestion of radon in water is suspected of being associated with an increased risk of tumors of several internal organs, primarily the stomach [4]. Inhalation of radon progeny accounts for about 89% of the individual risk associated with domestic water use, with almost 11% resulting from directly ingesting radon in drinking water [4]. Several authors [5–11] also pointed out that although radon in water is not a well-documented health risk, it does contribute to radon in indoor air, which has been established as a health threat. Furthermore, high concentrations of ^{222}Rn in groundwater also indicate the presence of radon's parent nuclides, ^{238}U and ^{226}Ra, in the water-rock system, which are known health risks when ingested in drinking water [12].

The knowledge of the geochemical and hydrogeological mechanisms that control the movement of ^{222}Rn through the groundwater system may be informative of the natural processes related to its high concentration associated with low transmissivity zones [13], with the uranium content of the source rock, severe chemical weathering, hydrothermal solution, deposition, or extensive fracturing [14], and with variations in stress in rocks associated with seismicity, where in some cases temporal variations have preceded large earthquakes [15-17].

Radon and decay product nuclei are present in indoor environments of spa facilities and have been identified as an agent of additional radiation burden both for bathers and working personnel [18, 19]. This additional burden has been studied by many researchers, resulting in the introduction of appropriate health regulations [19–21]. However, for the spa facilities existing in several areas in Brazil the measurements for radon and decay product nuclei indoors are incipient or non-existent. This is particularly true for the thermal spas utilizing waters of the huge Guarani aquifer located in the South American continent, which are extensively used for consuming purposes, among others. Thus, the aim of this paper is to evaluate the contribution of ^{222}Rn to the public exposure related to bathers utilizing the hot waters of a thermal spa located in Londrina city, Paraná State, Brazil. The implications of the data obtained in terms of health risks related to the presence of radon in water and air under the perspective of the actual international guidelines will also be discussed.

2 General features of the studied area

The Guarani aquifer of Triassic-Jurassic age has continental dimensions, extending over some 950,000 km^2 within the Paraná sedimentary basin, South America, and comprising southern Brazil (states of Mato Grosso, Mato Grosso do Sul, Goiás, Minas Gerais, São Paulo, Paraná, Santa Catarina and Rio Grande do Sul), eastern Paraguay, NW Uruguay and the northeastern extreme corner of Argentina (fig. 1).

The aquifer has an average thickness of 300-400m, and is composed of silty and shaly sandstones of fluvial-lacustrine origin (the Pirambóia and Rosário do Sul formations in Brazil and the Buena Vista formation in Uruguay), and variegated quartzitic sandstones accumulated by eolian processes under desertic conditions (the Botucatu formation in Brazil, Misiones formation in Paraguay, and Tacuarembó formation in Uruguay and Argentina) [22]. A thick basaltic package of the Serra Geral formation (up to 1,500 m) overlies this aquifer, reducing its exposed areas in non-continuous elongated strips, 10-100 km wide, along the edges of the proper Paraná basin, where the longest strip stretches between the states of São Paulo and Santa Catarina, in Brazil. The aquifer overlies previous formations ranging from the igneous basement to the Paleozoic sediments of the Passa-Dois and Tubarão Groups, being covered by Cretaceous sediments of the Bauru-Caiuá formations.

The potentiometric surface of the water shows a significant proportion of its total area having artesian conditions [23], and recharge occurring by direct infiltration of rainwater in the outcrop area, which is about 98,000 km^2 [24]. The percolating water moves from the phreatic exposed areas that surround the entire basin towards its central part, and, in spite of the great distances separating the existing exploitation centers, data obtained sporadically indicate hydraulic conductivity values of 10^{-4}-10^{-5} m/s, effective porosity values of 10-20%, storage coefficient values of 10^{-3}-10^{-6} and average transmissivity of 10^{-3} m^2/s [24]. The water is extensively used for drinking purposes, industrial activities and recreation (thermal swimming pools), with the yields of the wells varying from 10-150 m^3/h (phreatic exposed parts) up to 300-1000 m^3/h (confined artesian wells) [25].

3 Materials and methods

For the purpose of this investigation, the sampling was held in Londrina thermal spa situated at Londrina city, Paraná State, Brazil (fig. 1). The surface area of Londrina municipality is 1,651 km^2 and its population is approximately 480,000 inhabitants (according to the 2004 census). The spa is 6 km away from the city center and started its operation in 1991. The hot waters of the spa come from a 960m-deep tubular well, whose main characteristics, and their waters characteristics, are reported in table 1. The lithology cut by drilling corresponded to the Serra Geral Formation (0-846m), Botucatu Formation (846-884m), and Pirambóia Formation (884-960m).

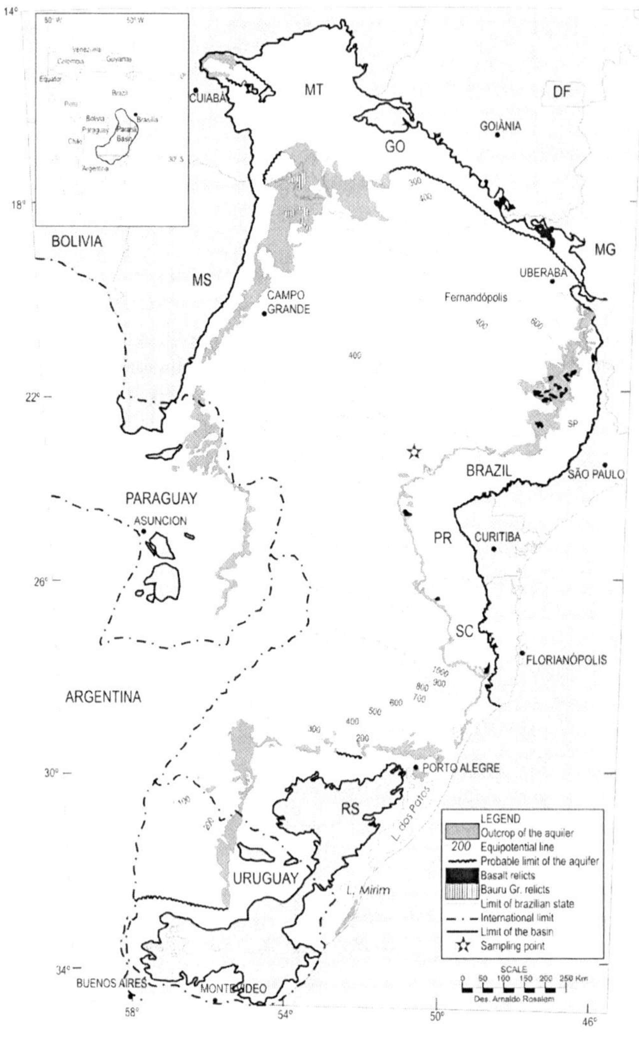

Figure 1: The outcrop of the Guarani aquifer at the Paraná sedimentary basin [22] and location of the sampling point for radon analyses.

The sampling campaign for radon analyses was performed between 23rd (18:50h) and 24th (10:30h) November 2006. The spa has facilities for immersion baths and the measurements were conducted in the room containing a bath (dimensions = 3.18-m long, 2.12-m wide, and 1-m deep) that receives the hottest water at a rate of ~0.4 l/s. The size of the room is approximately 6-m long, 4-m wide, and 4m-high, yielding a volume of about 100 m^3. The water temperature in the hottest bath varied between 42 and 45°C during this study, whereas the air temperature ranged from 26 up to 36°C.

Table 1: Description of the tubular well drilled at the Londrina thermal spa, Londrina city, Brazil, and chemical analyses of groundwater performed by [26].

Description		
Parameter	**Unit**	**Value**
Altitude of the top	m	450
Latitude	-	23° 19' 21" S
Longitude	-	51° 09' 49" W
Total length	m	960
Geostatic pressure	bar	224.8

Water analysis - Date of sampling = 01/16/2004					
Parameter	**Unit**	**Value**	**Parameter**	**Unit**	**Value**
Chemical oxygen demand	mg/l	< 1	Fluoride	mg/l	2.0
Biochemical oxygen demand	mg/l	< 1	Nitrate	mg/l	<0.04
pH	-	9.48	Nitrite	mg/l	<0.01
Conductivity at 25°C	μS/cm	470	Sodium	mg/l	105
Total alkalinity	mg/l	164.3	Potassium	mg/l	0.8
Total hardness	mg/l	2.1	Calcium	mg/l	0.7
Silica	mg/l	47.2	Magnesium	mg/l	0.07
Total Kjeldahl Nitrogen	mg/l	<0.01	Total iron	mg/l	<0.01
NH_3-Nitrogen	mg/l	<0.01	Aluminum	mg/l	<0.1
Organic-Nitrogen	mg/l	<0.01	Barium	mg/l	<0.5
Dry residue at 103°C	mg/l	308	Cadmium	mg/l	<0.01
Total Suspended Solids	mg/l	<5	Lead	mg/l	<0.05
Bicarbonate	mg/l	89.4	Total chromium	mg/l	<0.06
Carbonate	mg/l	54.6	Copper	mg/l	<0.01
Sulphate	mg/l	52	Manganese	mg/l	<0.01
Chloride	mg/l	14.2	Zinc	mg/l	<0.01

Water and air radon concentrations were measured using an Alpha Guard PQ2000PRO (Genitron GmbH) equipped with an appropriate unit (Aquakit), following a protocol proposed by the manufacturer [27]. Alpha Guard is an ionizing chamber that measures radon via alpha spectrometric techniques. For measurement with Aquakit, the water samples were forced to degas their radon content within a radon tight assembly, which consists of two glass vessels and the Alpha Guard unit. Alpha Guard monitored indoor radon in 1 min data sampling cycles simultaneously with air temperature. The indoor measurements were performed without interfering in the operation procedure of the spa, as about 20 bathers utilized the facilities for immersion baths during the experiments.

The determination of the radon concentration in the water samples through the Aquakit unit was based on the Rn-concentration indicated on the Alpha Guard radon monitor and on the use of the following equation:

$$1000\ c_w = c_a \times [k + (V_{sy} - V_{sa})/V_{sa}] - c_0$$

where: c_w = Rn-concentration in water sample (Bq/l); c_a = radon concentration (Bq/m^3) in the measuring set-up after expelling the radon (indicated by Alpha Guard); c_0 = radon concentration (Bq/m^3) in the measuring set-up before sampling (zero level, i.e. 0 Bq/m^3); V_{sy} = interior volume of the measurement set-up (1122 ml); V_{sa} = volume of the water sample (100 ml); k = radon distribution coefficient between a watery phase and the air volume existing above (0.16 for temperatures between 40 and 45°C).

Four water samples (1 kg) were also stored in glass bottles fitted with inlet and outlet stopcocks, conducted up to the laboratory, and subjected to a technique for quantifying ^{222}Rn based on the emanation procedure [28] and consisting of the 1) removal of radon from the sample, 2) transfer of radon to a scintillation flask, and 3) detection of radon by scintillation counting. The purpose of this sampling was to compare radon concentration data obtained by different methods.

4 Results and discussion

The thermal water radon measurement performed with Alpha Guard yielded an average value of 2.2 Bq/l, whilst the concentration varied between 0.06 and 5.9 Bq/l (average = 3.5 Bq/l) according to the data acquisition by scintillation counting. Future investigations are necessary to investigate if the differences are systematic, as they could indicate the need of recalibration of the system based on scintillation counting. Potential health hazards from radon in consuming water have been considered worldwide, with many countries adopting the guideline activity concentration of 100 Bq/l for drinking water quality recommended by [29]. The radon concentrations of the thermal waters from Londrina thermal spa vary, but, despite this, are greatly below the 100 Bq/l WHO limiting value. In addition, the thermal waters of the spa only occasionally are utilized for consuming purposes, as their main use is for bathing/recreation and, consequently, the health risk due to their ingestion is practically absent.

Figure 2 shows the variability of the indoor radon concentration in the room of the spa for immersion baths as evaluated by Alpha Guard in 24th November 2006 from 7:04 to 7:23 am. The average value corresponded to 71.4 Bq/m^3, which was higher than the mean values of 19.6 and 17.2 Bq/m^3 obtained, respectively, in the counting room of LABIDRO-Laboratory of Isotopes and Hydrochemistry (fig. 3), where the scintillation measurements were performed, and in LITOTECA (fig.4), that is a large room of DPM-Department of Petrology and Metallogeny utilized for storing different rock types with variable content of natural radionuclides.

The mechanisms which can cause ^{222}Rn release from the solid phase and consequently account for the observed Rn content of groundwater and air were discussed elsewhere [30, 31] and consists basically of the following processes: ^{222}Rn recoil following alpha-decay of ^{226}Ra atoms close to the surface of the solid particles (within the ^{222}Rn recoil range of 0.036μm); ^{222}Rn diffusion through the crystalline lattice from production sites below the rock surface; ^{222}Rn diffusion along crystal defects, grain boundaries or microfractures from greater depths below the rock surface; existence of a network of 100 - 200 Å wide nanopores in rocks and minerals, many of which intersect the grain surface, and give rise to a large internal surface area of the solids (in the range of about 10 m^2

per cm^3), orders of magnitude higher than the external surface calculated from grain size. Thus, the models developed for explaining the generation of radon in rocks and transfer to air and water have followed a more macroscopic approach [32] or have included many parameters that are difficult/impossible to measure practically, for instance, microscopic properties such as the surface roughness or inhomogeneous ^{226}Ra distribution in the solid [31, 33].

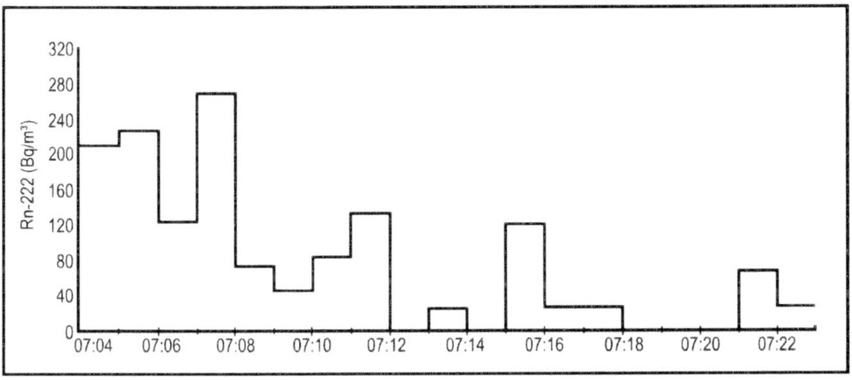

Figure 2: Characteristic variation of the indoor radon concentration in the room of the Londrina thermal spa for immersion baths. Date of the measurement: 24th November 2006.

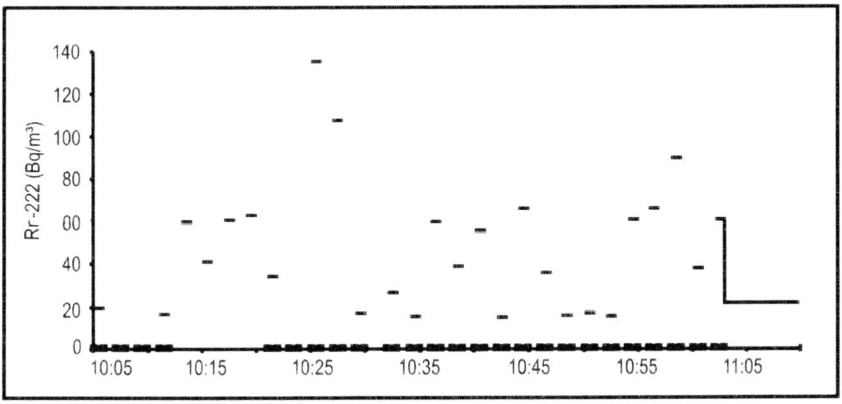

Figure 3: Characteristic variation of the indoor radon concentration in the counting room of LABIDRO, UNESP, Rio Claro. Date of the measurement: 15th December 2006.

The optimized action levels relating to chronic exposure involving radon in dwellings should, in most situations, fall within a yearly average concentration of 200 to 600 Bq/m^3 of ^{222}Rn in air [34]. On the other hand, the action level for remedial action relating to chronic exposure situations involving radon in workplaces is a yearly average concentration of 1000 Bq/m^3 of ^{222}Rn in air [34].

Therefore, the average indoor radon concentration of 71.4 Bq/m^3 in Londrina thermal spa is much lower than these limiting guideline values and, consequently, the inhalation of this gas is not a significant radiation burden both for bathers and working personnel of the spa.

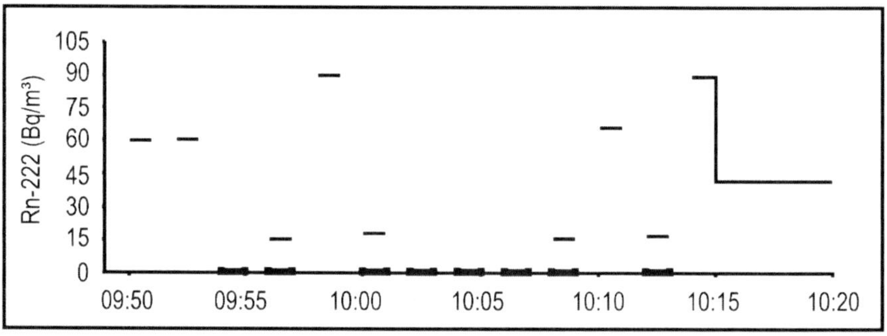

Figure 4: Characteristic variation of the indoor radon concentration in LITOTECA, UNESP, Rio Claro. Date of the measurement: 22nd December 2006.

As a conclusion, bathing and working in Londrina thermal spa does not impose any health risk related to the ingestion of radon in water and inhalation of radon in air both to bathers and personnel. However, this scenario may not be the same in other thermal spas utilizing the waters of Guarani aquifer, because intense variations of radon concentration have been previously identified [28]. Thus, further investigations in the aquifer are highly recommended in order to raise the radiometric data base to levels equivalent to those existing in more developed countries.

References

[1] Flügge, S. & Zimens, K.E., Die bestimmung von korngrossen und diffusionkonstanten aus dem emaniervermogen (Die theorie der emanier-methode). *Zeitschrift fur Physikalische Chemie*, B42, pp. 179-220, 1939.

[2] Petrie, A.S. & Cram, A.G., Design implications of the distribution of pollutants in collection and storage systems used in small rural water supplies. *Water Pollution V: Modelling, Measuring and Prediction*, eds. P. Anagnostopoulos & C.A. Brebbia, WIT Press: Southampton, pp. 503-512, 1999.

[3] Vogiannis, E., Nikolopoulos, D., Louizi, A. & Halvadakis, C.P., Radon variations during treatment in thermal spas. *J. Environ. Radioactivity*, 75, pp. 159-170, 2004.

[4] USEPA (United States Environmental Protection Agency), *Radon in drinking water health risk reduction and cost analysis*. Federal Register 64, Washington, pp. 9559-9599, 1999.

[5] Gesell, T.F. & Prichard, H.M., The technologically enhanced natural radiation environment. *Health Phys.*, 28, p. 361, 1975.

[6] Gesell, T.F. & Prichard, H.M., The contribution of radon in tap water to indoor radon concentrations. *The Natural Radiation Environment III*, eds. T.F. Gesell & W.M. Lowder, Proc. Symp., USDOE, Houston, Rep. Conf. 780422, 1, pp. 5-56, 1980.

[7] Partridge, J.E., Horton, T.R. & Sensintaffer, E.L., *A study of radon-222 released from water during typical household activities.* U.S. Environmental Protection Agency Tech. Note, ORP/EERF-79-1, 1979.

[8] Bruno, R.C., Sources of indoor radon in houses: a review. *J. Air Pollut. Control Assoc.*, 33, pp. 105-109, 1983.

[9] Prichard, H.M., The transfer of radon from domestic water to indoor air. *J. Am. Water Works Assoc.*, 79, pp. 159-161, 1987.

[10] Nazaroff, W.W. & Nero, A.V. Jr., *Radon and its decay products in indoor air*, John Wiley & Sons: New York, 1988.

[11] Nazaroff, W.W., Doyle, S.M., Nero, A.V. Jr. & Sextro, R.G. Radon entry via potable water. *Radon and its decay products in indoor air*, eds. W.W. Nazaroff & A.V. Nero Jr., John Wiley & Sons: New York, 1988.

[12] Aieta, E.M., Singley, J.E., Trussel, A.R., Thorbjarnarson, K.W. & McGuire, M.J., Radionuclides in drinking water: an overview. *J. Am. Water Works Assoc.*, 79, pp. 144-152, 1987.

[13] Lawrence, E.P., Poeter, E. & Wanty, R.B., Geohydrologic, geochemical, and geologic controls on the occurrence of radon in ground water near Conifer, Colorado, USA. *J. Hydrol.*, 127, pp. 367-386, 1991.

[14] Nelson, P.H., Rachiele, R. & Smith, A., Transport of radon in flowing boreholes at Stripa, Sweden. *J. Geophys. Res.*, 88, pp. 2395-2405, 1983.

[15] Shishkevich, C., Earthquake related variation of micro-components in thermal water of the Tashkent aquifer. *Geosci. Bull. Ser. A*, 2, pp. 69-91, 1971.

[16] Wollenberg, H.A., Smith, A.R., Mosier, D.F., Flexser, S. & Clark, M., Radon-222 in groundwater of the long valley caldera, California. *Pageoph.*, 122, pp. 327-339, 1984.

[17] Smith, A.R., Bowman, H.R., Mosier, D.F. & King, C.Y., Investigation of radon-222 in subsurface waters as an earthquake predictor. *IEEE Trans. Nucl. Sci.*, NS-23, pp. 694-698, 1976.

[18] Steinhäusler, F., Radon spas: source term, doses and risk assessment. *Radiation Protection Dosimetry*, 24, pp. 257-259, 1988.

[19] Datye, V.K., Hopke, K., Fitzgerald, B. & Raunemaa, A., Dynamic model for assessing Rn-222 and progeny exposure from showering with radon-bearing water. *Environmental Science and Technology*, 31, pp. 1589-1596, 1997.

[20] Bernhardt, G.P. & Hess, C.T., Acute exposure from Rn-222 and aerosols in drinking water. *Environmental International*, 22, pp. S753-S759, 1996.

[21] Fitzgerald, B., Hopke, K., Datye, V.K., Raunemaa, A. & Kuuspalo, K., Experimental assessment of the short- and long-term effects of Rn-222 from domestic shower water on the dose burden incurred in normally

occupied homes. *Environmental Science and Technology*, 31, pp. 1822-1829, 1997.

[22] Araújo, L.M., França, A.B. & Potter, P.E., Giant Mercosul aquifer of Brazil, Argentina, Uruguay and Paraguay: hydrogeologic maps of Botucatu, Pirambóia, Rosário do Sul, Buena Vista, Misiones and Tacuarembó Formations. *Proc. of the 9th National Meeting of Well-drillers*, Universidade Federal do Paraná: Curitiba, pp. 1-16, 1995.

[23] Rebouças, A.C., Groundwater in Brazil. *Episodes*, 11, pp. 209-214, 1988.

[24] Kimmelmann e Silva, A.A., Rebouças, A.C. & Santiago, M.M.F., ^{14}C analyses of groundwater from the Botucatu aquifer system in Brazil. *Radiocarbon*, 31, pp. 926-933, 1989.

[25] Gilboa, Y., Mero, F. & Mariano, I.B., The Botucatu aquifer of South America, model of an untapped continental aquifer. *J. Hydrol.*, 29, pp. 165-179, 1976.

[26] Hindi, E., *Physical-chemical analysis of waters from Londrina thermal spa*. Universidade Federal do Paraná: Curitiba, 2004.

[27] Genitron Instruments, *Alpha Guard PQ2000/MC50, Multiparameter Radon Monitor*, Genitron Instruments: Frankfurt, 2000.

[28] Bonotto, D.M. & Caprioglio, L. Radon in groundwaters from Guarani aquifer, South America: environmental and exploration implications. *Applied Radiation and Isotopes*, 57, pp. 931-940, 2002.

[29] WHO (World Health Organization), *Guidelines for drinking water quality: radiological aspects*, available at http:www.who.int/water_sanitation_ health/dwq/gdwq3/en/, 2004.

[30] Andrews, J.N. & Wood, D.F. Mechanism of radon release in rock matrices and entry into groundwaters. *Inst. Mineral. Metal. Trans.*, B81, pp. 198-209, 1972.

[31] Rama & Moore, W.S., Mechanism of transport of U-Th series radioisotopes from solids into groundwater. *Geochim. Cosmochim. Acta*, 48, pp. 395-399, 1984.

[32] Andrews, J.N. & Lee, D.J., Inert gases in groundwater from the Bunter Sandstone of England as indicators of age and palaeoclimatic trends. *J. Hydrol.*, 41, pp. 233-252, 1979.

[33] Krishnaswami, S. & Seidemann, D.E. Comparative study of ^{222}Rn, ^{40}Ar, ^{39}Ar and ^{37}Ar leakage from rocks and minerals: implications for the role of nanopores in gas transport through natural silicates. *Geochim. Cosmochim. Acta*, 52, pp. 655-658, 1988.

[34] IAEA (International Atomic Energy Agency) *International basic safety standards for protection against ionizing radiation and for the safety of radiation sources*, Safety Series 115, Vienna, 353 pp., 1996.

Environmental hazard and water quality: the River Platani basin

V. Liguori & G. Manno
Dipartimento di Ingegneria Strutturale e geotecnica,
Facoltà di Ingegneria, Università degli Studi di Palermo, Sicilia, Italy

Abstract

The River Platani, situated in the western side of Sicily, is one of the greatest rivers of the island. It runs for about 103 Km and the basin extends to about 1,784.9 Km^2. It rises near Santo Stefano Quisquina (Ag); the river flows to Capo Bianco (Ag) ends in the Mediterranean Sea. The morphology of the basin is predominantly characterized by rises of modest entities with slopes sweet or calanques. In the containing gypsum and carbonatic stony heaps are diffused the karst phenomena. In the Platani basin some mines are located of rock salt and potassium salts; today the mines are closed after a long activity and they interact with the geomorphology of the territory and on the water quality of the river. An example is given by the ex mine "Muti-Coffari" (Ag), in fact the mine determines an evident incidence on the physical-chemical characteristics of the water and the fluvial ecosystem. Where the "sinkholes" are present, caused by the incessant thinning of the vault and pillars of the mine's tunnel, meteoric water penetrates inside, flooding all the underground levels; the waters, through different chemical process, attach the evaporitics rocks and they have a concentration of salts. Consequently, because of the flooding of the tunnels, the saturated salt waters escape from the entrance of the mines to flow into the River Plantain. Through the monitoring of the principal branch of the River Platani it can be deduced that the river can be considered constituted by two separate ecosysystems: the first goes from the source to the point of immission of the small affluent coming from the mine; the second extended from the salt mine up to the mouth. Observing the graphs products on the chemical-physical parameters evident as the element of separation is constituted by the immission of saturated salt water. After the immission of the Torrente Salina, the values of the sulphates, of the chlorides, and of the sodium, sensitively increase. The environmental aspect that derives is a hyper saltiness that affects the fluvial ecosystem, as a matter of fact a desertification of fertile areas where once there were very fertile cultivations.
Keywords: river basin, ecology, environmental risk, water quality.

WIT Transactions on Biomedicine and Health, Vol 11, © 2007 WIT Press
www.witpress.com, ISSN 1743-3525 (on-line)
doi:10.2495/EHR070161

1 Introduction

The watershed of the Platani River is situated in the western centre of Sicily, fig. 1, and has a total surface of 1.784,9 Km^2. It extends along in a NE-SW direction (in the map of Sicily). It includes 46 communes pertaining to territory limits to the provinces of Agrigento, Caltanissetta and Palermo, see fig. 2.

The River Platani starts around the premises of S. Stefano Quisquina (province of Agrigento) around Pizzo Confessionario. It flows for 103 Km, ending into the Mediterranean sea near Capo Bianco with a front of about 4 Km.

The basin starts from the Sicani mountains, which is the highest peak located in the north-western sector between the provincial territories of Palermo and Agrigento (Serra della Moneta, 1,188 m o.s.l.; Serra Quisquina, m 1,169 m o.s.l..; Pizzo Stagnataro, 1,346 m o.s.l.) and in the north-eastern sector near Valledolmo (Pizzo San Pietro, 1,018 m o.s.l., Serra di Puccia, m 1,052 o.s.l.; Monte Catuso, m 1,042 o.s.l.).

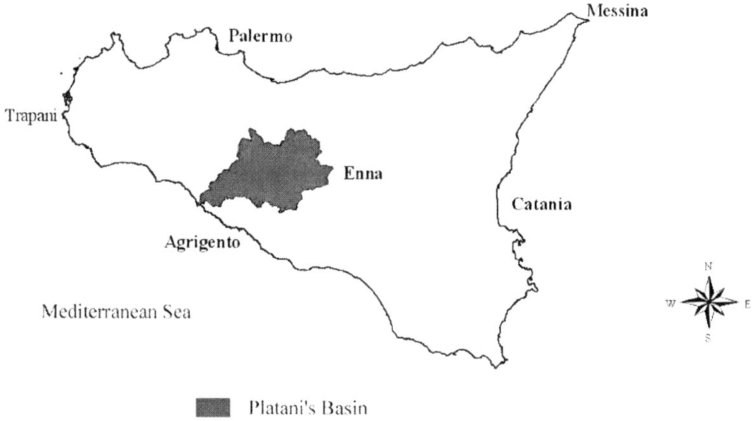

Figure 1: Location of the Platani basin in Sicily.

The highest parts of the mountains are located in the north-western side of the basin: the mountain range of Monte Gemini (1,392.4 m o.s.l.) and Monte Cammarata (1,578 m o.s.l.).

The basin flows beside a road called Strada Statale 189 and the railway track Palermo-Agrigento. It flows to the territory of Castronovo di Sicilia (province of Palermo), where the lake has created a dam called "Diga Fanaco" ($24.4 \cdot 10^6$ m^3), a barrage of the Platani River.

The lake supplies water to the various communes of the province of Agrigento.

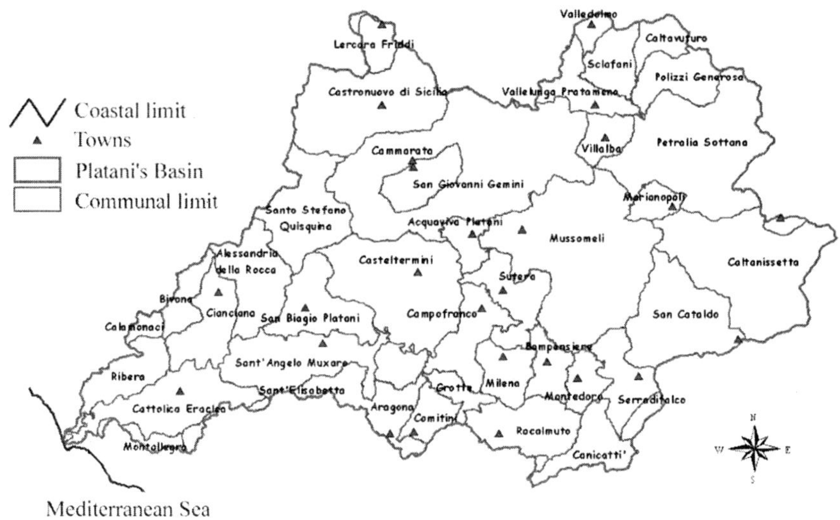

Figure 2: Boundary limits.

2 Geological and geomorphological aspects

The basin of the Platani River, on the geological side, is characterized by two sectors:

1 North-western side the lithological terms belong to Catena Appennino-Maghrebide forming the Monti Sicani.
2 Southern side formed mostly of post orogenetic lithology prevalently belonging to the "Formazione Gessoso Solfifera" upper Miocene and mostly argillaceous sandy calcarenitical terms plio-quaternary.

The Monti Sicani are the southern sector of the western segment of the "Catena Appenninico Maghrebide"; it rises as a deformation of "Dominio Sicano" formed by Mesozoic carbonatic rocky units and by "Flysh Numidico".

The "Catena Appennino Maghrebide" is the product of the mio-pliocenic deformation of different carbonate platforms and pelagic basins, deposit are piled up with ramp-flat and duplex style and located during the mosozoic-tertiary along the northern African continental margin, Renda and Nigro [1].

In the southern area of the basin appears the lithology belonging to the "Formazione Gessoso Solfifera", the lithological succession is: diatomites, evaporitical limestones, gypsums, salts with clay intercalations, marls and limestones. This formation rests in discordance on pre-evaporitic deposits "Formazione Terravecchia" (Upper Tortonian - Lower Messinian) and it is covered in discordance, with calcilutite constituent "Trubi" (Lower Pliocene) Catalano and Argenio [2].

The evaporitic rocks settled during the Messinian in coincidence with the paleogeographic event of the closing of the Mediterranean basin. This event happened after the continental collision between Spain and Africa as a coincidence the closing of the straits of Gibraltar. The closing of the Mediterranean sea caused an hidrological deficit, lowered the sea level, wide areas surfaced and the creation in the deeper areas of basins where the evaporates were deposited, Agnesi et al [3].

The water of the Platani River, originated from Monte Cammarata crossing the southern side of the basin, is constituted mostly of evaporitic rocks, (rich in gypsum and halite). So the water became particularly brackish like the nearby "Imera meridionale" River.

The average altitude level of the basin is 439 m o.s.l. The morphology of the basin changes, moving from the northern side of the start, depending on the lithologies that characterized the landscape.

The general aspect of the northern side is mountainous with carbonatic relief more or less sheer, with slope incised with ripid valley lines that flow together in the principal stream. In the central side of the basin the landscape becomes hilly and this influences the different characteristics of erosion of the lithologies in outcrop: the harder morphologies on the rocky cluster, while the slightest morphology are bound with terms of argillaceous and marly.

Proceeding along the SW direction to the start of the basin zone, the predominant element morphological is caused by an alluvional valley floor. Here the rivers have a course, mostly like a meander, up until it reaches the sea near to NW called Capo Bianco.

Relative to the use of the soil, inside the river basin there are vineyards, citrus groves, olive groves, simple irrigous and arboreus seminative, gardens, annual cultures and permanent cultures.

The landscape is also mainly covered with broadleaf trees, conifers, mixed forest maquis, areas with shrubby woody vegetation and with uncultivated zones. The use of the soil is 77% seminative and 13% with tree cultures.

The course of the precipitation in the river basin is various, according to the change of altitude. Proceeding through the mountain area of Cammarata, Santo Stefano Quisquina, Castronovo di Sicilia, and up to the cliff the temperatures increase while the precipitations diminish, giving rise to frequent and long periods of dry weather.

3 Mines

The Sicilian southern subsoil, formed by evaporated rocks, have, over the years, become areas of interest in the past for its numerous mines used mostly for the extraction of sulphur, and in recent times for the extraction of potassic and sodic salts. Most of the salt mines are located in the province of Enna, Caltanissetta and Agrigento.

The evaporated rocks have generated large deposits for the Formazione Gessoso Solfifera mostly found in the watershed of the Platani River; they are still nowadays the object of interest for the mining extraction.

Table 1 shows the mines and the caves belongings to each territory at different Communes.

Table 1: List of anthropic activities.

Commune	Caves	Mines	Solfatara
Aragona		1	
Caltanissetta	1		4
Casteltermini		3	
Cattolica Eraclea	1		
Cianciana		5	
Comitini		1	3
Milena			1
San Biagio Platani	1		
San Cataldo		1	1

The territory, therefore, has suffered and still suffers for the modifications caused by the various geomorphologic conditions generated for the exploration of mining on the surface and underground, evidenced by looking at the already exhausted cultivations. In the territories where there were mining activities a deep and heavy dynamic mechanisms has developed that sometimes is observed on the surface showing the unforeseeable and uncontrollable phenomena that man can control.

This phenomena, the most common called subsidence, is more evident in areas where extractive activities have been carried out, especially mineral salts. This event caused the formation of great "sinkholes" and landslides in tandem with the underground workings, with enormous damage to the surface.

The salt has a mechanical behavior that is commonly defined as not linear, and depends on its chemical composition, " granulmetrics of crystals", are particularly visco-elastic and have a plastic behavior and are sensitive to the underground microclimate. The subsidence for the presence of the cavities can be emphasized for the presence of seismic, alluvional phenomena, and the erosion of the versant.

Other negative effects on the environment linked to the mining activities, are:

1. mobilization of the melted refusal materials that accumulate in the dump in some parts of the versant with an incline variable;
2. the alteration of the superficial and underground hidrology and the harvest in the dug areas of meteoric water consequently has an emission with brackish waters or for interception of water stratus;
3. the supercharging of the hydrographical net with fine and rough detritus that can cause pollution;
4. modifications of the morphology and the destruction of the vegetation with modification of the landscape.

It is the second effect that causes the changes to the Platani River, an effect caused by the brackish waters that come out from the Mine "Muti-Coffari", with the consequent risk to the environment and which modifies the surrounding territory and water risk for the fluvial ecosystem of the Platani River. The salt mine is an example that constitutes the risk for the natural environment, linked to the already existing anthropic cavities (abandoned mines). The mine "Muti-Coffari", is located in "Contrada Salina", in the territory of Cammarata, in the province of Agrigento where the lithologies in outcrop are gypsum and clay, Liguori *et al* [4]. Now the mine has been stopped because of exhaustion. In the winter of 1994 the mine suffered a sinkhole that has produced a sinking of the plan of 30 meters involving the first two galleries of the mine, fig. 3. The river of mud, water and salt coming out from the mine, fortunately did not sweep up the nearby bridge of the Strada Statale n.189 but channeled itself below the river bed. However, the waters eroded the land for a depth of 1.5 meter, also affecting the supporting structure of the subway of the Strada Statale 189.

The overlooking zones were the mines were located has started a trigger of complex landslides (rock slumps followed from mud flow) whose evolution has created numerous surface depressions, very visible on the north side of the Vallone Salina.

Moreover this phenomena can be considered the cause of the chemical alteration of the hydrological characteristics of the Platani's River. In fact the water of the Vallone Salina enters from a natural well and falls in the mine, dissolving the salts. The water that is not infiltrated in the subsoil comes out from the entrance of the mine and flows in the Platani River rendering its water salty and polluted. The presence of the mine determines an obvious record on the state of water since it pours, above all in winter, and the salt continues to pollute the Platani. The halite that flows in the river, drying up the soil, causes the death of fish, alters the ecosystem and generates desertification of the fertile areas. The most involved areas from the effects caused by the hypersalinity of the river are those of Acquaviva Platani. Here waters (of the Platani) cannot be used for the irrigation of citrus groves and orchards placed along the sides of the river, Campofranco and Sutera.

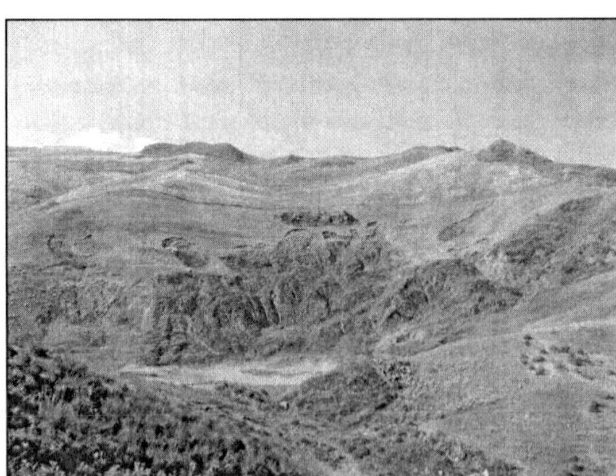

Figure 3: Sinkhole of winter 1994.

4 Qualitative monitoring of River Platani

In the month of December 2001 the monitoring of the area was organized to ascertain the qualitative state of the waters of River Platani, Mortellaro [5].

Along the principal course of the river, from the start up to the lake Fanaco, with 13 stations of sampling to test the water, the sampling, as shown in table 2 in which both the analysis in the field (measure of the dissolved O_2, temperature of the air and the water) and chemical analysis of the waters that have been checked in a laboratory, have been carried out.

The location of the stations has been selected on the basis of the peculiarities found in the river, in relation to particular situations of antropic impact which clearly have influenced the quality of the waters: presence of inhabited centers, presence of urban and industrial emissions, immission of principals tributaries.

Table 2: Sampling station.

ID	Sampling Station	ID	Sampling Station
1	Landslide on the Platani (c.da S.Andrea)	8	Acquaviva Platani station
2	Bridge Vecchio: Castronovo	9	Fonnuto Pass: SS189
3	After the valley of the freshet Morello	10	Bridge S.Biagio Platani - S.Angelo Muxaro
4	Cammarata - Village Regalmici Road	11	Bridge Raffadali–Cianciana
5	Crossroads Tumarrano	12	Bridge Cattolica Eraclea-Cianciana
6	1 km downstream of the Mancuso Bridge: SS189	13	Mouth of the River Platani
7	After the valley of the mine salt		

In some cases the locations of the selected sites to test the waters have been changed because they were very difficult to reach, but only after being sure that the distance of the points of sampling from the above-mentioned immissions was enough to guarantee the full remixing of the waters, with the purpose to estimate the quality of the water receptor and not that of the emissions.

Station n°1 was located near the "Contrada S.Andrea" where the River Platani sets again its natural course, after having been canalized for 150meter in an artificial canal. The canal takes the waters from the artificial lake that was created following the landslide, to the lake Fanaco.

Station n°2 has been selected in "Ponte Vecchio". This is the first bridge built on the River Platani (1951) and it is disfigured by the presence of a modern bridge. It is evident that the presence of the foam was probably due to the dumping of the commune of Castronovo of Sicily and Lercara.

Station n°3 has been situated after the flow in the valley of the "Vallone Morello".

Station n°4 has been situated near by the bridge on the road that branches from the Strada Statale 189 to the road that goes to "Borgo Regalmici".

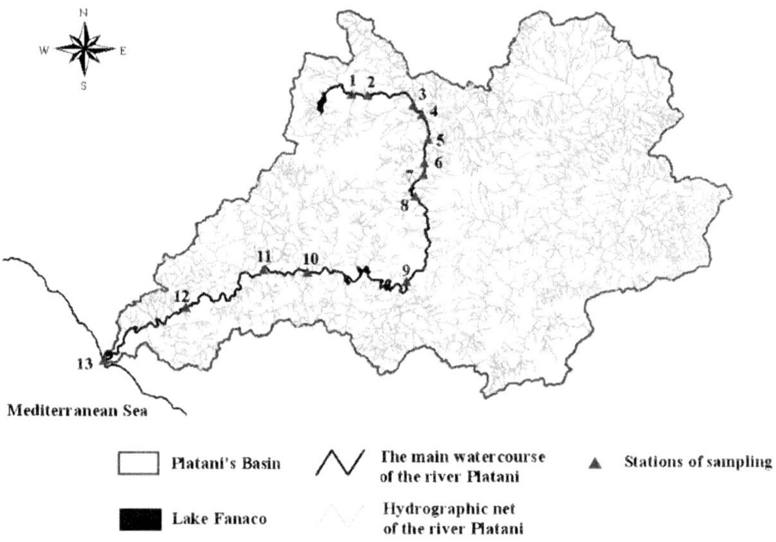

Figure 4: Sampling station.

Station n°5 has been selected near by the bridge on the flood called the "Torrente Tumarrano". Station n°6 has been situated in a location 1 km downstream of the Ponte Mancuso, since the stream under the bridge was hardly attainable for the presence of enclosure and high vegetation. Besides, the stream was polluted by the wastewater coming from Cammarata. The sample has been taken after having guaranteed a dilution of the waters.

Station n°7 has been situated in the location of the ex salt mine, called "Muti – Coffari". The presence of the salt along the edges and on the bed of the "Vallone Salina" coming from the mine flows on the right bank of the River Platani.

Station n°8 has been situated near the Acquaviva Platani station, after it has gone under the viaduct that goes to the Strada Statale 189.

Station n°9 is selected near to the "Passo Fonnuto".

Station n°10 has been situated near to the bridge that connects S. Biagio Platani with S. Angelo Muxaro.

Station n°11 has been situated near to bridge of the Strada Statale 118 that connects Cianciana with Raffadali. Along the bed of the Platani River there are brushwoods and some part of pebbles and gravel.

Station n°12 has been situated near to the bridge to the road that connects Cattolica Eraclea with Cianciana. The presence of foam has been revealed, due probably to the dumping of water from the commune of Cattolica Eraclea.

Station n°13 has been situated near to the mouth of the Platani River where there is the headquarters of a Reserve called "Riserva Naturale Orientata", situated in a territory called "Capo Bianco".

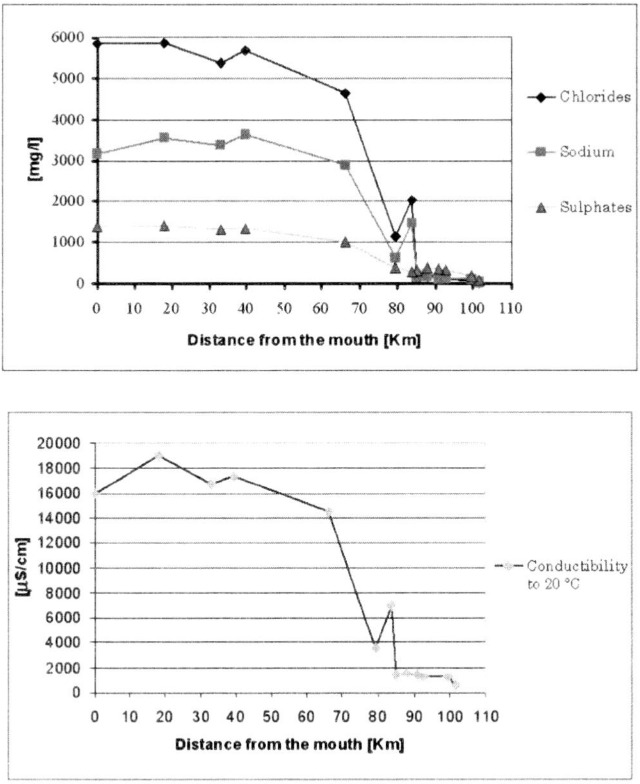

Figure 5: State of salts, sulfates and conducibility along the main course.

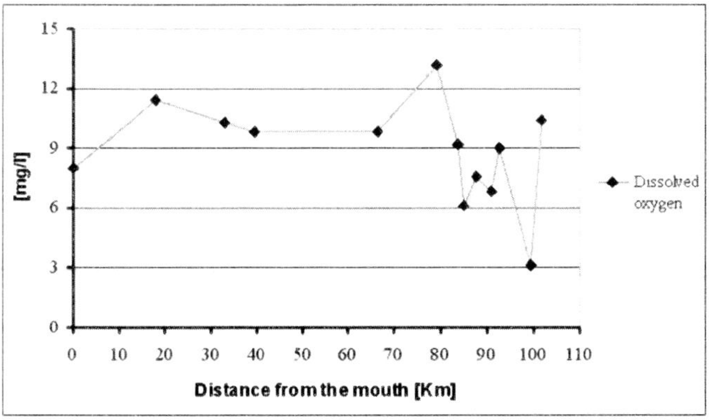

Figure 6: State of the dissolved oxygen along the main course.

During the experiment the following parameters have been monitored: external temperature, temperature of the water, dissolved oxygen, BOD, COD, TOC, N, P, conductibility, surface-actives, Cl^-, SO_4^{--}, Na^+ e K^+; Ca^{++} e Mg^{++}; pH, fecals coliforms and streptococcus, totals coliforms. The chemical-physics analyses are representative of the existing conditions in the river at the time of the collecting, while biological analyses are the most significant datum of the environmental state. To underline clearly the course of the measured concentrations along the principal course some graphs have been created relating to the salts, the conductivity, the sulfates, the dissolved oxygen, the streptococcus and coliforms, and the nutrients.

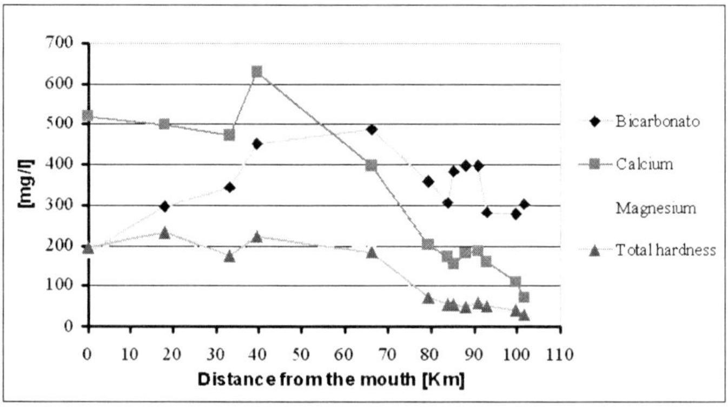

Figure 7: State of the HCO_3^-, Ca^{++}, Mg^{++} along the main course.

The ammonia values, nitrite and nitrates, fig. 8, are indicative of the presence of wastewater and the effectiveness for the depurative treatments.

Observing the following graphs, in particular all those of salts and of conductivity, it can be deduced that the river is constituted by two separate ecosystems. The first ecosystem includes the mountain part of the watershed from Lake Fanaco up to the "Torrente Salina". The second one goes from "Vallone Salina" up to the mouth of the Platani River. The element of separation is the immission of "Vallone Salina" in the River Platani fig. 9-10.

The values of chlorides, sodium sulfates and the remarkably effects that the conductivity increase after the impluvium coming out of the mine are shown in fig. 4.

Calcium and magnesium gradually increase beginning from the same point of immission, fig. 7.

The station of testing: Ponte Vecchio, in the commune of Castronovo can be considered another critical site.

The dissolved oxygen, fig. 6, keeps varying with values among 6 and 13 mg/l. The only value that is quite far from that is the one in correspondence of the station of the "Ponte Vecchio", where the measure is 3,10 mg/l. This is due to the presence of the dumpwater of the Castronovo and Lercara.

The course of the phosphates and the total phosphorus, fig. 8, shows a peak in correspondence of the Ponte Vecchio, and is almost constant in the other points.

In the same sampling station an elevated concentration of fecals streptococcus, fecal and total coliforms has been recorded, fig. 8.

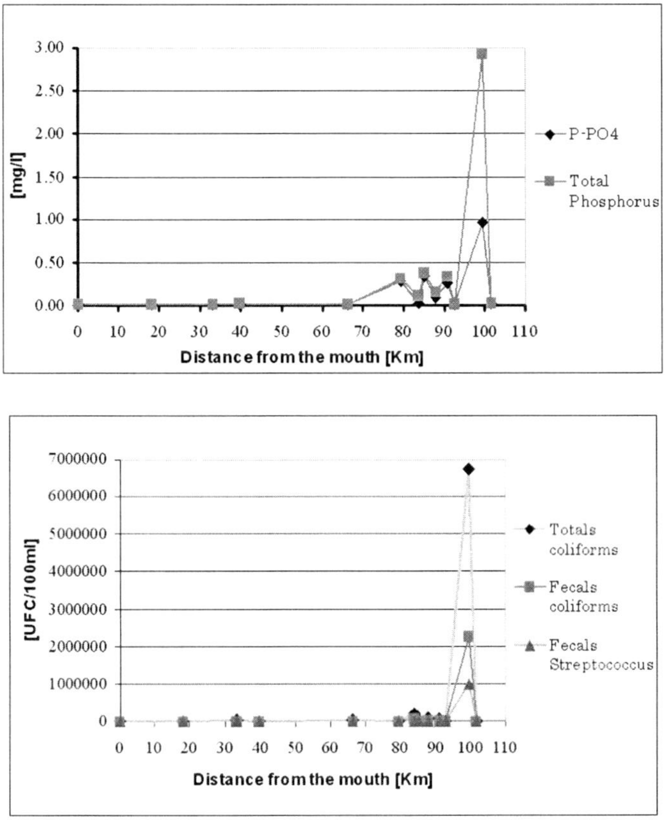

Figure 8: State of the phosphorus and compounds and coliforms, streptococcus along the main course.

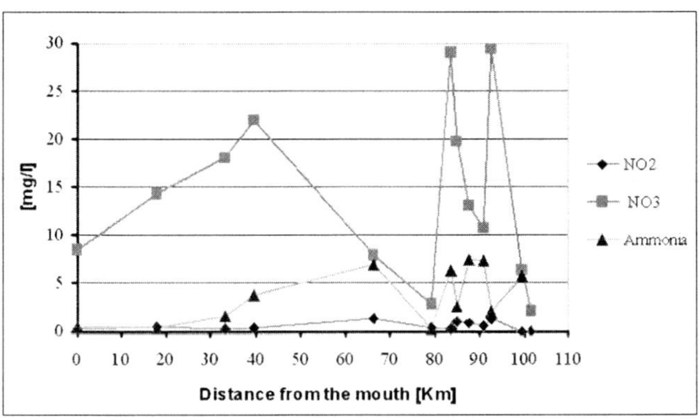

Figure 9: State of the nitrogen's compounds along the main course.

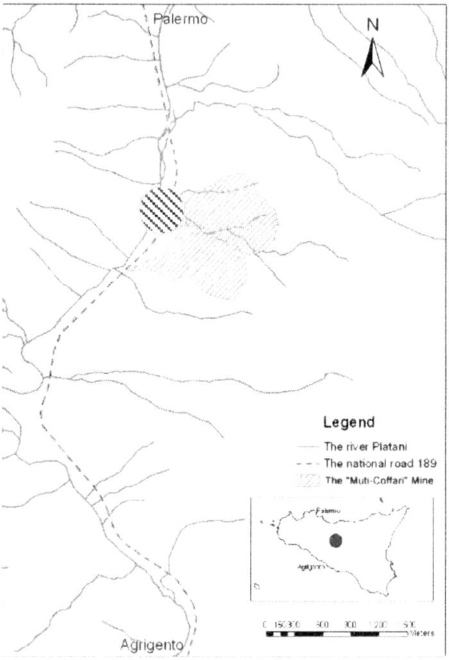

Figure 10: Location of the valley of the salt water ("Muti-Coffari" mine).

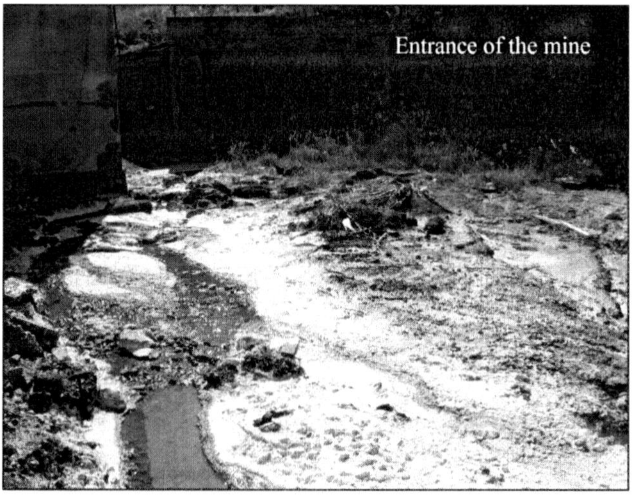

Figure 11: Entrance of the "Muti-Coffari" mine from where exit the salt water.

5 Conclusions

The river is formed by two separate ecosystems. The first ecosystem is included in the mountain part of the watershed from the Lake Fanaco up to the Torrente Salina. The second goes from the Torrente Salina up to the mouth of the Platani River. The element of separation is formed and set up by the immission of the Torrente Salina that changes the conditions of waters rendering them saline and altering the fluvial ecosystem.

The presence of the mine "Muti-Coffari" effects the state of waters of the River Platani, altering the physical-chemical characteristics.

The salt that flows into the river dries the cultivations, causes the reduction of fish numbers and leads to their death, alters the ecosystem and produces desertification of the fertile areas since it is not possible to use the waters of the Platani River for the irrigation. The mine constitutes also a serious risk for the environment as it alters the morphology of the surrounding territory that is subjected to subsidence phenomena, with the creation of sinkholes and landslides.

The ex salt mine represents an elevated environmental level of danger and a remarkable risk: for the fluvial ecosystem, for the natural environment and for the nearby infrastructures, such as the Strada Statale 189 Palermo-Agrigento.

References

[1] Renda, P., Nigro F., *Evoluzione geologica ed assetto strutturale della Sicilia centro-settentrionale,* Boll. Soc. Geol. It. , pp. 375-388, 1999.

[2] Catalano, R., D'Argenio, B., *Schema geologico della Sicilia,* Mem. Soc. Geol. It. , 24, pp. 9-41, 1982.

[3] Agnesi, V. et al, *Gypsum-karst caves versus surface land forms to define a morfphoevolutive model in Central Southern Sicily (Southern Italy),* Sixth International Conference on Geomorphology, Zaragoza, 2005.

[4] Liguori, V., Manno, G., Mortellaro, D., *Evaporite karst in Sicily,* Sixth International Conference on Geomorphology, Zaragoza, 2005.

[5] Mortellaro, D., *Studi preliminary per la redazione di un piano di tutela delle acque ai sensi del D. Lgs 152/99. Applicazione al bacino del fiume Platani,* Tesi di laurea, Università di Palermo, 2001.

The contribution of drinking water fluoride to the risk of dental fluorosis in Estonia

E. Indermitte[1,2], A. Saava[1], S. Russak[3] & A. Kull[2]
[1]*Department of Public Health, University of Tartu, Estonia*
[2]*Institute of Geography, University of Tartu, Estonia*
[3]*Department of Stomatology, Tartu University Clinicum, Estonia*

Abstract

Fluoride is one of the few chemicals of natural origin that have been shown to cause significant health effects in people through drinking-water. The association between the fluoride level in drinking water and the degree of dental fluorosis has been documented worldwide. The permissible maximum health-based fluoride limit in drinking water is 1.5 mg/l. The aim of this paper is to assess human exposure to drinking water fluoride in Estonia and determine the contribution of drinking water fluoride content to the dental fluorosis risk. The paper is based on the survey of drinking water supply in Estonia drawn from the database of the National Health Protection Inspectorate and supplemented by a special study to determine the fluoride content of water in public water supplies all over Estonia. The retrospective case study to determine the risk of fluorosis was carried out. The subjects of the study were 12 years old, living in six districts of the town of Tartu with different fluoride content in drinking water. In total 368 children were investigated. Fluoride content in the drinking water of the Estonian population varied in a large scale. The permissible maximum limit was exceeded in 14.4% of water samples. High levels of fluoride are due to a natural geogenic source. The proportion of the population exposed to a high fluoride level in drinking water was small (4.2%), mainly consumers of small water supply systems in West-Estonia, where the only drinking water source is the Silurian-Ordovician aquifer system. Association between prevalence of dental fluorosis among 12-year old schoolchildren and fluoride content in drinking water was observed. The obtained data allowed the assessment of the risk of dental fluorosis for the Estonian population. Control of drinking water quality is critical in preventing fluorosis.
Keywords: drinking water, Estonia, fluoride, fluorosis, health risks.

WIT Transactions on Biomedicine and Health, Vol 11, © 2007 WIT Press
www.witpress.com, ISSN 1743-3525 (on-line)
doi:10.2495/EHR070171

1 Introduction

Levels of chemicals in environmental media and population exposure to these levels are critical to protect public health from environmental health risks [1]. Fluoride is one of the few chemicals of natural origin that has been shown to cause significant effects in people through drinking-water. The long-term moderate-level chronic exposure to fluoride in drinking-water at or over the current WHO guideline value (1.5 mg/l) can cause incurable but potentially preventable fluorosis which affects the teeth and bones [2]. The association between fluorides in drinking water and the degree of dental fluorosis has been documented worldwide [2–4]. Dental fluorosis is characterized by staining and pitting of the teeth. In more severe cases, all the enamel may be damaged. Millions of people around the world both in developing and developed countries are exposed to excessive amounts of fluoride through drinking water contaminated from natural geological sources. As a result, many suffer conditions ranging from mild dental fluorosis to crippling skeletal fluorosis. Therefore, the control of drinking water quality is critical in preventing dental diseases.

In Estonia groundwater from several aquifers is the main drinking water source in most towns and rural settlements. Fluoride concentrations in ground water were found to vary in a large range: from 0.01 to 6.95 mg/l [5]. Since drinking water is typically the most significant source of fluoride [2] an in depth exposure assessment to fluoride is urgently called for.

On the other hand, health problems arising from different fluoride levels in drinking water have been detected in Estonia [6]. Faced with an incurable but preventable condition (fluorosis) from fluorides in drinking water, the risk of fluorosis due to high fluoride levels in drinking water is an irrefutable argument for risk assessment on fluorides in drinking water.

2 Materials and methods

2.1 Study area

Estonia is the smallest Baltic country with an area of 45.227 km^2 and population of 1.351 (01.01.2004) million people, situated on the East coast of the Baltic Sea and lying in North-western part of the East-European Platform. Administratively Estonia is divided into 15 counties (Figure 1). 82.9% of Estonian population is well provided with public water supplies, what is a very high share if we will consider that urban population makes up to 69.3% of population and rural population (30.7%) is highly scattered with average population density of 10.5 in/km^2. There are 1233 public water supplies in the country. The prevalence of small water supplies is characteristic for Estonia. Up to 86% of supplies serve less than 500 inhabitants [5].

Deep groundwater of several aquifers abstracted by drilled tube wells in towns and rural settlements is the main source of drinking water. Five aquifer systems are exploited depending on location (Middle-Devonian, Middle-Lower-

Devonian, Silurian-Ordovician, Ordovician-Cambrian and Cambrian-Vendian). They differ from each other in distribution and chemical composition [7]. The groundwater is used directly without treatment. In two towns (capital Tallinn and Narva) surface water after treatment and disinfection is used as main source of drinking water.

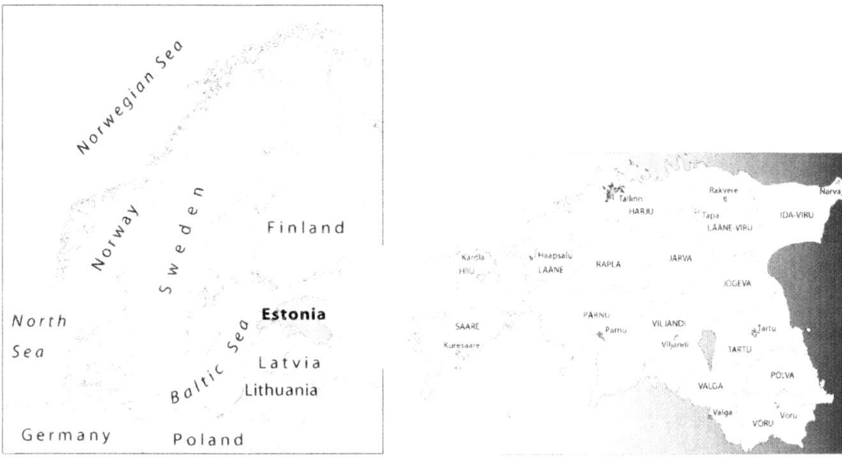

Figure 1: Location of study area.

2.2 Exposure data

The determination of fluoride content in drinking water of inhabitants of the whole of Estonia was performed in 2004. Data on access of population to water supplies and number of water consumers by supplies were obtained from Estonian Health Protection Inspectorate database on drinking water "JVESI". All water supplies serving at least 100 consumers were visited and the sites for sampling were selected. In case the supply system operated several drilled tube wells, additional samples were taken from different locations according to the influential area of the wells. Altogether 735 samples were collected in 47 towns and 471 rural settlements in all 15 counties throughout Estonia.

Water samples for fluoride analyses were collected from tap water closest to the consumer. The analyses were carried out according to the Standards Methods for the Examination of Water and Wastewater by the SPADNS colorimetric method during 48 hours [8].

The results of analyses were grouped into 3 categories according to the health effects of fluoride level in water:

1) high-fluoride content drinking water (over 1.50 mg/l) – causing adverse health effects (primarily dental fluorosis);
2) medium-fluoride content drinking water (0.51-1.50 mg/l) – having protection against dental caries with the least risk of producing dental fluorosis or other toxic effects;
3) low-fluoride content drinking water (up to 0.50 mg/l) – insufficient to prevent caries.

2.3 Case study

A special retrospective case study to determine the contribution of drinking water fluoride to the dental fluorosis risk (odds ratio – OR) was carried out among 12-year old schoolchildren who were born and living in Tartu city where the content of fluoride in drinking water varies by regions. Tartu is the second largest city in Estonia, covering an area of 39 km^2 with the population of 101 740 inhabitants. The groundwater without any treatment is used to supply drinking water. Over 100 drilled deep tube wells are connected to the public water supply network. They rely on Devonian, Silurian and Ordovician-Cambrian hydrogeological aquifers with different quality of water. The data on fluoride concentration in water were obtained from the water quality database of drilled tube wells in 1986-1997 compiled for the Tartu Agenda 21 [9]. Since the municipal drinking water distribution system combines water from several groundwater aquifers, the fluoride concentration in tap water at consumer varies depending on the district of the influence of the tube well. For the study we took care to select only districts that were supplied by definite tube wells of known fluoride concentration. In result six districts were defined purposively for the study (Figure 2). These districts are of approximately the same eco-environmental and ethnic conditions as well as socioeconomic standards.

The sampling population was a part of the over-Estonian survey of dental health of schoolchildren conducted in 1999-2000 according to the uniformed methodology of World Health Organisation [10]. The 12-year old children served as a target group. Consent from the children, as well as from local authorities was obtained prior to examination. The children were asked about the duration of their residence at the present address. Schoolchildren were localized according to their current home address and their correspondence to drinking water districts was determined. Only those schoolchildren who had reported continuous residence since birth in corresponding districts were included in the study. As a result the total sample size was 368 children.

Clinical intra-oral examination was conducted at the schools by a trained examiner with an assistant recording the observations. Dental fluorosis was assessed on vestibular, occlusal and lingual surfaces. The white flecks, fine white and brown lines in the enamel were registered as a mild degree of fluorosis. Very chalky, opaque enamel, mottling and loss of portions of the outer enamel were diagnosed as severe fluorosis.

Data was digitized using Excel programme and a Statistical Package for Social Science (SPSS 10.0 for Windows). The prevalence of dental fluorosis was calculated as frequency of occurrence among study population (%). The risk of dental fluorosis was expressed as the odds ratio of disease (OR).

3 Results

3.1 Exposure of population to fluorides through drinking water

Fluoride content in drinking water in Estonia varied on a large scale: 0.01-6.95 mg/l with a mean of 0.88 ±0.90 mg/l. In 306 (41.6%) samples the fluoride content was low (<0.5 mg/l). Medium concentrations (0.5-1.5 mg/l) were measured in 323 (44.0%) samples. The Estonian national limit – 1.5 mg/l – was exceeded in 106 (14.4%) samples. Fluoride content in drinking water varied greatly both between and within counties (Table 1).

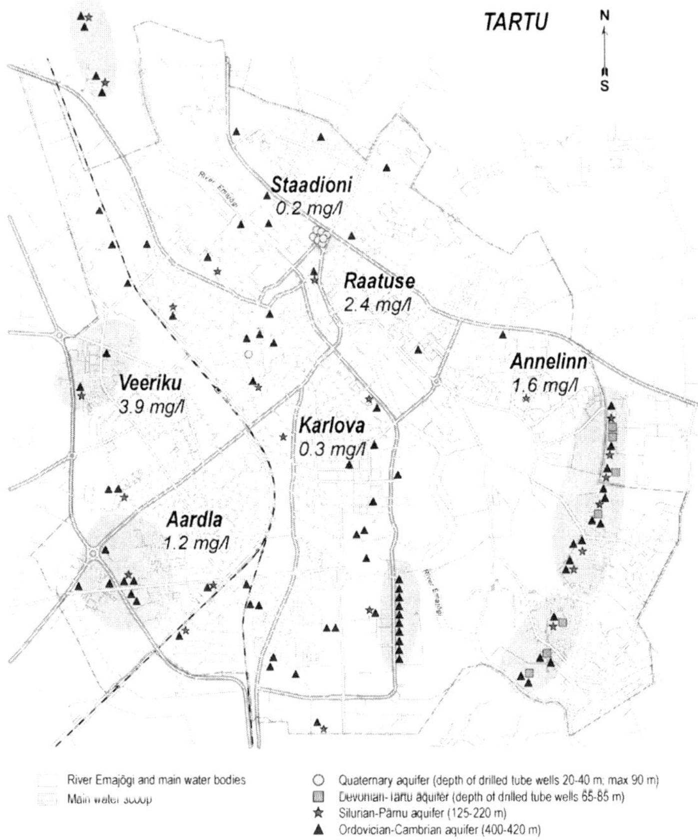

Figure 2: Location of Tartu districts covered by retrospective case study.

The exposure analysis revealed that only 38.1% of study population (400 040 inhabitants) was consuming water with medium fluoride concentration, low-fluoride water was consumed by 57.8% (607 544 in) and high-fluoride water by 4.1% (42 571 in) of the study population. The situation differed to a large extent in different towns and counties. The population of Tallinn (396 000 in) and Narva (68 000 in) used mainly surface water with naturally very low fluoride content. The second largest city Tartu (101 000 in) was provided mainly with medium-fluoride water. While most of the population (over 60%) in Harju, Pärnu, Saare, Hiiu, Viljandi and Lääne counties was exposed to medium-fluoride water, the whole population in Võru county (100%) was exposed to low-fluoride water. Over half of population was consuming low-fluoride water also in Valga,

Järva and Põlva counties. Most of people consuming high-fluoride water were living in Pärnu county, followed by people in Rapla, Tartu, Järva and Lääne counties. The main risk from consuming high-fluoride water is dental fluorosis, but also other toxic effects of fluorides are of serious concern [2, 11].

Table 1: Approximate number of people consuming drinking water with different levels of fluoride in 2004 by counties.

Name of county	Number of water samples	Range of fluoride content mg/l	Number of people consuming drinking water with different fluoride level		
			Low-fluoride	Medium-fluoride	High-fluoride
Harju	119	0.01 – 2.06	364 979	86 324	3 978
Hiiu	17	0.38 – 1.92	50	5 372	1 228
Ida-Viru	48	0.21 – 1.29	108 207	57 952	0
Jõgeva	38	0.06 – 3.28	9 125	8 267	1 571
Järva	49	0.05 – 3.12	16 621	3 560	5 026
Lääne	29	0.54 – 5.60	0	13 965	4 110
Lääne-Viru	65	0.10 – 1.81	21 370	29 884	225
Põlva	31	0.08 – 1.10	9 835	5 885	0
Pärnu	63	0.08 – 6.95	980	44 765	8 562
Rapla	42	0.12 – 3.68	4 667	12 901	5 354
Saare	28	0.22 – 5.50	1 360	18 805	2 140
Tartu	73	0.10 – 3.48	27 165	81 165	5 222
Valga	30	0.06 – 1.58	17 303	1 247	1 500
Viljandi	56	0.05 – 2.56	4 621	29 948	3 655
Võru	47	0.08 – 0.45	21 261	0	0
Total	**735**	**0.01 – 6.95**	**607 544**	**400 040**	**42 571**

3.2 Dental fluorosis risk

The dental fluorosis risk (odds ratio – OR) was studied among 12-year-old schoolchildren who were born and living in Tartu city where content of fluoride in drinking water varies in a large scale by districts depending on the water source (groundwater aquifer) from which the supply system feeds on.

Table 2 represents the mean value, standard deviation and range of fluoride content in drinking water sources (tube wells) by the study districts in 1986-1997. It is the period when the study population was born and grown up.

The distribution of study subjects according to residence in six districts and prevalence of dental fluorosis is shown in the same Table 2.

The number of children was different by districts. Boys and girls were equally represented in the total sample (47% and 53%, respectively). The prevalence of dental fluorosis among Tartu schoolchildren was 30.2%, being 26.3% among boys and 33.7% among girls. The difference between boys and girls was not statistically significant. In most cases (89%) the mild degree of fluorosis was diagnosed. Only twelve children (3 boys and 9 girls) had severe fluorosis. They lived in the high-fluoride districts.

Results obtained by districts showed that the percent of children with dental fluorosis increased with the increase of fluoride content in the drinking water source (Table 2). Strong association between water fluoride level and prevalence of fluorosis allowed the calculation of the odds ratio (OR) of dental fluorosis in relation to district of residence and the fluoride content in the drinking water (Table 3).

The risk of dental fluorosis was over 6 times higher among children of Annelinn district (IV) where the average fluoride content exceeded the permissible level as compared to Staadioni district (I). In districts V and VI the risk was even higher. Currently, the wells producing high-fluoride water are excluded from the public water supply system. In districts II and III where the fluoride content in water was below the limit, there was no significant risk of dental fluorosis as compared to district I where the fluoride content in water was the lowest.

Table 2: Fluoride content (mg/l) of drinking water sources in Tartu, 1986-1997 and prevalence of dental fluorosis among 12-year old schoolchildren.

District		No of water samples	Fluoride content in water (mg/l)		No of children	Children with fluorosis
No	Name		mean	range		No / %
I	Staadioni	25	0,18	0,10 – 0,30	34	3 / 8,8
II	Karlova	20	0,29	0,10 – 0,70	38	6 / 15,8
III	Aardla	28	1,19	0,80 – 1,50	100	21 / 21,0
IV	Annelinn	35	1,59	1,30 –1,90	149	57 / 38,3
V	Raatuse	24	2,41	1,85 – 3,20	17	8 / 47,1
VI	Veeriku	8	3,89	3,35 – 4,40	30	16 / 53,3
	Total	**140**	**1,34**	**0,10 – 4,40**	**368**	**111 / 30,2**

Table 3: Risk of dental fluorosis among schoolchildren in different districts of Tartu (compared to Staadioni district).

No of district	Name of district	Content of fluoride in water mg/l	Odds ratio	Confidence interval (CI 95%)
I	Staadioni	0,2	1,00	
II	Karlova	0,3	1,94	0,37 – 12,91
III	Aardla	1,2	2,75	0,73 – 15,30
IV	Annelinn	1,6	**6,40***	1,85 – 33,95
V	Raatuse	2,4	**9,18***	1,66 – 61,76
VI	Veeriku	3,9	**11,81***	2,65 – 70,32

* statistically significant.

4 Discussion

The research approach and sampling scheme of this study was designed to evaluate Estonian population exposure to fluoride from drinking water and assess the contribution of drinking water fluoride to dental fluorosis. This study cannot comment on overall exposure to fluoride, although drinking water is usually the largest contributor to fluoride intake [2, 12].

The study covered all 15 counties in Estonia embracing 93.7% of population having access to public water supplies. The overall access to public water supplies was 82.9%, but the variation between cities and rural settlements is large [5]. The prevalence of a large number of small water supplies complicates the improvement of water quality.

Groundwater is the most important source of drinking water. Only few studies on occurrence and distribution of fluoride in groundwater have been carried out in Estonia [13–15]. Quite often the tap water originates from different sources and is mixed in water supply systems. Our data from the analysis of drinking water samples collected throughout Estonia provide the necessary information for assessment of human exposure to fluoride.

Based on current study, the great majority (about 96%) of Estonian population was drinking water with fluoride below 1.5 mg/l. Over half (57.8%) of population was exposed to water containing very low fluoride levels (up to 0.5 mg/l). Only 4.1% of the population was exposed to high-fluoride content (over 1.5 mg/l) drinking water. Nearly 4 000 people was exposed to very high fluoride levels (over 4.0 mg/l). They lived mainly in West Estonia (Lääne, Rapla and Pärnu counties), where the only drinking water source is Silurian-Ordovician aquifer system. The high levels of fluoride are due to geogenic sources [13].
Elevated fluoride concentrations were also found in some water supplies of central Estonia (Tartu, Viljandi and Järva counties). This is the area where hydraulically connected Devonian and Silurian strata form the Devonian-Silurian aquifer system. The content of fluoride is related with the depth of the wells [13].

The prevalence of dental fluorosis among schoolchildren was studied in Tartu where the fluoride content in drinking water varied between districts significantly. Other conditions (climate, quality of outdoor air, living conditions, dietary habits and oral hygiene) were considered to be distributed evenly inside the city. This study assumed that the fluoride exposure of each child in the district corresponded to the average fluoride level in drinking water of that district. Because of the lack of resources it was not possible to determine the individual exposure of subjects via drinking water.

The present results and those of previous studies [6] strengthen the notion that there is a systematic and positive relationship between the fluoride content in drinking water and the prevalence of dental fluorosis. It has been determined that fluoride concentration in excess of 1.6 mg/l and over exposes residents to high fluorosis risk quantified as odds ratio.

5 Conclusions

This study provides an overview of the fluoride content in drinking water and the extent of human exposure to different levels of fluoride through drinking water for the whole of Estonia. As drinking water is usually the main source of fluoride intake, the levels of fluoride in tap water is very important in determining total fluoride exposure.

Human exposure analysis revealed that majority of people (about 96%) consumed water with a fluoride content below the maximum permitted level (1.5 mg/l). Very small portion of population (4.1%) was exposed to high-fluoride drinking water. Very high naturally occurring fluoride concentrations (up to 7 mg/l) were common in West Estonia where the main drinking water source is the Silurian-Ordovician aquifer system.

A systematic and positive relationship between the prevalence of dental fluorosis and the exposure to fluoride through drinking water was determined. The fluoride in excess of 1.6 mg/l in drinking water increased the dental fluorosis risk over 6 times. The information of population about the levels of fluoride in drinking water is an important key element in health risk prevention.

The results of the current study as well as other available data from water quality should be taken into account when developing strategies for safe drinking water supplies.

Acknowledgements

This study has been supported by the Target Funding Projects No. 0180052s07 and No. 0182648s04 of the Ministry of Education and Science of Estonia and by Estonian Society of Stomatology.

References

[1] Pirkle, J.L., Osterloh, J., Needham, L.L. & Sampson, E.J., National exposure measurements for decisions to protect public health from environmental exposures. *Int J Hyg. Environ. Health,* **208(1-2)**, pp. 1-5, 2005.

[2] Farwell, J., Bailey, K., Chilton, J., Dahi, E., Fewtrell, L. & Magara, Y., *Fluoride in drinking-water.* World Health Organization (WHO), IWA Publishing, London-Seattle; 2006.

[3] Angelillo, I.F., Torre, I., Nobile, C.G. & Villari, P., Caries and fluorosis prevalence in communities with different concentrations of fluoride in water. *Caries Res.,* **33(2)**, pp. 114-122, 1999.

[4] Moturi, W.K., Tole, M.P. & Davies, T.C., The contribution of drinking water towards dental fluorosis: a case study of Njoro Division, Nakuru District, Kenya. *Environ. Geochem. Health,* **24**, pp. 123-130, 2002.

[5] Indermitte, E., Saava, A. & Kull, A., The survey of drinking water supply in Estonia from the point of view of public health. *The Sustainable City IV. Urban Regeneration and Sustainability,* eds. U. Mander, C.A. Brebbia

& E. Tiezzi, Wessex Institute of Technology Press: Southampton, Boston, pp. 817 – 826, 2006.

[6] Saava, A., Health hazards due to drinking water. *Proc Latvian Acad Sci* **52**, eds. I. Rašals et al, Latvian Academy of Sciences: Riga, pp. 162-167, 1998.

[7] Karise, V., Metsur, M., Perens, R., Savitskaja, L. & Tamm, I. Eesti põhjavee kasutamine ja kaitse [Use and protection of groundwater in Estonia]. Eesti Põhjaveekomisjon: Tallinn (in Estonian), pp. 81, 2004.

[8] APHA, *Standard methods for the examination of water and wastewater, 2nd edn.*, American Public Health Association: Washington, DC, 1998.

[9] Alakivi, U., Frey, T., Maastik, A. & Mander, U., (eds). *Tartu Agenda 21*, Tartu, 1999.

[10] WHO, *Oral Health Surveys. Basic Methods. 4th ed*, World Health Organisation: Geneva, 1997.

[11] Colquhoun, J., Why I changed my mind about fluoridation. *Fluoride*, **31**, pp. 103-18, 1998.

[12] Erdal, S. & Buchanan, S.N., A quantitative look at fluorosis, fluoride exposure, and intake in children using a health risk assessment approach. *Environ. Health Persp,* **113(1)**, pp. 111-117, 2005.

[13] Karro, E. & Rosentau, A., Fluoride levels in the Siluarian-Ordovician aquifer system of western Estonia. *Fluoride,* **38(4)**, pp. 307-311, 2005.

[14] Kuik, L., Joogivee fluori- ja joodisisaldus Eesti NSV-s [Fluoride and iodine content of drinking water in Estonian SSR]. *Kurortoloogilised Uurimised,* **2**, pp. 39-45 (in Estonian), 1963.

[15] Karro, E., Indermitte, E., Saava, A., Haamer, K., Marandi, A. Fluoride occurrence in publicly supplied water in Estonia. *Environmental Geology,* **50(3)**, pp. 389 – 396, 2006.

Vanadium and lithium contamination in freshwaters of the Conchos River in Chihuahua, Mexico

H. Rubio-Arias[1], C. E. Quintana[2], K. Wood[3], R. A. Saucedo[1] & R. Bautista-Margulis[4]
[1]*Campo Experimental La Campana-Madera, INIFAP, México*
[2]*Facultad de Zootecnia, de la Universidad Autónoma de Chihuahua, México*
[3]*New Mexico Water Resources Research Institute, USA*
[4]*Universidad Juarez Autônoma de Tabasco, México*

Abstract

The hydraulic Conchos Watershed is essential for the inhabitants of the state of Chihuahua, Mexico. Nevertheless, evidence shows that the water that flows in the Conchos River is contaminated. The objective was to determine if Vanadium (V) and Lithium (Li) were present in the water of the Conchos River. During 2004 and 2005 six points were located in different tributaries for obtaining water samples. The points were Zaragoza (Z), Satevo (S), Florido (F), Parral (P), Chuviscar (CH) and Ojinaga (O). The samples were collected at 2-monthly intervals. Both elements were determined using an Inductively Coupled Plasma-Optical Emission Spectrometer (ICP-OES). Variation in V pollution was observed between sampling location as well as in sampling dates. In 2004 highest values of V were observed in June (Z had 0.498 mg L^{-1}; S had 0.479 mg L^{-1}; F had 0.449 mg L^{-1}; P had 0.437 mg L^{-1}; CH had 0.412 mg L^{-1}; O had 0.473 mg L^{-1}) and in August samples (Z had 0.542 mg L^{-1}; S had 0.502 mg L^{-1}; F had 0.452 mg L^{-1}; P had 0.451 mg L^{-1}; CH had 0.447 mg L^{-1}; and O had 0.609 mg L^{-}). In 2005 maximum V-values were noted in February samples reaching 0.545 mg L^{-1} in Z; 0.502 mg L^{-1} in S; 0.687 mg L^{-1} in P; 0.411 mg L^{-1} in CH; and 0.582 mg L^{-1} in O. Lithium was detected at all points. The highest values were reported in October 2004 in O (0.707 mg L^{-1} in October and 0.496 mg L^{-1} in August) and P with 0.383 mg L^{-1}. In 2005, maximum concentrations of Li were observed in O reaching 0.344 mg L^{-1} in February, 0.507 mg L^{-1} in April and 0.396 mg L^{-1} in June.
Keywords: vanadium, lithium, Chihuahua, Mexico, metals.

WIT Transactions on Biomedicine and Health, Vol 11, © 2007 WIT Press
www.witpress.com, ISSN 1743-3525 (on-line)
doi:10.2495/EHR070181

1 Introduction

The Vanadium (V) and Lithium (Li) are heavy metals that might be present in different concentrations in water of different ecosystems in the earth. The V constitutes about 0.01% of the earth′ crust [1] while Li, the lightest metal is present in an average of 65 ppm on earth. In the particular case of V, the human is exposed to low levels of this element in different forms, but in the food a person may intake 10-20 micrograms daily, suggesting to be an essential element. For instance, fish contributed with an 11-34% of daily V ingestion in the inhabitants of the Adriatic coast [2]. In addition, some studies have shown that V is essential for goats and chicks [3]; nevertheless, the essentiality of V is still an open question, when is showed that is toxic to some animals [4] like rainbow trout [5]. Likewise the V, the Li appears to be an essential trace element for some animals, hypothesizing a fundamental role in human by analogy. An interesting fact is that both elements have been considered for the treatment of human diseases, like diabetes, utilizing vanadium salts [6, 7] and the disease known as bipolar disorder using lithium [8–10]. The V is also believed to control high blood pressure [11].

Most surface waters contain some levels of V as well as Li. Highest concentration of V was reported in surface water of the Mount Fuji in Japan where 14.8 and 16.4 $\mu g\ L^{-1}$ were detected in twp springs and a range of 17.7 to 48.8 $\mu g\ L^{-1}$ was observed in the water of five rivers [12]. Japan has so much volcano activity, so this fact may explain the V presence in the water as reported by Aiuppa *et al.*, [13] that found that much of the V presence might be a natural process, however, in other areas, anthropogenic activity must be responsible for V presence the environment [14]. With respect to Li, generally this element is found in low concentrations in surface waters. In rivers of the United States of America was reported in concentrations of about 0.002 mg L^{-1} [15] while in study evaluating four segments of the Conchos River in Chihuahua, Mexico was found a range concentration of 14.3-119.9 $\mu g\ L^{-1}$ [16].

This paper gives an overview of the vanadium and lithium levels in waters flowing in six tributaries of the Río Conchos of the State of Chihuahua, Mexico over a two years period. To our knowledge, this is the first time that these two elements are determined in the whole watershed. These results will help to different authorities, as well as the decision makers of different levels to analyze potential harmful effects of vanadium and lithium on human health, wildlife, environment or, in general, the suitability of the Conchos water for beneficial utilization.

2 Materials and methods

Water flow of the Rio Conchos originates in the mountain zone of the state of Chihuahua, Mexico, identified as the Sierra Tarahumara. The Conchos′ stream flow descends from the 2,700 meters above sea level (masl) through the great plains with 1,000-1,500 masl, and finally, the flow joins the Rio Bravo/Rio Grande water in the city of Ojinaga at 720 masl. The Rio Bravo/Rio Grande serves as the natural boundary between Mexico and the United States of America. The most important tributaries of the Rio Conchos are; the Rio Florido and the Rio Parral in the south of the state, the San Pedro and the Conchos in the central part, and the Río Chuviscar that flows in the middle of the city of Chihuahua. The flow of the tributaries located in the south is stored in the Boquilla Dam with a capacity of 2,903 million m^3, the flow of the tributaries in the central part is stored in Las Virgenes Dam with a capacity of 348 millions of m^3, and the El Granero Dam with a capacity of 356 millions of m^3 stored the flows before joining the Rio Bravo/Rio Grande.

Six points along the Rio Conchos watershed were selected to obtain water samples during the years of 2004 and 2005. The water samples were obtained in a 2-month interval in each point; therefore, water samples were obtained in February, April, June, August, October and December every year. Point 1 was located in the Río Chuviscar (latitude 28° 49′ 23.7"; longitude 105° 54′ 57.0"; 1,279 masl) about 15 km east of the city of Chihuahua. Point 2 was located in the Rio San Pedro (latitude 27° 57′ 13.2"; longitude 106° 06′ 35.9"; 1,375 masl), approximately 5 km of the Satevo Town and before the water is capted in the Virgenes Dam. Point 3 was located about 2.5 km of Valle de Zaragoza town (latitude 27° 28′ 15.5"; longitude 105° 42′ 25.4"; 1,329 masl). The sampling point 4 was identified in the Rio Parral (latitude 27° 40′ 03.4"; longitude 105° 12′ 33.8"; 1,228 masl) about 30 kn of the city of Parral. Point 5 was located in the Rio Florido (latitude 27° 40′ 36.6"; longitude 105° 08′37.4"; 1,225 masl) about 10 km south of the city named Camargo. Sampling point 6 was established near the city of Ojinaga (latitude 29° 34′ 02.1"; longitude 104° 26′ 46.1"; 786 masl) about 3 km above the junction with the flow of Rio Bravo/Rio Grande.

Water samples were collected in sterilized containers, preserved in a cool place and inmediatelly transported to the laboratory of the Faculty of Zootechnic of the Autonomous University of Chihuahua where they were placed at about 4°C. The vanadium and lithium extraction of the water samples was done according to the Mexican Norm [17]. The concentration of both metals was using ICP optical emission spectrometry (Perkin Elmer 2100) in the laboratory of the National Institute for Research in Forestry, Agriculture and Livestock (INIFAP-Mexico).

An Analysis of Variance (ANOVA) was performed on values for both elements to determine year effect, bi-month effect, and location effect as well as the following interactions; bi-month*year, year*location and location*bi-month. In addition, descriptive statistics was used to visualize differences in concentration considering sampling points as well as bimonthly samples.

3 Results and discussion

In Figure 1 are showed the levels of V detected during the 2004 sampling. Its can be noted that the maximum level of V was observed in Ojinaga while minimum levels were noted in Parral and Florido rivers. In the particular case of Ojinaga, the highest level of V was observed in August (0.609 mg L^{-1}) and June (0.473 mg L^{-1}). The trend showed in 2004 is consistent in all sampling location

and all sampling dates, meaning that most of V presence in the water of the Conchos River is noted in summer time during the rainy season. In the six location points, the maximum level of V was detected in August; thus in Zaragoza the concentration was 0.542 mg L^{-1}; in Satevo, 0.502 mg L^{-1}; in Florido,
0.452 mg L^{-1}; in Parral, 0.451 mg L^{-1}; and in Chuviscar, 0.447.

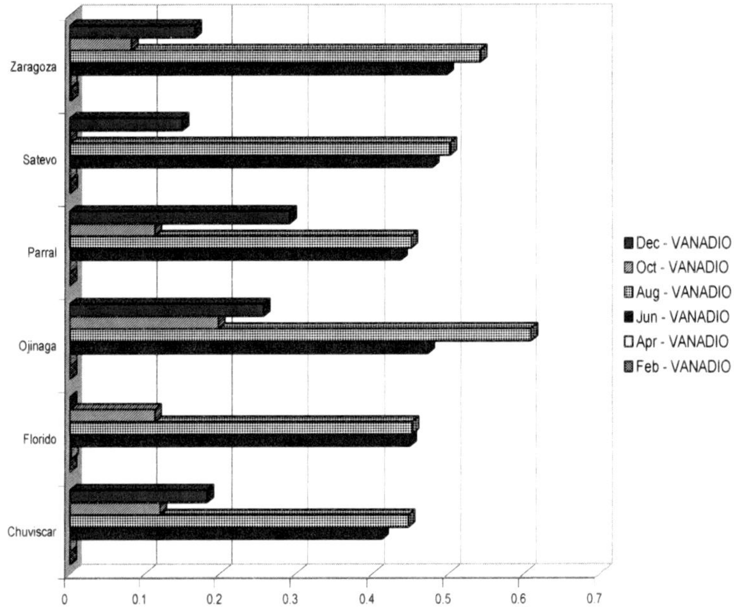

Figure 1: Levels of vanadium detected in six locations of the Rio Conchos in Chihuahua, Mexico during six months of the year 2004.

The water samples collected in 2005 resulted in different findings. In Figure 2, it is pointed out the levels of V during the 2005 sampling. It is obvious that maximum concentration of this element was observed in Parral during the sample of February with a concentration of 0.687 mg L^{-1} followed by the amount noted in Ojinaga where it was detected about 0.582 mg L^{-1}. During this year, the maximum V concentration was detected in the February samples; hence, in Zaragoza it reached 0.545 mg L^{-1}; in Satevo, 0.502 mg L^{-1}; and in Chuviscar 0.411 mg L^{-1}. Moreover, it can be observed that V was not detected in Florido samples and that the minimum amount of this element was detected in the locations Satevo. With respect to this element, statistical differences were found by year, bi-month, and the interaction of year*bi-month samples (Table 1). These principal effects are noted in Figure 1 and Figure 2.

There is a lack of historical information concerning the V levels in the Conchos River. The existence of this sort of data would help to analyze weather the V amounts in the water have been constant or have increased in a certain period of time. If we assume no anthropogenic pollution in the whole watershed; then, the levels of V should be similar. Therefore, it could be said that we do not have information to said that there have been an anthropogenic effect in the Conchos River with respect to V levels. In general, the results presented here are higher that the findings of other environments. For instance, in the Tercero River in Argentina it was noted a level of V up to 0.109 mg L^{-1} [18]. In the Colorado River in the USA it was noted a V range of 0.2-49.2 µg L^{-1} [19] while in Yangtze River in China it was detected 0.24 to 64.5 µg L^{-1} [20].

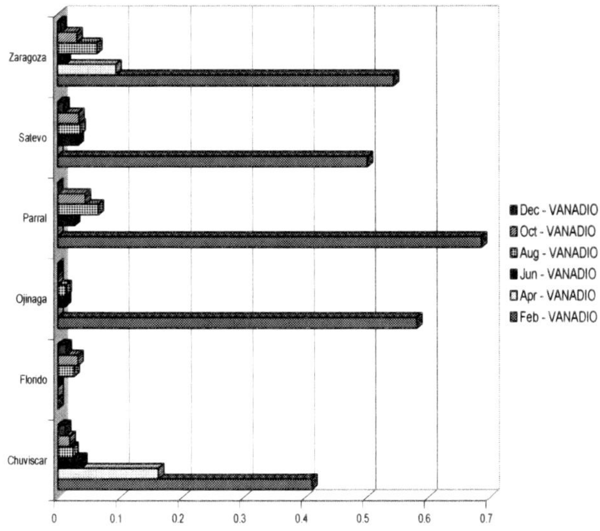

Figure 2: Levels of vanadium detected in six locations of the Rio Conchos in Chihuahua, Mexico during six months of the year 2005.

In Figure 3 it is presented the levels of Li detected in six locations of the Río Conchos during six monthly samples of 2004. The maximum levels were observed in Ojinaga with an amount of 0.707 mg L^{-1} during the October samples and in Zaragoza with 0.680 mg L^{-1} in the August sample. In general, the Ojinaga point reached the major levels of Li when it was observed values of 0.496 mg L^{-1} in August samples and of 0.437 mg L^{-1} in December samples. In Figure 4 it is presented the levels of Li detected in six locations of the Río Conchos during six monthly samples of 2005. It is obvious that maximum levels were observed in the sampling locations of Ojinaga and Chuviscar. These two sampling locations are closed to the cities of Ojinaga and Chihuahua. In the particular case of Ojinaga, it is a border city between the United States of America and Mexico where most drainage and runoff flows to the Conchos River. With respect to Chihuahua city, it has about a million inhabitants and some drainage flows in the Chuviscar tributary. According to the findings of this study it can be

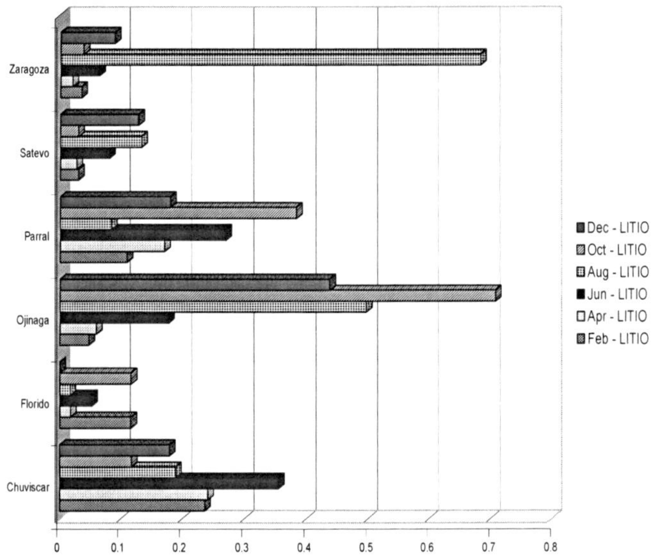

Figure 3: Levels of lithium detected in six locations of the Rio Conchos in Chihuahua, Mexico during six months of the year 2004.

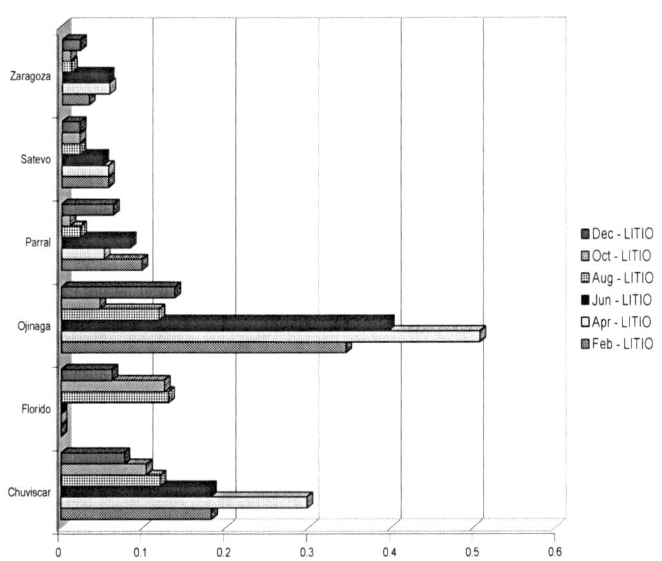

Figure 4: Levels of lithium detected in six locations of the Rio Conchos in Chihuahua, Mexico during six months of the year 2005.

Table 1: Analysis of Variance for vanadium and lithium concentration in water of San Pedro River of Chihuahua, México.

Vanadium					
Source	DF	Adj SS	Adj MS	F	P
Year	1	0.211250	0.211250	27.01	0.000
Location	5	0.065353	0.013071	1.67	0.178
Bi-month	5	0.663218	0.132644	16.96	0.000
Year*Bi-M	5	1.732206	0.346441	44.29	0.000
Year*location	5	0.020908	0.004182	0.53	0.748
Location*bi-M	25	0.134716	0.005389	0.69	0.821
Error	25	0.195554	0.007822		
Total	71	3.023204			
Lithium					
Source	DF	Adj SS	Adj MS	F	P
Year	1	0.08954	0.08954	3.88	0.060
Location	5	0.50326	0.10065	4.36	0.005
Bi-month	5	0.03046	0.00609	0.26	0.929
Year*Bi-m	5	0.17617	0.03523	1.53	0.217
Year*location	5	0.04409	0.00882	0.38	0.856
Location*bi-m	25	0.25435	0.01017	0.44	0.977
Error	25	0.57706	0.57706		
Total	71	1.67492			

hypothesized that Li amount is due to anthropogenic effects. With respect to Lithium concentration statistical differences were found only for location (Table 1) and none of the interactions tested were significant.

The results of the present study with respect to the level of Li are higher than previous studies reported by Bradford [21] who found Li levels of about 0.05 mg L^{-1} in water of California, USA and for Feder [22] who reported Li levels of less than 10 μ L^{-1} in Missouri, USA. Nevertheless, the most important aspect of these findings is the potential toxic effect in some organisms that live in water of the Conchos River when it is analyzed that Emery et al., (1981) supported a toxic effect of some insect larvae with levels of 0.4 mg L^{-1}. In addition, these researchers (Emery et al. [23]) hypothesized a toxic effect in rainbow trout with levels of Li of 0.6 mg L^{-1}.

Acknowledgements

The authors would like to express appreciation for funds from the Fundación Produce Chihuahua. In addition, we are very grateful to the Faculty of zootechnic of the Autonomous University of Chihuahua whose staff actively and significantly contributed to the whole project.

References

[1] Budavari, S., O'Neil, M.J., Smith, A., Heckelman, P.E., Kinneary, J.F. eds. 1996. The Merck index-an encyclopedia of chemicals, drugs and biologicals, 12th ed. Whitehouse Station, N.J., Merck & Co., Inc. 1691-1692

[2] Sepe, A., Ciaralli, L., Ciprotti, M., Giordano, R., Funan, E., Constantino, S. 2003. Food Addit. Coontam 20(6): 543-552. Determination of cadmium, chromium, lead and vanadium in six fish species from the Adriatic Sea.

[3] Nielsen F, Uthus E (1990) The essentiality and metabolism of vanadium. In: Chasteen N, ed. *Vanadium in biological systems.* Dordrecht, Kluwer Academic Press, pp. 51–62.

[4] Scibior, A., Zaporowska, H., Ostrowski, J. 2006. Selected haematological and biochemical parameters of blood in rats after subchronic administration of vanadium and/or magnesium in drinking water. Arch. Environ Contam Toxicology 51(2):287-295.

[5] Stendahl, D.H., and Sprague, J.B. 1982. Effects of water hardness and pH on vanadium lethality to rainbow trout. Water Research 16(10):1479-1488

[6] Badmaev, V., Prakash, S., Majeed, M. 1999. Vanadium: a review of its potential role in the fight against diabetes. J. Altern Complement Med 5:273-291

[7] Clark, T.A., Heyliger, C.E., Edel, A.L., Goel, O.P., and Pierce, G.N. 2004. Co-delivery of a tea extract prevents morbidity and mortality associated with oral vanadate in streptozotocin-induced diabetic rats. Metabolism, 53(9):1145-1151

[8] Tondo, L., Baldessarini, R.J., Floris, G. 2001. Long-term clinical effectiveness of lithium maintenance treatment in types I and II bipolar disorders. Br. J. Psychiatry Suppl.41:184-190.

[9] Geddes JR, Burgess S, Hawton K, Jamison K, Goodwin GM. Long-term lithium therapy for bipolar disorder: systematic review and meta-analysis of randomized controlled trials. *Am J Psychiatry.* 2004;**161**:217–222

[10] Kruger, S., Alda, M., Trevor Young, L., Goldapple, K. et al. 2006. Risk and resilience markers in bipolar disorder: brain responses to emotional challenge in bipolar patients and their healthy siblings. The American Journal of Psychiatry 162(2):257-264.

[11] Bhanot, S., McNeill, J.H., Bryer-Ash, M. 1994. Vanadyl sulphate prevents fructose-induced hyperinsulinemia and hypertension in rats. Hypertension 23:308-312

[12] Hamada, T. 1998. High vanadium content in Mount Fuji groundwater and its relevance to the ancient biosphere. In: Nriagu J. ed. Vanadium in the environment Part 1: Chemistry and biochemistry. New York, NY. John Wiley & Sons. 97-123

[13] Aiuppa, A., Bellomo, S., Brusca, L., Alessandro, W.D., and Federico, C. 2003. Natural and anthropogenic factors affecting groundwater quality of an active volcano (Mt. Etna, Italy). Applied Geochemistry 18(6):863-882

[14] Hope, B.K.1994. A global biogeochemical budget for vanadium. The science of Total Environment 141(1):1-10

[15] Kszos, L.A. and Stewart, A.J. 2003. Review of lithium in the aquatic environment: distribution in the United States, toxicit and case example of groundwater contamination. Ecotoxicology 12(5):439-447

[16] Gutierrez, M., and Borrego, P. 1999. Water quality assessment of the Rio Conchos, Chihuahua, Mexico. Environment International 25(5):573-583.

[17] NOM, 1981.Norma Mexicana NMX-AA-051-SCFI-1981. Análisis de agua, determinación de metales. Método espectrofotométrico de Absorción Atómica.

[18] Lerda, D.F. and Prosperi, C.H. 1996. Water mutagenicity and toxicology in Rio Tercero (Córdoba, Argentina). Water Research 30(4):819-824.

[19] Linstedt, K., Kruger, P. 1969. Vanadium concentrations in Colorado River basin waters. Journal of the American Water Works Association 61:85-88

[20] Zhang L, Zhou K (1992) Background values of trace elements in the source area of the Yangtze River. *The science of the total environment*, 125:391–404.

[21] Bradford, G.L. 1963. Lithium survey of California's water resources. Soil Science 96:77-81

[22] Feder, G.L. 1972. Geochemical survey of Missouri, open file report, United States Geological Survey

[23] Emery, R.D., Klopfer, C. and Skalski, J.R. 1981. The incipient toxicity of lithium to freshwater organisms representing a salmonid habitat PNC-3640, UC-11. Pacific Northwest Laboratory; Richland, WA, USA. 364 p.

Arsenic concentrations in the San Pedro River of Chihuahua, Mexico

R. Gutiérrez-Espinoza[1], H. Rubio-Arias[2], R. Quintana[1], J. A. Ortega[1] & C. Pinedo[1]
[1]*Faculty of Zootechnic, Autonomous University of Chihuahua, Mexico*
[2]*Experimental Research Center La Campana-Madera, INIFAP, Mexico*

Abstract

There is a general belief that high levels of arsenic are found in waters of the northern states of Mexico. In order to test this hypothesis, research was conducted with the objective of determining arsenic levels in waters of the San Pedro River located in the state of Chihuahua, Mexico. From October 2005 to August 2006 on a monthly basis, water samples were collected at five points along the San Pedro River. Three repetitions were collected at each point resulting in a total of 165 water samples. Total arsenic concentration was L^{-1} detected in an Inductively Coupled Plasma-Optical Emission Spectrometer (ICP-POE) model 2100 by Perkin Elmer. The arsenic concentrations in waters of the San Pedro River ranged from 0.0110 mg L^{-1} to 0.587 mg L^{-1} with a mean of 0.104 mg L^{-1} ± 0.234 mg. Most samples were over the maximum permissible value established as Mexican and international standards. A quadratic projection was observed between the basic points through the fifth point; these results might be influenced by the decrease of flow and the decrease of the drainage level. These results confirm the hypothesis that waters in northern Mexico contain high levels of arsenic that potentially might be harmful to the whole ecosystem and being potentially dangerous to human development and health.
Keywords: arsenic, Chihuahua, Mexico, San Pedro, pollution.

1 Introduction

Arsenic (As) is a metalloid generally considered toxic that may be present in a variety of water environments. This metalloid is ubiquitous, meaning that it may be found in air [1], water [2, 3], soil [4], plants [5], as well as in other living

WIT Transactions on Biomedicine and Health, Vol 11, © 2007 WIT Press
www.witpress.com, ISSN 1743-3525 (on-line)
doi:10.2495/EHR070191

organisms [6]. This elements is considered teratogenic [7], carcinogenic [8, 9] and has been associated with different diseases [10, 11]. An extreme case is Bangladesh were millions people drink water with an arsenic concentration higher than 10 μg L^{-1} that is much higher than the guidelines recommended by the World Health Organization [12]. Moreover, recent research has hypothesized that the ingestion of arsenic by humans has been associated with the potential increase of Type 2 diabetes in inhabitants living in high-arsenic areas [13–15]; nonetheless, in other studies carried out in the United States this effect has not been proven [16]. The good news concerning this element is that some arsenic compounds might be positively utilized to treat some kinds of leukaemia [17] and that there is no evidence of food chain biomagnification [18].

Among the inhabitants of northern Mexico, the word arsenic is considered synonymous with the word poison. In addition, there is a general believe that waters contains high levels of this element. Even though there are some studies in Mexico that show different levels of arsenic in a variety of water environments [19, 20], no information is available concerning levels of arsenic in the San Pedro River. The San Pedro River is one tributary of the Conchos River that is considered the most important for the inhabitants of the state of Chihuahua. Along the San Pedro River there are several communities that have experienced unprecedented human development as a result of industrial, agricultural and livestock activities.

For this reason it is important to know the water quality that flows in this river. Therefore, the objective was to determine the arsenic levels in the water of the San Pedro River located in the state of Chihuahua, Mexico. The results will shed light on the potential effects of arsenic in the health of the inhabitants settled along the river, as well as to give an idea about the toxic levels for the whole environment.

2 Materials and methods

The research was carried out from October 2005 to August 2005. Five points along the San Pedro River were located to collect a monthly water sample (Figure 1). The locations were; La Presa, Rosales, Meoqui, El Torreon and La junta de los Rios. The water samples were collected monthly from October 2005 through August 2006. Three water repetitions were obtained; hence, a total of 165 water samples were collected for the whole study.

The water samples were collected in polyethylene bottles that were previously rinsed with nitric acid and deionised water. Once the water samples were collected, they were placed in an ice box to be transported to the laboratory of the Faculty of Zootechnic of the Autonomous University of Chihuahua where they were placed at about 4° C. Arsenic extraccion was done according to the Mexican Norm [21] using nitric acid digestion. Arsenic concentration levels were measured using an Inductively Coupled Plasma-Optical Emission Spectrometry (ICP-OES) Perkin Elmer 2100 property of the laboratory of the National Research Institute for Forestry, Agriculture and Livestock in Chihuahua, Mexico.

The results were compared with some Mexican standards, with the U.S. Environmental Protection Agency (EPA) and some standards and reference doses for humans (EPA). Two probability graphs were designed to show confidence intervals considering monthly samples as well as locations samples.

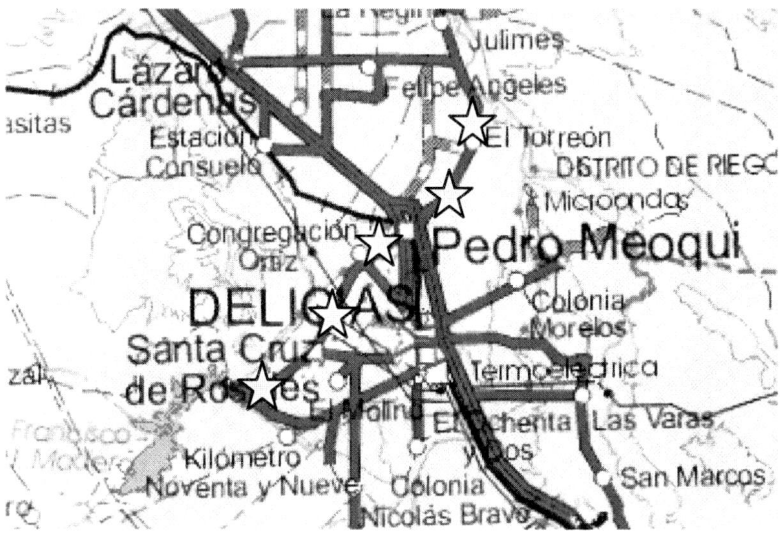

Figure 1: Sampling points in the San Pedro River to estimate arsenic pollution.

3 Results and discussion

The samples collected in October 2005 resulted in a concentration of 0.08 mg L^{-1} for La Presa, 0.11 mg L^{-1} for Rosales, 0.13 mg L^{-1} for Meoqui, 0.15 mg L^{-1} for El Torreon and 0.14 mg L^{-1} in Junta de los Rios. It can be noted an increase of the arsenic concentration as the water flows down from the upper part (La Presa location) to the lower part (Junta de los Rios). The concentrations of all samples in the five locations were higher than the values specified in the Mexican Norm (0.01 mg L^{-1}) as well as the EPA for potable water (0.01 mg L^{-1}). In addition, the concentration values of four locations were higher than the values established in the Mexican Norm for agricultural uses (0.10 mg L^{-1}). The second sample of November 2005 resulted in lower concentrations of arsenic in the five locations as compared with the October samples. Hence, the result for La Presa was 0.10 mg L^{-1}, for Rosales 0.07 mg L^{-1}, for Meoqui, 0.07 mg L^{-1}, for El Torreon 0.04 mg L^{-1} and a concentration of 0.05 mg L^{-1} in Junta de los Rios. All samples were higher than the values of the Mexican Norm as well as those established in the International standards for potable water. The third sample collected in December 2005 resulted in the following concentrations: 0.03 mg L^{-1} in La Presa, 0.06 mg L^{-1}in Rosales, 0.09 mg L^{-1} in Meoqui, 0.05 mg L^{-1} in El Torreon and 0.07 mg L^{-1} in Junta de los Rios.

The results of the arsenic concentration in the waters of San Pedro River at five locations in the State of Chihuahua, Mexico during 2006 are shown in Table 1. In general, the location La Presa was less contaminated compared with the other four sampled locations. The maximum concentration over the whole study was noted in March on El Torreon with 0.2533 mg L^{-1}. This concentration is much higher that that established in the Mexican Norm for waters used in agriculture (0.10 mg L^{-1}) and for livestock production (0.20 mg L^{-1}). With a few exceptions, the results are higher than the values indicated in Mexican and International Norms for potable water.

Although the inhabitants settled in communities close to the river did not drink water directly, the use of such water is common for different activities especially in rural areas. These findings must be an alert to the people living in the area or close to the area, because the arsenic was considered an important element in the development of leukemia [22] that was detected in an abnormally large number of children if Nevada, USA [23].

Table 1: Mean concentration of arsenic in five locations of the San Pedro River during the 2006 sampling (mg L^{-1}).

Location	January	Feb	March	April	May	June	July	August
La Presa	0.0726	0.0633	0.0753	0.0766	0.0736	0.0920	0.1353	0.0376
Rosales	0.1213	0.0740	0.1370	0.1130	0.1320	0.1123	0.1246	0.0860
Meoqui	0.0923	0.1100	0.1343	0.1106	0.1316	0.1396	0.1536	0.1436
El Torreon	0.1163	0.1260	0.2533	0.1246	0.1156	0.1333	0.1143	0.0916
Junta de los Rios	0.1160	0.1183	0.1616	0.0940	0.1380	0.1263	0.0903	0.0933

It is recognized that arsenic is primarily released into water due to intemperism of soil and rocks as well as from geothermal sources [24]. The other source is from anthropogenic activities mainly agricultural applications [25]. These findings did not find evidence of anthropogenic sources in the water of the San Pedro River and agree with results of previous studies in a tributary close to the San Pedro River [20]. These researchers found an arsenic range of 19.7-60.0 mg L^{-1} in three segments of the Rio Conchos.

Even though the arsenic concentrations in the waters of the San Pedro River apparently are not of human concern because it is not drank directly, the results reported here might be considered an alert for the aquatic environment when it is considered that Cantu *et al.*, [26] reported that large-mouth bass (*Micropterus salmoides*) had deformed fins, jaws heads and eyes in a water environment with 0.54 mg L^{-1}. In addition, the ambient water quality criteria for arsenic for protection of human health have been established at a safe level of 0.14 μg L^{-1} [27].

The results in this study were much higher than this specific value. It should be noted that people living in the communities along the San Pedro River consume fish collected from the river, and there is no information about the level of contamination in edible tissues of these fish. Finally, the other concern that should be evaluated for the San Pedro River is the water quality supplied for the wells that are in operation for human needs. This is important because there are evidences that the groundwaters in the aquifer of that area have arsenic levels that are higher than the levels permitted in Mexican and International norms [28].

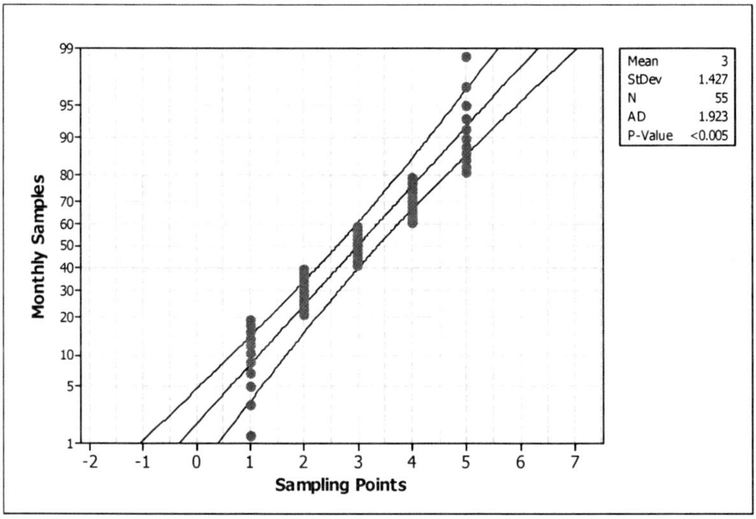

Figure 2: A 95% Confidence Intervals of the arsenic concentration in five sampling points in the San Pedro River in Chihuahua, Mexico.

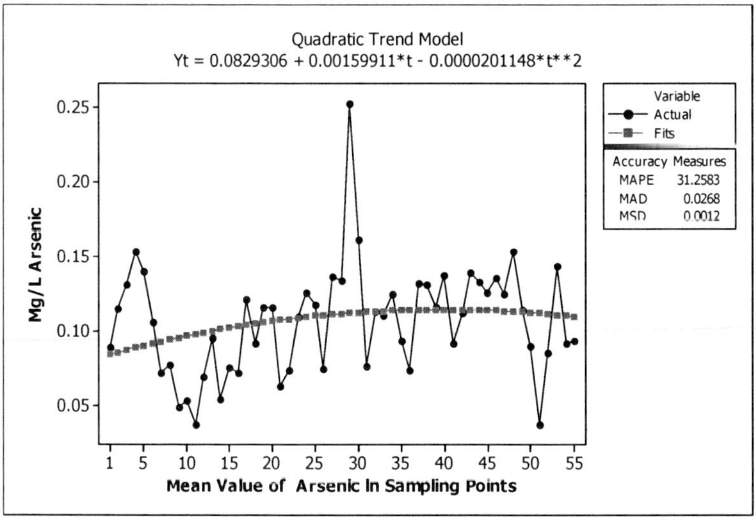

Figure 3: Quadratic trend of the arsenic concentration in the San Pedro River in Chihuahua, Mexico.

In Figure 2 the Confidence Intervals are shown for the five sampling locations in a monthly period. Moreover, in Figure 3 it is noted a quadratic trend in the different locations as well as the monthly samples concerning the arsenic concentration in the San Pedro River.

4 Conclusions

The data obtained in this study confirm our hypothesis that waters of the San Pedro River contain arsenic levels that are above levels recommended for Mexican as well as international standards. Therefore, we suggest future studies concerning the effects of these arsenic levels on human health and ecosystem effects, and especially to determine if arsenic pollution is due to natural or anthropogenic sources.

References

[1] Chu-Fang, Wang, Cheng-Yuan, Ch., Su-Fen, T., & Hung-Lung, Ch. 2005. Characteristics of Road Dust from Different Sampling Sites in Northern Taiwan. Journal of the Air & Waste Management Association 55(8):1236-1244

[2] Rubio, A.H., Wood, K., & Alanis, H.E. 2004. Water pollution in the Rio Conchos of northern Mexico. Development and application of computer technics to Environmental studies X. Ed. G. Latini, G. Passerini, and C.A. Brebbia. Wit press. 167-176.

[3] Rubio, A.H., Saucedo, T.R., Lara, M.C., Wood, K., & Jimenez, J. 2005. Water quality in the Laguna de Bustillos of Chihuahua, Mexico. Water Resources Management III. Ed. M. de Conceicao Cunha and C.A. Brebbia. Wit press. 155-160

[4] Rubio, A.H., Saucedo, T.R., Wood, K., Nuñez, A., & Jimenez, J. 2005. Metal contamination of a riparian area in the conchos watershed of Chihuahua, Mexico. Water Resources Management III. Ed. M. de Conceicao Cunha and C.A. Brebbia. Wit press. 269-275

[5] Prasad, M.N.V. & de Oliveira Freitas, H.M. 2003. Metal hyperaccumulation in plants-Biodiversity prospecting for phytoremediation technology. Electron. J. Biatechnol. 6, 285-321.

[6] Baos, R., Blas, J., Bortolotti, G.R., Marchant, T.A., & Hiraldo, F. 2006. Adrenocortical Response to Stress and Thyroid Hormone Status in Free-Living Nestling White Storks (Ciconia ciconia) Exposed to Heavy Metal and Arsenic Contamination. Environmental Health Perspectives 114(10):1497-1501

[7] WHO. 2001. Arsenic and Arsenic Compounds. Environmental Health Criteria 224. 2nd ed. Geneva: World Health Organization. Available: http://www.who.int/ipcs/publications/ehc/ ehc_224/en/ [accessed 10 February 2007.

[8] Chen, C.J., Kuo, T.L., & Wu, M.M. 1988. Arsenic and cancer. Lancet 1: 414-415

[9] IARC, 2004. International Agency for Research on Cancer. Some Drinking-Water Disinfectants and Contaminants, Including Arsenic. IARC Monogr Eval Carcinog Risks Hum 84.
[10] Hopenhayn-Rich, C., Biggs, & M.C., Smith, A.H. 1998. Lung and kidney cancer mortality associated with arsenic in drinking water in Cordoba, Argentina. Int. J. Epidemiol 27:561569.
[11] NRC, 2001. National Research Council. Arsenic in Drinking Water: 2001 Update. Washington, DC: National Academy Press
[12] Smith, A.H., Lingas, & E.O., Rahman, M. 2000. Contamination of drinking water by arsenic in Bangladesh: A public health emergency. Bull WHO 78(9):1093-1103.
[13] Rahman M, Tondel M, Ahmad SA, & Axelson 0.1998. Diabetes mellitus associated with arsenic exposure in Bangladesh. Am J Epidemiol 148:198-203.
[14] Longnecker MP, & Daniels JL. 2001. Environmental contaminants as etiologic factors for diabetes. Environ Health Perspect 109(suppl 61:871-876.
[15] Tseng CH, Tseng CP, Chiou HY, Hsueh YM, Chong CK, & Chen CJ. 2002, Epidemiologic evidence of diabetogenic effect of arsenic. Toxicol Lett 133:69-76.
[16] Zierold KM, Knobeloch L, & Anderson H. 2004. Prevalence of chronic diseases in adults e> posed to arsenic-contaminated drinking water. Am J Public health 94:1936-1937.
[17] NIH, 2007. National Institute of Health. Arsenic compound improves survival of adults with uncommon form of leukemia. ProQuest document ID:1201354551. Accessed February 13, 2007
[18] USEPA, 2003. United States Environmental Protection Agency. Technical summary of information available on the bioaccumulation of arsenic in aquatic organisms. EPA-822-R-03-032. Office of science and Technology & Office of water. Washington, D.C. USA.
[19] Holguín, C., Rubio, A.H., Olave, M.F., Saucedo, T, R., Gutiérrez, M., & Bautista, M.R. 2006. Calidad del agua del Río Conchos en la región de Ojinaga, Chihuahua: Parámetros fisicoquímicos, metales y metaloides. Universidad y Ciencia 22(1): 51-63.
[20] Gutiérrez, M., & Borrego, P. 1999. Water quality assessment of the rio conchos, Chihuahua, Mexico. Environmental International 25(5): 573-583
[21] NOM, 1981. Norma Oficial Mexicana. Norma NMX-AA-051-SCFI-1981. Análisis de agua-determinación de metales, método espectrofotométrico de absorción atómica
[22] Robinson, L., T. Sinks, A. Smith, M. Smith, M. Guinan, R. Todd, L. Brown, & B. Dudding, 2001. Acute Lymphoblastic (Lymphocytic) Leukemia - Review and Recommendations of the Expert Panel. Nevada State Health Division.
[23] Steinmaus, C., Lu, M., Todd, R.L. & Smith, A.H. 2004. Probability Estimates for the Unique Childhood Leukemia Cluster in Fallon, Nevada,

and Risks Near Other U.S. Military Aviation Facilities. Environmental Health Perspectives 112(6):766-771.

[24] Lacayo, M.J., Cruz, A., Calero, S., Lacayo, J., & fomsgaard, I. 1992. Total arsenic in water, fish and sediments from Lake Xolotlan, Managua, Nicaragua. Bull. Environ. Contam. Toxicol. 49:463-470

[25] Eisler, R. 1994. A review of arsenic hazards to plants and animals with emphasis on fishery and wildlife resources. In: Arsenic in the environment, Part II: Human health and ecosystem effects. J.O. Nriagu Ed. John Wiley & Sons, N.Y. 185-259.

[26] Cantu, R., Stacell, M., & Webb, M. 1991. Observation of abnormalities in largemouth bass fry exposed to arsenic contaminated water. Texas Parks and Wildlife Department. Austin, Texas, USA.

[27] USEPA, 1980. United States Environmental Protection Agency. Ambient Water Quality Criteria for arsenic. EPA 440/5-80-021. Office of water regulations and Standards. Washington, DC, USA. Available at: www.epa.gov/ost/pc/ambientwqc/arsenic80.pdf

[28] Kelly, M.E. 2001. El Rio Conchos: Un informe preliminary. Texas Center for policy studies. Marzo 2001. Austin, Texas, USA.

Nitrate pollution in the Delicias-Meoqui aquifer of Chihuahua, Mexico

M. S. Espino[1], H. O. Rubio[2] & C. J. Navarro[1]
[1]*Faculty of Engineering, Autonomous University of Chihuahua, Mexico*
[2]*Faculty of Zootechnic, Autonomous University of Chihuahua, Mexico*

Abstract

Nitrate concentration higher than 10 mg L^{-1} in drinking water can cause health problems, especially in infants. Nitrates from a variety of surface and subsurface sources, such as fertilizers, are soluble in water and can leach into groundwater causing quality degradation. Groundwater from Delicias-Meoqui aquifer supplies drinking and irrigation water to six municipalities in the state of Chihuahua. A part of the area overlying this aquifer corresponds to the irrigation district DR-005, one of the most important hydro-agricultural works in Mexico. An evaluation was conducted using historical water quality data from 134 drinking water wells to make a preliminary diagnosis concerning nitrate presence in that aquifer. Water analyses showed that 34% of samples have nitrate concentrations equal or higher than the 10 mg L^{-1} drinking water standard. Most of these samples were from the Delicias, Saucillo and Meoqui municipalities, with approximately 180,000 inhabitants total. Undoubtedly, the high nitrate concentrations can be attributed to pollution within the irrigation district DR-005 where nitrogen fertilizers in large quantities are applied, dissolve in water and move with it through the soil profile down to groundwater. This preliminary evaluation will contribute to the development of preventative strategies that can protect groundwater in proximity to agricultural production systems from nitrate contamination.
Keywords: nitrate, fertilizers, leaching, groundwater pollution, Delicias-Meoqui aquifer, Chihuahua, México.

WIT Transactions on Biomedicine and Health, Vol 11, © 2007 WIT Press
www.witpress.com, ISSN 1743-3525 (on-line)
doi:10.2495/EHR070201

1 Introduction

Nitrate is constituted by the NO_3^- anion and its presence in the environment results from the decomposition of nitrogen compounds. High concentrations of nitrates in drinking water can cause human health problems [1]. When nitrate undergo reduction to nitrite (NO_2^-), a process which occurs in the digestive tract by faecal microorganisms, blood oxygen transport is disabled causing the disease named metahemoglobinemia [2, 3]; also known, as baby blue syndrome concerning infants [4]. Other researches have associated nitrate with certain type of lymphoma [2] and have suggested the risk of acquiring cancer in areas where water with high levels of nitrate is consumed [5]. Pertaining to animal special cases, it has been demonstrated than consumption of these nitrogen compounds can cause birth defects [6, 7].

The presence of nitrate in water is seasonal and variable [8]. Because of their negative charge these ions may have great mobility [9] and can pollute surface water and groundwater. Rubio *et al.*, [10] found nitrate levels up to 10.53 mg L^{-1} in water samples of the Río Florido, which is a Río Conchos tributary. These values are higher than the International and Mexican standards of 10 mg N-NO_3^- L^{-1} in drinking water that were established to prevent human health problems [11, 12].

Aquifers can become polluted from nitrogen leaching from urban or rural wastewater, as is the case of fertilizers that are commonly applied in agricultural irrigation. A study in the United Sates of America showed that 11% of sampled wells had nitrate concentrations higher than 10 mg L^{-1} [13]. In the special case of the state of Chihuahua, groundwater is the main hydrological resource both for drinking water supply and for industrial and agricultural irrigation. The Delicias-Meoqui Aquifer (DMA) is located in the central-east portion of the hydrologic region RH-24 of Río Conchos-Bravo watershed [14]. Leaching of nitrogen residues are favored by several factors including the high permeability of aquifer, the low slope on the Delicias-Meoqui valley and the periodical application of large quantities of fertilizers in the DR-005. Presently, it is possible to find some data about nitrate concentration in drinking water wells for those localities within the DMA area. Nevertheless, a comprehensive evaluation of the influence of irrigation activities on groundwater quality does not exist.

The objective of this study was to perform a preliminary diagnosis of the presence of nitrate in the Delicias-Meoqui aquifer based on existing historical data of groundwater quality. The results will establish the basis for planning a more detailed study which includes a formal monitoring program and the geochemical evaluation of water quality parameters. These will contribute to the determination of strategies that would diminish the risk of aquifer contamination.

2 Materials and methods

The climate in the study area is arid, with extreme temperatures and with an average precipitation of 319 mm $year^{-1}$ [15]. The aquifer is constituted by alluvial material of medium to high permeability. Its recharge occurs by pluvial precipitation over the area and surrounding hills, irrigation returns, and percolation water from the Conchos and San Pedro rivers. Groundwater flow agrees with these rivers' path, south to north [14]. About 1,000 wells pierce the DMA; most of them, are used for agricultural irrigation. However, part of the extracted volume is used to satisfy the drinking water requirements of the population living in Delicias, Meoqui, Julimes, Rosales, Saucillo and La Cruz municipalities.

A part of the area occupied by this aquifer corresponds to the irrigation district (DR-005) which is one of the most important hydro-agricultural works in the country. Crop production including wheat, corn, alfalfa, sorghum, soybeans, chilli, onion, walnut and vegetables occupies approximately 90,000 ha of irrigated land. Typical agricultural activities include the use of nitrogen and phosphate compounds as fertilizers, such as anhydrous ammonia, urea and ammonium phosphate. The doses vary between 100 and 270 kg ha^{-1} [16].

Historical data concerning aquifer characteristics and groundwater quality were reviewed and analyzed a total of 134 wells. The source for this information was federal and state governmental agencies. Water groups were established by means of hydrochemical tools using data available for 2003, 2004, and 2005. Also, qualitative aspects related with relevant substances for human health were evaluated in drinking water sources of the area.

In the area is notorious calcium and sodium sulfate as well as calcium and sodium bicarbonate, on agree with geological characteristics of arid zones. Important elements like arsenic, fluoride and nitrate are present in several groundwater sources in concentrations that exceeded the drinking water quality guidelines. Some of these wells had high levels of dissolved solids and sulfate too. Arsenic and fluoride exist on groundwater of several states of Mexico, as in many regions of the world. It's a consequence of nature of rocks which are in contact with water. The arsenic and/or fluoride high levels in drinking water problem of 43 communities in the region of study has been attended by Chihuahua state authorities by means the establishment of local treatment systems. They are based on reverse osmosis principle to demineralize the water fraction which is ingested by consumers.

3 Results and discussion

The quality data review on 134 drinking water samples demonstrated that 34% of the wells had concentrations equal or exceeding 10 mg $N\text{-}NO_3^-$ L^{-1} (Table 1). Communities of Delicias, Saucillo and Meoqui are particularly important because they have 50%, 40% and 29% of wells above or at the permissible limit for nitrate, respectively. These communities have a total population of more than 180,000 inhabitants. Of the 46 localities with nitrate above or in the limit, only 15 have a demineralization treatment system [17]. These results are of practical importance considering that high levels of nitrate in drinking water have been associated with urothelial diseases, including cancer [18] and a type of lymphoma [19].

Examination of data showed four distinct zones of high levels of nitrate. These areas are shown in Figure 1, and are described below. Zone 1: The northwest portion of aquifer, with some localities within the Meoqui municipality (Diez de Mayo, Sta. Rita de Casia, Barranco Blanco, Potrero del Llano, Felipe Angeles). Zone 2: An area between Meoqui (Loreto, Francisco Portillo, Nuevo Loreto) and Delicias (Cuauhtémoc, La Gomeña, Morelos, Ampliación Mercedes). Zone 3: Some localities near Delicias (Colonia Campesina, Ciudad Delicias, Vicente Guerrero, Santa Fe) and Saucillo (Sta. Rosa, Las Varas, Orranteño). Zone 4: Several localities south of Saucillo (Armendáriz, San Francisco de Mezquital, Vicente Guerrero, Ciudad Saucillo, Puerto del Toro).

These four identified areas represent non-point or dispersed pollution zones within the irrigation district DR-005 influence area. According to official reports [14], this is the principal recharge area for the aquifer; therefore, the zone where water is added to the groundwater system (Figure 2). The total recharge includes rain infiltration, the water irrigation returns of surface water and the leakages from domestic pipelines. Its value reaches 217.39 Hm^3/year. It can be noticed in Figure 2 that the higher values of recharge zone (where 81% of total aquifer recharge occurs) are found in zones Z-5, Z-6 and Z-9, which corresponds geographically to the surface occupied by the irrigation district DR-005.

Table 1: Summary of drinking water wells with high nitrate concentration.

MUNICIPALITY	Number of wells: Total	Number of wells: With high nitrate concentration (*)	Percentage of wells with high nitrate concentration (%)
Julimes	9	1	11.1
Rosales	16	4	25.0
La Cruz	8	0	0.0
Meoqui	31	9	29.0
Saucillo	30	12	40.0
Delicias	40	20	50.0
TOTAL	134	46	34.3

(*) Nitrate concentration $\geq$ 10 mg $N\text{-}NO_3^-$/L.

In comparison with Figure 1, we notice that this region also corresponds with the nitrate leaching zone. Hence, it is possible to establish a close relationship between groundwater quality and nitrate pollution from irrigation activities. Interestingly, a study by Nolan [20] concluded that six variables will predict the presence of more than 4 mg L^{-1} of nitrate in the ground water: nitrogen fertilizer, percent cropland-pasture, population density, percent well-drained soils, depth of the seasonally high water table and the presence or absence of a bedrock fracture zone within an aquifer. These variables are maximized in the Delicias-Meoqui aquifer, where the nitrate in groundwater represents a potential hazard to human health as well as for the whole ecosystem.

A prominent result is that 50% of drinking water wells within the Delicias municipality (115,000 inhabitants) tested is above the nitrate permissible limits. This area corresponds to the most exploited part of the aquifer, with local flow lines moving in radial direction to higher nitrate concentration sites [14]. The high incidence of nitrate in the Delicias area can be associated with nitrogen compounds leached from irrigation as well as from livestock facilities which are common in the area. Another important nitrate source in the rural areas may be septic systems and in urban zones the leakage from sanitary sewers and effluents from treated and raw sewage discharged at surface water bodies.

Necessary actions to reduce potential risks of pollution in the DMA include the application of fertilizers at tested agronomic doses to avoid nitrogen leakage into the groundwater saturated zone. Also, a careful management during storage and cleaning of fertilizer containers is needed, as well as removal of organic wastes from livestock, adequate maintenance of sanitary sewers, and an advanced wastewater treatment that removes nitrogen residues capable of polluting groundwater.

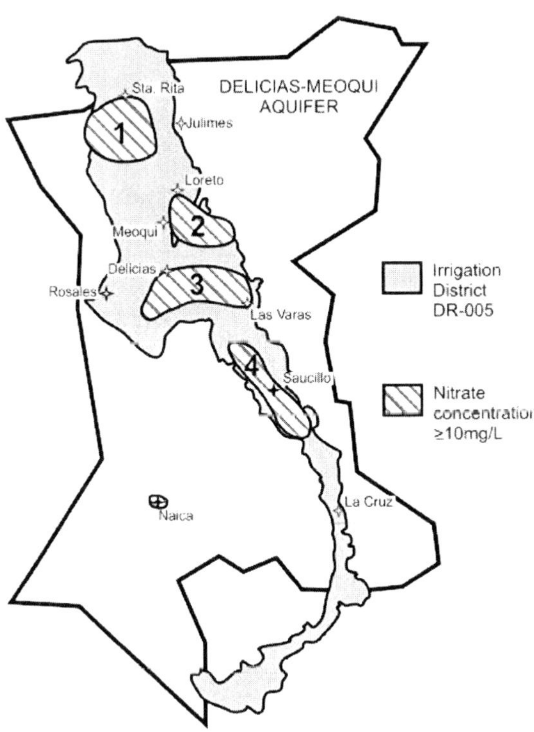

Figure 1: Zones in Delicias-Meoqui aquifer with high nitrates levels.

The authors recommend additional studies that would link health records with the water quality records for each community to estimate the average long-term exposure to nitrate in drinking water, among other findings. The advantage to this study would be that health institutions already have information concerning the health problems of the inhabitants of the study zones. At the same time, research utilizing denitrification walls to remove nitrate in ground water should be carried out in the studied area. This technology has been proved to be effective in Canada [21] and New Zealand [22].

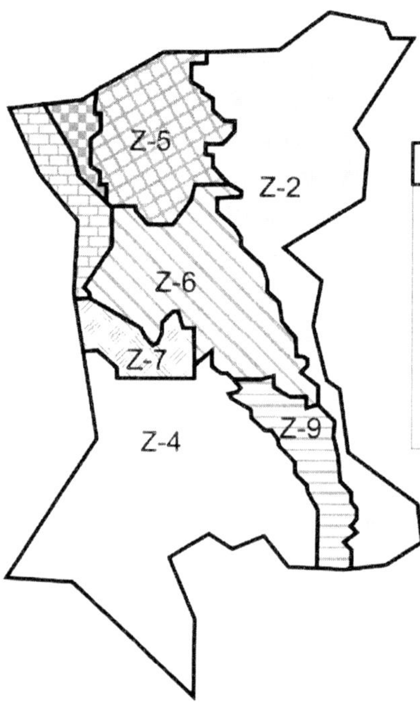

ZONE	$Hm^3/year$
Z-2	10.27
Z-3	1.51
Z-4	11.3
Z-5	57.82
Z-6	96.11
Z-7	12.08
Z-8	6.31
Z-9	21.99

Figure 2: Map of recharge zones in Delicias-Meoqui aquifer (National Water Commission-Mexico, 2005).

4 Conclusions

A high percentage of drinking water wells located at Delicias-Meoqui aquifer link nitrate contamination to fertilizers applied on the irrigation district DR-005. The knowledge of specific requirements of fertilizers dose is needed to avoid nitrogen entering the groundwater.

An intense research about the contribution of irrigation to DMA pollution is needed, as is actualizing water quality information and its relationship with geology, the hydrologic variables, human activities influence and the evaluation of agricultural and irrigation techniques.

Results of this and further studies will contribute to the development of preventive strategies and mitigating measures to protect aquifer from nitrate contamination and to improve knowledge on the management of groundwater resources in proximity to agricultural production systems.

Acknowledgements

This study was partly supported by the Professors Improvement Program (PROMEP) of the Public Education Ministry (Secretaría de Educación Pública) in Mexico. The information provided by the Water National Commission (Comisión Nacional del Agua) and the Central Board of Water and Sanitation of the State of Chihuahua (JCAS) is greatly appreciated.

References

[1] Legault, T., Stewart, B., & Lebedin, J. 2000. In-situ remediation of nitrate in groundwater: Phase 1: Site characterization [online]. Agriculture and Agri-Food Canada. World Wide Web: http://www.agr.gc.ca/pfra/water/nitremed_e.htm

[2] Kross, B.C., Oison, M.L., Ayebo, A. & Johnsons, J.K. 1995. Humans. In J.E. Rechcigl (Ed.), Boca Raton, FL: Lewis Publishers. 153-214

[3] Ayebo, A., Kross, B.C., Vlad, M., & Sinca, A. 1997. Infant metahemoglobinemia in the Transylvania Region of Romania. Int. J. of Environ. Health 3(1):20-29.

[4] Lamond, R.E., Powell, G. M. & Devlin, D. 1999. Nitrate and groundwater [online]. Kansas State University Agricultural Experiment Station and Cooperative Extension Service. World Wide Web: http://www.oznet.ksu.edu

[5] Cuello, C., Correa, P., Haenszel, W, Gordillo, G., Brown, C., Archer, M. & Tannenbaum, S. 1976. Gastric cancer in Colombia I: Cancer risk and suspected environmental agents. Journal of National Cancer Institute. 57(5):1015-1020

[6] Dorsch, M.M., Scragg, R.K., McMichael, A.J., Baghurst, R.A., & Dyer, K.E. 1984. Congenital malformations and maternal drinking water supply in rural South Australia: A case-control study. American Journal of Epidemiology 119:473-486

[7] Super, M., Heese, H., Mackenzie, D., Dempster, W.S., Dupless, J. & Ferreira, JJ.1981. An epidemiologic study of well water nitrates in a group of southwest African Namibian infants. Water Research 15:1265-1270.

[8] Chapman, P.J., Reynolds, B. & Wheater, H.S. 1996. Experimental investigation of potassium and nitrate dynamics in a headwater stream in Mid-Wales. Chemistry and Ecology. 13:1-19.

[9] Baker, J.L., & Laflen, J.M. 1982. Effect of crop residue and fertilizer management on soluble nutrient runoff losses. Transactions of the American Society of Agricultural Engineers 25:344-348.

[10] Rubio, A.H., Wood, K. & Alanis, H.E. 2004. Water pollution in the Rio Conchos of northern Mexico. Development and application of computer techniques to Environmental Studies X. Ed; G. Latini, G. Passerini, C.A. Brebbia. Witpress. 67-176.
[11] NOM, 1996. Modificación a la norma oficial Mexicana NOM-127-SSAI-1994. Salud ambiental. Agua para uso y consumo humano. Límites permisibles de calidad y tratamientos a que debe someterse el agua para su utilización. Diario Oficial.
[12] USEPA, 2002. United States Environmental Protection Agency. Edition of the drinking water Standards and Health Advisories. EPA 822-R-02-038, USEPA, office of water, Washington, D.C.
[13] Squillace, P.J., Scott, P.J., Moran, M.J., Nolan, B.T., & Kolpin, D.W. 2002. VOCs, pesticides, nitrate, and their mixtures in groundwater used for drinking water in the United States. Environmental Science and Technology 36:1923-1930
[14] CNA, 2005. Comision Nacional del Agua. Actualización del Estudio Geohidrológico del Acuífero Meoqui-Delicias, Chihuahua. Subdirección General Técnica. Gerencia de Aguas Subterráneas.
[15] INIFAP, 2006. Instituto Nacional de Investigaciones Forestales, Agrícolas y Pecuarias. Estadísticas climatológicas básicas del estado de Chihuahua. (período 1961-2003). Libro Técnico No. 1. CIRNOC-Chihuahua. P. 151.
[16] INEGI, 1999. Instituto Nacional de Estadística, Geografía e Informática y Gobierno del Estado de Chihuahua. Estudio Hidrológico del Estado de Chihuahua
[17] JCAS, 2006. Junta Central de Agua y Saneamiento del Estado de Chihuahua (JCAS). Personal, May 1999
[18] Volkner, B.G., Ernst, B., Simon, J., Kuefer, R., Bartsch, G. Jr., Bach, D., & Gschwend, J.E. 2005. Influence of nitrate levels in drinking water on urological malignancies: a community-based cohort study. BJU Int. 95(7):972-976.
[19] Gulis, G., Czompolyova, & M., Cerhan, Jr. 2002. An ecological study of nitrate in municipal drinking water and cancer incidence in Trnava District, Slovakia. Environ Res. 88(3):182-187
[20] Nolan, B. 2001. Relating nitrogen sources and aquifer susceptibility to nitrate in shallow ground waters of the United States. Ground Water 39, no. 2: 290-299
[21] Robertson, W.D., & Cherry, J.A. 1995. In situ denitrification of septic-system nitrate using reactive porous media barriers: Field trials. Ground Water 33:99-111.
[22] Schipper, L.A., & Vojvodic-Vukovic, M. 2001. Five years of nitrate removal, denitrification and carbon dynamics in a denitrification wall. Water Res. 35:3473-3477.

Environmental impacts of wastewater from low-rank coal handling processes in terms of mutagenicity and acute toxicity

T. Nakajima, K. Kuzumaki, H. Hasegawa, H. Takanashi & A. Ohki
Department of Bioengineering, Faculty of Engineering, Kagoshima University, Kagoshima, Japan

Abstract

Two low-rank coals, a sub-bituminous coal (BA) and a lignite (LY), were treated by hot water extraction (HWE) and hydrothermal treatment (HTT), and the environmental impacts of water-soluble matters eluted from coal by the HWE and HTT processes were evaluated in terms of TOC, mutagenicity, and the acute toxicity against freshwater organisms. When HWE was performed at 80°C, the degree of TOC for LY was much higher than that for BA. However, for HTT, the two coals gave comparable TOC values in L/S ratio of both 100 and 3. The HWE and HTT eluents of two coals were assessed by the Ames mutagenicity assay with *Salmonella typhimurium* TA100 and TA98 strains, and no notable mutagenicity was observed in the presence or absence of metabolic activation. When the mutagenicity of the 300°C-HTT eluent of LY was analyzed, no notable mutagenicity was also observed. For the HWE and HTT eluents of LY, the acute toxicity test was carried out by use of *Daphnia magna* and *Oryzias latipes*. When the 80°C-HWE eluent was tested, almost no toxicity was observed for *D. magna* and *O. latipes*. However, when the HTT eluents were examined, the toxicity increased as the elevation of the HTT temperature, and the toxicity of organic matters dissolved in the 350°C-HTT eluent was comparable to that of reference phenolic compounds. From the FTIR analysis of organic matters eluted in the HTT eluents, it is found that the toxicity is caused by the presence of aromatic compounds with hydrophilic substituents, such as carboxyl and hydroxyl groups.
Keywords: low-rank coal, wastewater, water-soluble organic matters, mutagenicity, ames assay, acute toxicity.

WIT Transactions on Biomedicine and Health, Vol 11, © 2007 WIT Press
www.witpress.com, ISSN 1743-3525 (on-line)
doi:10.2495/EHR070211

1 Introduction

In coal handling processes, there are many cases in which coal contacts with water. Various water-soluble hazardous matters may be eluted from coal into effluent in coal washing processes, storage pile exposed to rain and/or water spray, and transport in coal-water slurry. In previous studies, many organic compounds, such as phenols, polycyclic aromatic hydrocarbons (PAHs), and humic substances, have been detected in coal washing water [1], natural coal storage pile runoff [2, 3], simulated coal storage pile runoff [4-6], coal slurry transport wastewater [7-9], and wastewaters from hydrothermal treatment (HTT) of low-lank coals [10]. These wastewaters, if released into natural water, may have deleterious damage to aquatic ecosystem and human life. There have been only a few studies about the evaluation of environmental impacts, particularly mutagenicity for water-soluble organic matters eluted from coal [7, 11, 12].

In this study, an Indonesian sub-bituminous coal and an Australian lignite were subjected to HWE and HTT, the leaching of organic matters was measured by total organic carbon (TOC), and the environmental impacts of these water-soluble organic matters were evaluated in terms of mutagenicity and acute toxicity against some freshwater organisms.

2 Materials and methods

2.1 Coals

An Indonesian subbituminous coal (BA), and an Australian lignites (LY) were used in this study. Table 1 presents the analyses of these coals. The particle sizes of coals were under 149 μm (100 mesh).

Table 1: Analytical data of coal.

Coal	Proximate (wt%, dry base)			Ultimate (wt%, dry ash free)				
	I.M.	Ash	V.M.	C	H	N	O	O/C
BA	10.70	2.30	44.80	71.20	5.20	1.10	22.10	0.23
LY	24.90	0.60	39.80	69.57	5.00	0.60	26.20	0.28

I.M., inherent moisture; V.M., volatile matter.

2.2 Hot water extraction (HWE) procedure

Powdery coal (1.0 g) was placed in a filter paper thimble (ADVANTEC No. 84, i.d. 28mm x 100 mm), and the thimble and 100 ml of deionized water were set in a Soxhlet extractor (Buchi B-811). The procedure of HWE was the same as that described in our previous paper [11].

2.3 Hydrothermal treatment (HTT) procedure

The powdery coal was mixed with 200 ml water and the mixture was placed in an autoclave (Suzuki Rika Seisakusho 200H). The liquid per solid ratio (L/S) was 3, 20, and 100 in this study. The atmosphere in the autoclave was purged by N_2. The autoclave was heated at a rate of 3-4°C/min to a desired temperature and the temperature was kept for 1 h. After cooling, the eluent was separated from coal by filtration, and analyzed.

2.4 Measurement of TOC

The determination of total organic carbon (TOC) in the eluents was conducted by catalytic oxidation followed by IR spectrometry for CO_2 measurement using an automatic TOC analyzer (Shimadzu TOC-V CSH).

2.5 FTIR analysis

The organic matters dissolved in the HWE and HTT eluents were freeze-dried into powdery form. The powdery organic matters (0.01 g) were mixed with KBr (1.0 g) in a motor with pestle and a portion of the resulting mixture was molded into a disc. The disc was analyzed by a FTIR spectrophotometer (JASCO FT/IR-420).

2.6 Mutagenicity assay

The organic matters dissolved in the HWE and HTT eluents were 100 times concentrated into a dimethyl sulfoxide (DMSO) solution by a solid phase extraction (SPE) method using an adsorbent cartridge (Sep-Pak Plus CSP-800, Nihon Waters) according to a literature [13]. The mutagenicity of the eluent was evaluated by the Ames *Salmonella* mutagenicity assay according to the authorized method [14]. Two *Salmonella typhimurium* strains TA100 and TA98, which were obtained from the National Institute of Public Health, Japan, were used. The preincubation method using TA100 and TA98 strains with or without metabolic activation by a rat liver homogenate S9 mix was employed. S9 mix was purchased from Oriental Yeast Co., Ltd. Dose-response tests were carried out using three dose-steps and one negative control (DMSO). Positive control tests were concurrently performed with a DMSO solution of 4-nitroquinoline-1-oxide (4NQO) for the -S9 condition and that of 2-aminoanthracene for the +S9 condition to confirm the activity of the strain. After incubation at 37°C for 48 h, colonies on the plate were scored, and the numbers of net revertant colonies per plate (net rev./plate) were obtained as the difference with negative control.

2.7 Toxicity test for freshwater organisms

In order to evaluate the acute toxicity of HWE and HTT eluents against freshwater organisms, *Daphnia sp.* acute immobilization test and fish acute toxicity test were conducted in accordance with the OECD guideline for testing of chemicals using *Daphnia magna* (OECD TG202) [15] and *Oryzias latipes*

(OECD TG203) [16]. The HWE eluent was produced by the 80ºC-HWE (L/S=100), while the HTT eluents were produced by the 200-350ºC-HTT (L/S=20). In *Daphnia sp.* acute immobilisation test, the adequately diluted eluents were exposed to *D. magna* for 48 h, and the concentrations of organic matters which produced 50% immobilization of *D. magna* (EC_{50}; mg-C/l) was calculated by probit analysis. In fish acute toxicity test, the adequately diluted eluents were exposed to *O. latipes* for 96 h, and the concentrations of organic matters which produced 50% mortality of *O. latipes* (LC_{50}; mg-C/l) was calculated by the same method.

3 Results and discussion

3.1 TOC in eluent

Two coals BA and LY were subjected to the HWE procedure, and the TOC and pH in the eluents were measured. In Table 2, the TOC values obtained are listed. The eluent of LY gave a higher TOC value (42.8 mg-C/l) than that for BA (13.3 mg-C/l) in the 80ºC-HWE. For pH value, considerably low pH was observed in the LY eluents. It is evident that the organic matters eluted from LY contain more acidic components, compared to that from BA in the HWE eluent.

When the 350ºC-HTT was performed in L/S=100 and 3, the results are also recorded in Table 2. For comparison with 80ºC-HWE eluents in the same L/S (100) condition, the 350ºC-HTT eluents of BA and LY gave much higher TOC values than the 80ºC-HWE eluents. For the HTT eluents, there is not so big difference between BA and LY in the degree of TOC. Practical HTT process is usually carried out in L/S=3-4. When the 350ºC-HTT was performed in L/S=3, the degree of TOC in the BA and LY eluents were 4220 and 5910 mg-C/l, respectively. Racovalis et al. [10] reported that LY produced 6000-7000 mg-C/l of TOC when 350ºC-HTT was carried out in L/S=3. The TOC values obtained in this study (L/S=3) is reasonable compared with their results. For the pH value of 350ºC-HTT eluent, almost same pH was observed in both of the eluents.

Table 2: TOC and pH in the HWE and HTT eluents.

Coal	Procedure	L/S	TOC (mg-C/l)	pH
BA	80ºC-HWE	100	13.3	6.6
	350ºC-HTT [a)]	100	489	-
	350ºC-HTT	3	4220	4.8
LY	80ºC-HWE	100	42.8	4.7
	350ºC-HTT [a)]	100	535	-
	350ºC-HTT	3	5910	4.1

a) From [12].

3.2 Effect of HTT conditions upon leaching

The effect of HTT temperature upon the degree of TOC in the HTT eluent was investigated, and the results are shown in Figure 1. When the 200°C-HTT (L/S=3) was performed for LY, the TOC in the eluent was 440 mg-C/l, and the degree of TOC was increased as the temperature was raised. In case of BA, the degree of TOC was about the same as that for LY in the 200°C-HTT eluent, and that was greatly increased as the temperature was raised from 300 to 350°C. In our previous paper [17], we reported that the oxygenic functional group, such as COOH and OH presented in coal was diminished as the elevation of HTT temperature. Also, the autoclave pressure was greatly increased between 300 and 350°C (from 96 to 180 kg/cm^2). It is proposed that the decomposition of these functional groups is greatly enhanced when the 350°C-HTT is performed, and therefore the leaching of organic matters from coal is greatly increased.

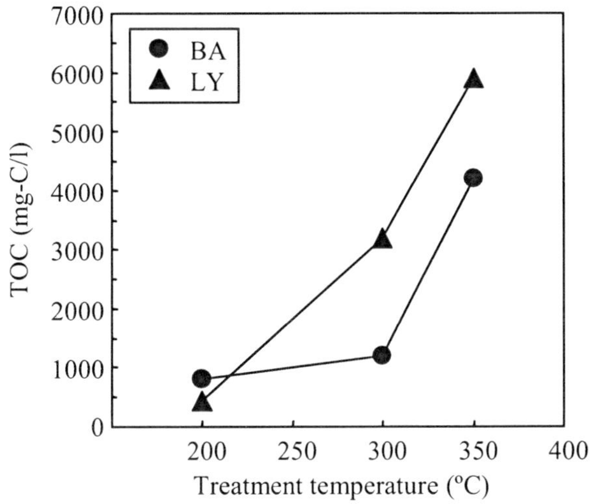

Figure 1: Effect of treatment temperature upon TOC in HTT eluent (L/S=3).

3.3 Ames *Salmonella* mutagenicity assay

The organic matters dissolved in the HWE eluent of coals were concentrated into DMSO by an SPE method [13]. The resulting DMSO solution was analyzed by the Ames *Salmonella* mutagenicity assay using TA100 and TA98 strains according to the authorized method [14]. To check the activity of the *Salmonella* strains used, positive controls using 4NQO for -S9 condition and 2-aminoanthracene for +S9 condition were performed, and the both TA100 and TA98 strains were adequately responsible to these mutagenic compounds.

In Figure 2, dose responses of the HWE eluents of BA and LY coals are indicated. For both of the eluents, there were almost no linear responses and no significant differences between the number of revertant colonies per plate for the maximum dose and that for the negative control, either in the presence or in the absence of metabolic activation (S9). Therefore, it is evident that the HWE eluents of BA and LY coals do not give significant mutagenicity. When the mutagenicity of the 300°C-HTT (L/S=100) eluent obtained from LY was analyzed, no notable mutagenicity was also observed.

Also, the effect of HTT temperature upon the mutagenicity of eluent was investigated under TA100-S9 conditions, when LY lignite was extracted by 200 to 350°C-HTT (L/S=3). From the dose responses listed in Table 3, although a little larger number of revertant colonies was observed for 300 and 350°C-HTT eluents compared to 200°C-HTT eluent, no significant mutagenicity was detected. It is concluded that no notable mutagenicity was observed for either HWE or HTT eluents.

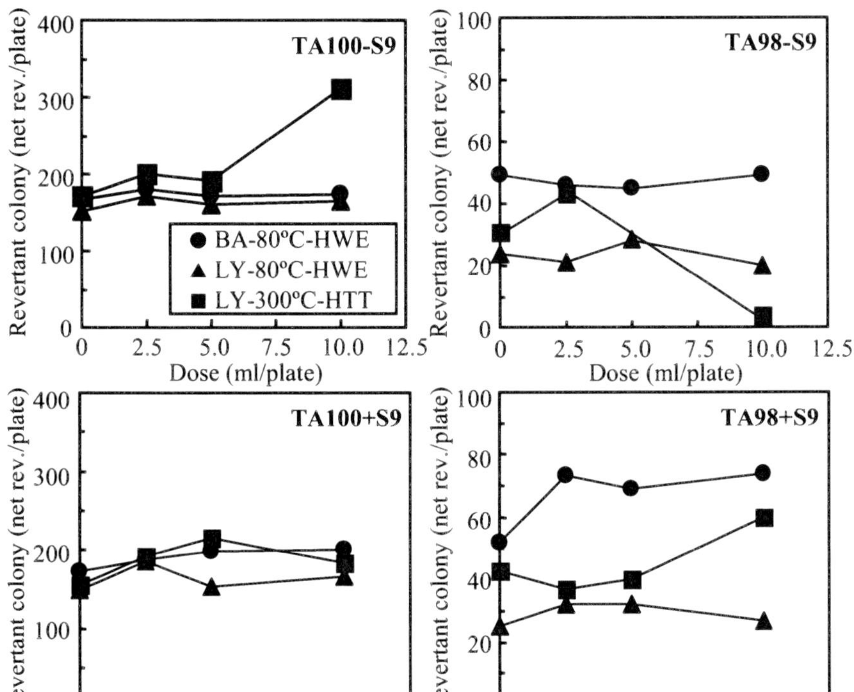

Figure 2: Ames mutagenicity assay of HWE and HTT eluents.

3.4 Toxicity test for fresh water organisms

When the HWE and HTT of coal were performed, not only organic matters but also inorganic matters will be leached out. When the concentrations of some toxic metals (As, B, Cd, Cr, Cu, Mn Pb, and Zn) in the HWE and HTT eluents obtained from LY lignite were measured, it was found that the concentrations of these hazardous metals were below the detection limits and the leaching of the metals was negligible in the HWE and HTT eluents (data not shown). Hence, the acute toxicity of HWE and HTT eluent was evaluated only for the organic matters in the eluents.

Table 3: Effect of HTT temperature upon mutagenicity of HTT eluent (L/S=3)[a].

Coal	Dose (ml/plate)	Number of revertant colony (net rev./plate)		
		200°C	300°C	350°C
LY	0 (Control)	149	149	149
	2.5	146	172	169
	5.0	165	194	167
	10.0	168	228	220

a) Mutagenicity was assayed under TA100-S9 conditions.

Table 4: Acute toxicity test of HWE and HTT eluent for *D. magna* and *O. latipes*.

Test sample	*D. magna*	*O. latipes*
	48 h-EC_{50} (mg-C/l)	96 h-LC_{50} (mg-C/l)
80°C-HWE eluent	a)	a)
200°C-HTT eluent	14.6	66.5
300°C-HTT eluent	13.2	21.6
350°C-HTT eluent	5.7	7.6
Phenol	15.8	25[b)]
p-Cresol	8.5	14[b)]
Catechol	1.2[b)]	3.5[b)]
4-nonyl phenol	0.059[b)]	0.24[b)]

a) Practically non-toxic.
b) From [18].

Toxicity tests were carried out using *D. magna* and *O. latipes* as test organisms for characterizing the HWE and HTT eluents of LY. In Table 4, the 48 h-EC_{50} value for *D. magna* and the 96 h-LC_{50} value for *O. latipes* were listed, when the 80°C-HWE and 200 to 350°C-HTT eluents are examined. It has been reported that wastewaters obtained from low-rank coal handling processes contain various phenolic compounds [5, 6, 19]. Therefore, the EC_{50} and LC_{50} value of four reference phenolic compounds which may present in the HWE and HTT eluent were also listed in Table 4. The EC_{50} and LC_{50} value obtained from each assay were described as mg carbon per litter (mg-C/l).

When the HWE eluent was tested, almost no acute toxicities were observed for either *D. magna* or *O. latipes*. For the HTT eluents, significant acute toxicities which were comparable to those of the reference phenolic compound were detected for each organism. The 48 h-EC_{50} values for *D. magna* decreased in the order, Phenol ≈ 200°C-HTT eluent > 300°C-HTT eluent > *p*-Cresol ≈ 350°C-HTT eluent > Catechol > 4-nonyl phenol. The 96 h-LC_{50} values for *O. latipes* were also decreased in about the same order.

The organic matters dissolved in the HWE and HTT eluents were freeze-dried, which were analyzed by FTIR, and aromatic ring peak (ca. 1610 cm^{-1}), aliphatic and aromatic carboxyl peak (ca. 1750 and 1710 cm^{-1}, respectively), and hydroxyl peak (ca. 3450 cm^{-1}) were observed in the FTIR spectrum. As shown in Figure 3, the organic matters dissolved in the HWE eluent gave aromatic ring peak and weak aliphatic carboxyl peak. For the organic matters form HTT eluents, aromatic ring peak and the aromatic carboxyl peak was found in their spectrum, and the intensity of the aromatic carboxyl peak was increased as the elevation of HTT temperature. These results suggest that the organic matters dissolved in the HTT eluents under higher temperature conditions possess more aromatic carboxyl groups. Consequently, the HTT eluents under higher temperature conditions give more toxicity provably due to the elution of toxic aromatic compounds with hydrophilic substituents, such as carboxyl and hydroxyl groups.

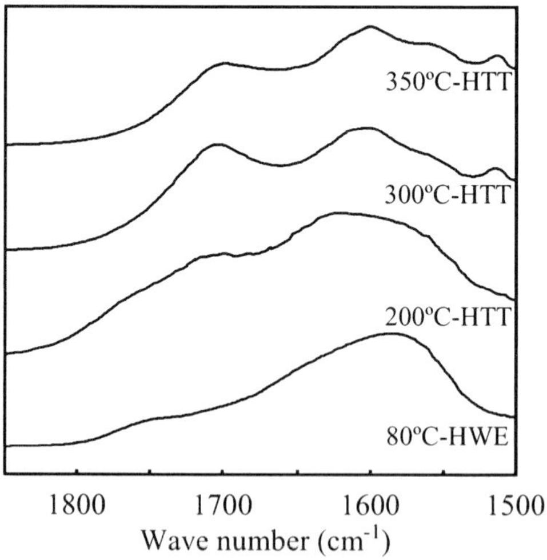

Figure 3: FTIR spectra of organic matters dissolved in HWE and HTT eluent of LY lignite.

4 Conclusions

A sub-bituminous coal BA and a lignite LY were subjected to the HWE and HTT processes, and the leaching of organic matters from coal was evaluated by TOC. When the HTT process was carried out, much higher TOC was obtained compared to HWE, and the degree of TOC increased as the increase of HTT temperature. When the HWE and HTT eluents of two coals were assessed by the Ames mutagenicity assay, no notable mutagenicity was observed in the presence or absence of metabolic activation. The 300°C-HTT eluent of LY also gave no notable mutagenicity. For the HWE and HTT eluents of LY, the acute toxicity test was carried out. When the 80°C-HWE eluent was tested, almost no toxicity was observed. However, when the HTT eluents were examined, the toxicity increased as the elevation of the HTT temperature. From the FTIR analysis of organic matters eluted, it is found that the toxicity is caused by the presence of aromatic compounds with hydrophilic substituents, such as carboxyl and hydroxyl groups.

References

[1] Berrueta, A., Fernandez, L.A., Vicente, F., Fluorescence study of the solubilization of benzo [a] pyrene: application to its detection in coal washing waters. *Anal. Chem. Acta.*, 243 (1), 115-119 (1991).

[2] Atwater, J.W., Jasper, S.E., Parkinson, P.D., Mavinic, D.S., Organic contaminants in Canadian coal wastewaters and associated sediments. *Water Pollution Research Journal of Canada*, 25 (2), 187-200 (1990).

[3] Curran, K.J., Irvine, K.N., Droppo, I.G., Murphy, T.P., Suspended solids, trace metal and PAH concentrations and loadings from coal pile runoff to Hamilton Harbour, Ontario. *J. Great Lakes Res.*, 26 (1), 18-30 (2000).

[4] Stahl, R.G., Liehr, J.G., Davis, E.M., Characterization of organic compounds in simulated rainfall runoffs from model coal piles. *Arch. Environ. Contam. Toxicol.*, 13 (2), 179-90 (1984).

[5] Fendinger, N.J., Radway, J.C., Tuttle, J.H., Means, J.C., Characterization of organic material leached from coal by simulated rainfall. *Environ. Sci. Technol.*, 23 (2), 170-177 (1989).

[6] Fendinger, N.J., Radway, J.C., Tuttle, J.H., The effect of environmental storage conditions on the organic content of simulated coal leachates. *Arch. Environ. Contam. Toxicol.*, 19 (2), 249-256 (1990).

[7] Reid, M.C., Davis, J.W., Sayler, G.S., Minear, R.A., Dissolved organic carbon of coal slurry transport water. *Water Res.*, 19 (19), 1199-1203 (1985).

[8] Reid, M.C., Davis, J.W., Minear, R.A., Sayler, G.S., Fulvic acid constituents of coal slurry transport wastewater. *Water Res.*, 22 (1), 127-131 (1988).

[9] Sayler, G.S., Minear, R.A., Reid, M.C., Davis, J.W., Enhanced reuse potential of coal slurry transport water: Toxic organics assessment and removal. *PB Rep. PB-84-230432*, p.75 (1983).

[10] Racovalis, L., Hobday, M.D., Hodges, S., Effect of processing conditions on organics in wastewater from hydrothermal dewatering of low-rank coal. *Fuel*, 81 (10), 1369-1378 (2002).

[11] Nakajima, T., Kanda, T., Fukuda, T., Takanashi, H., Ohki A., Characterization of eluent by hot water extraction of coals in terms of total organic carbon and environmental impacts. *Fuel*, 84 (7-8), 783-789 (2005).

[12] Nakajima, T., Nakamata, S., Takanashi, H., Ohki, A., Bioassay for environmental impacts of water-soluble matters eluted from coal. Proceedings of the International Conference on Coal Science and Technology, Okinawa, Japan, paper No. 2P504 (2005).

[13] Takanashi, H., Urano, K., Hirata, M., Hano, T., Ohgaki, S., Method for measuring mutagen formation potential (MFP) on chlorination as a new water quality index. *Water Res.*, 35 (7), 1627-1634 (2001).

[14] Ministry of Labor Japan, Mutagenicity assay for the occupational safety and health act. Test guideline and GLP, Occupational Health Service Center, Tokyo, (1991), (in Japanese).

[15] OECD, Test guideline 202, *Daphnia sp.* Acute immobilisation test and reproduction test (adopted April 4, 1984), In section 2 Effects on biotic systems, OECD guidelines for the testing of chemicals, Paris, (1984).

[16] OECD, Test guideline 203, Fish acute toxicity test. In section 2 Effects on biotic systems, OECD guidelines for the testing of chemicals, Paris, (1992).

[17] Xie, X.-F., Ohki, A., Morimatsu, K., Nakajima, T., Oda, H., Maeda, S., Surface properties of coals upgraded by hydrothermal treatment. *J. Jpn. Inst. Energy*, 77 (6), 478-484 (1998).

[18] Chemicals Evaluation and Research Institute, Japan, Hazard data book of existing chemicals, available from web site, http://www.cerij.or.jp/db/sheet/hazard_databook.htm.

[19] Yukawa, K., Hirashima, T., Tsunekawa, M., Suyama, T., Sasaki, K., Fukushima, M., Kobayashi, H., Hirai, T., Characterization of liquid products obtained from hot water-drying treatment of low rank coal and their ability of Cr(VI) reduction. *Shigen to sozai*, 119 (4-5), 161-169 (2003), (in Japanese).

Section 5
Risk prevention and monitoring

Climate change, migratory species and pandemic influenza

K. Duncan
University of Toronto, Canada

Abstract

Environment and health dominate international journals, newspapers, and global search engines with climate change and avian flu usurping world headlines. Global mean temperature is projected to increase 1.1-6.4°C over the coming century, a rise greater than any increase experienced by humans during the past 10,000 years. Climate change is a growing concern to the World Health Organization (WHO) because of its potentially serious health consequences, including an increase in illness and death related to extreme temperature events, weather events, and infectious disease.

A more pressing issue for the WHO is pandemic flu, which leading influenza experts fear is inevitable, if not imminent; for example, evidence suggests that influenza A H5N1 is now endemic in parts of Asia, is affecting new mammalian hosts, is expanding its geographic range, and is increasingly pathogenic.

Future climate change is likely to impact migratory bird species, their breeding and non-breeding areas, migration routes, and stopover sites. This paper will therefore first discuss environmental controls for key migratory species, and how climate change may influence their survival and distribution, and possibly affect the spread of highly pathogenic influenza. This paper will then discuss other possible impacts of climate change on pandemic influenza.
Keywords: global climate change, pandemic influenza, migratory birds, climatic impacts.

1 Introduction

Global mean temperature is projected to increase 1.1-6.4°C over the coming century, a rise greater than any increase experienced by humans during the past 10,000 years (IPCC [1]). Climate change is a growing concern to the World

Health Organization (WHO) because of its potentially serious health consequences, including an increase in illness and death related to extreme temperature events, weather events, and infectious disease (Duncan [2]).

A more pressing issue for the WHO is pandemic flu, which leading influenza experts fear is inevitable, if not imminent; for example, evidence suggests that influenza A H5N1 is now endemic in parts of Asia, is affecting new mammalian hosts, is expanding its geographic range, and is increasingly pathogenic (Duncan [3]). Between February, 2006, and April, 2006, 32 countries, located in Africa, Asia, Europe, and the Middle East, reported their first cases in birds. This spread marks the fastest and most extensive geographical spread of any highly pathogenic influenza virus since the disease was first described in 1878. The virus has now affected some of the world's most densely populated and impoverished regions – areas poorly served by health care and surveillance systems (Duncan [4–5]).

Future climate change is likely to impact migratory bird species, their breeding and non-breeding areas, migration routes, and stopover sites. This paper will therefore explore the environmental controls for key migratory species, and how climate change may influence their survival and distribution, and possibly affect the spread of highly pathogenic influenza.

2 Environmental health

Restoring health to the world's ecosystems must be an essential component in the strategy to reduce human vulnerability to emerging and re-emerging diseases (Chivian [6]); McMichael [7]; and WHO [8]). Unfortunately, environmental factors (including high concentrations of poultry production, especially in areas with high human population densities, and poultry production in major wild bird flyway zones) have, in part, given rise to the pandemic influenza threat (IISD [9]).

It is important to address the environment because the control of many infectious diseases requires an understanding of the causative agent, the vector, the host and the environment in which transmission occurs. The most pressing environmental issue facing humankind is climate change, and as a result, it warrants exploration, as does its possible impacts on the spread of influenza.

2.1 Climate change

According to the Intergovernmental Panel on Climate Change (IPCC)'s *Fourth Assessment Report*, 'warming of the climate is now unequivocal, as is now evident from observations of increases in global air temperatures, widespread melting of snow and ice, and rising global average sea level.' More disturbing is the fact that most of the observed warming is likely due to increased concentrations of GHGs (IPCC [1]).

Continued GHG emissions at or above current rates would cause further warming 'and induce changes in the global climate system that would very likely be larger than those observed during the 20th century'. Global mean temperature is projected to increase 1.1-6.4°C over the coming century (IPCC [1]), a rise greater than any increase experienced by humans during the past 10,000 years (Houghton et al. [10–12]). Anthropogenic warming and sea level rise would continue for centuries due to the timescales associated with climate processes and feedbacks, even if GHGs were to be stabilized (IPCC [1]). Susceptibility to climate change differs across countries, populations, regions and sectors (Cohen and Miller [12] and McCarthy et al. [13]).

3 Influenza

Influenza, like climate change, is receiving worldwide attention, as countries, organizations, and individuals prepare to mitigate its effects. Briefly, influenza is a unique respiratory viral disease infecting the whole respiratory tract, namely, the nose, sinuses, throat, lungs, and even the middle ear. The disease is spread from person-to-person by airborne droplets produced when an infected individual coughs or sneezes. Acute symptoms of influenza, including fever, headache, shivering, muscle pain, cough, and pneumonia, are the result of the virus replicating in the respiratory tract where infected cells die and slough off (Collier and Oxford [14]).

The influenza virus exists in three forms, called A, B, and C, but only A and B cause significant disease in humans. Despite the virus's three forms, all influenza viruses look similar. They are roughly spherical particles, 80-120 nm in diameter, containing a nucleoprotein core of RNA and a lipid envelope from which two distinct forms of glycoprotein project – the rod-shaped haemagglutinin (H) and the mushroom-shaped neuraminidase (N). A third protein structure, called the matrix (M1) protein layer, lines the surface of the virus, and contains M2 molecules (Hill and Knowlton [15]).

Today there is no effective cure, which works against all influenza viruses. Current prevention for influenza is by annual vaccination, particularly for high-risk groups such as those with respiratory disease, heart disease, renal trouble, and diabetes (Collier and Oxford [14]). Vaccination is given by intra-muscular injection, 6-8 weeks before the influenza season. In general, most studies suggest that vaccines reduce the frequency of severe illness, "but do less to reduce the overall frequency of infection" (Collier and Oxford [14]). The closer the vaccine is in structure to the antigenic composition of the circulating strain of virus, the more effective it is. Vaccine efficacy varies greatly from about 20% to as high as 90% depending on the patient group. Protection rates of 70-90% can be achieved in young healthy adults when vaccine and epidemic strains are closely matched (Hill and Knowlton [15]).

Influenza infection can be attenuated with the use of antiviral drugs, such as oseltamivir (Tamiflu), amantadine and rimantidine. Over-the-counter medication is also available to help ease fever and sore throats, reduce coughing, unblock sinuses, etc. Unfortunately, none of these drugs has an effect on the underlying influenza infection (Hill and Knowlton [15]; and Duncan [16]).

3.1 Avian Influenza

Avian influenza refers to a large group of influenza viruses that primarily affect birds. On rare occasions, these bird viruses can infect other species, including humans (Horimoto and Kawaoka [17]). An influenza pandemic occurs when a new influenza subtype emerges that has not previously circulated in humans. Avian Influenza virus H5N1, which causes cyanosis of the un-feathered skin, diarrhea, excessive lacrimation, edema of the head and face, respiratory distress, sinusitis, and even sudden death, is a strain with pandemic potential, since it might ultimately mutate into a strain that is contagious among humans (OIE [18, 19]; and Liu et al. [20]). Once this mutation occurs, it will no longer be a bird virus – it will be a human influenza virus.

3.1.1 Epidemiology

The principal vectors in the spread of H5N1 are the migration of wild birds harboring the virus – H5N1 infections have been found in dead bar-headed geese (*Anser indicus*), brown-headed gulls *(Larus brunnicephalus*), great black-headed gulls (*Larus ichthyaetus*), great cormorants (*Phalacrocorax carbo*), and ruddy shelducks *(Tadorna ferruginea)*–, and trade in domestic poultry. From April to June, 2005, more than 6000 migratory birds, comprised mainly of the above species, died of H5N1 infection at the Qinghai Lake Nature Reserve in China's Qinghai Province. More recently, migratory ducks have been shown to be asymptomatically carrying the H5N1 virus in Hong Kong and elsewhere in China (Chen et al. [21]).

Low pathogenic avian influenza (LPAI) viruses have been isolated from at least 105 wild bird species of 26 different families. Although many wild bird species may harbor influenza viruses, birds of aquatic and wetland environments, such as the Anseriformes (particularly ducks, geese, and swans) and Charadriiformes (particularly gulls, terns, and waders) constitute the major natural LPAI virus reservoir. Anseriformes and Charadriiformes are distributed globally, except in the most arid regions of the world (Olsen et al. [22]).

When wild migratory birds mix with domestic flocks through sharing of habitat, there is an enhanced potential for genetic re-assortment of avian influenza viruses, resulting in novel genotypes, which could trigger a human influenza pandemic. Once avian influenza is established in domestic poultry, it is a highly contagious disease. Infected birds excrete virus in high concentration in their feces and in nasal and ocular discharges. Once introduced into a flock, the virus is spread from flock to flock by contaminated equipment, egg flats, feed trucks, movement of infected birds, service crews, etc. (FAO [23–25]). Airborne transmission may occur if birds are in close proximity and with appropriate air movement (OIE [18]).

3.1.1.2 Migration Migration, a common strategy for birds occupying seasonal habitats, may range from short local movements to intercontinental migrations. Migratory birds can carry pathogens, particularly those that do not significantly affect the birds' health status. Many Anseriformes and Charadriiformes are known to perform regular long-distance migrations, thereby potentially distributing LPAI viruses between countries or even continents.

Birds breeding in one geographic region often follow similar migratory flyways: for example, the East Asian–Australian flyway from eastern Siberia south to eastern Asia and Australia. However the major flyways are simplified models of complex ecological-behavioral relationships, and there are numerous exceptions where populations perform differently from the common patterns (Lincoln et al. [26]; and Migratory Bird Center [27]).

Migrating birds rarely fly the full distance between breeding and non-breeding areas without stopping over and refuelling. Many species therefore aggregate at favorable stopover or wintering sites, resulting in high local densities. These sites may be important for transmission of LPAI viruses between wild and domestic birds, and between different species (Olsen et al., [22]). One gram of contaminated manure can contain enough HPAI virus to infect one million birds (IISD [9]).

Unfortunately, the understanding of the global distribution of LPAI viruses in wild bird populations is still limited despite intense surveillance studies that have been performed in Eurasia and North America (Olsen et al. [22]).

4 Weather and migration

Weather can influence breeding success (through chilling or starving young) foraging conditions, and necessary behaviors, such as courtship. Extreme weather events, such as droughts and prolonged freezing, can have catastrophic effects on bird populations; El Niño events, which warm the waters off the west coast of South America, cause fish populations to crash, and ultimately, adult mortality among seabirds in the Pacific.

Weather has a profound influence on bird migrations. For a first example, temperature affects the rate of pre-migratory preparation. Maintaining body temperature under cold stress reduces the energy that might be stored as fat in preparation for the migratory journey. Therefore an earlier, warmer spring accelerates the preparation, while a cooler, later spring inhibits the process, and delays species arrival. During both spring and fall migrations, the primary stimulus for departure is the wind. In the spring, the wind is from the south, and in the fall, it is from the north in North America.

Areas of high and low pressures also affect migration. During fall migration, birds flying south usually travel the day after passage of a cold front with its brisk north winds and dropping temperatures; as wind direction becomes more variable and wind velocity decreases as high pressure begins to dominate, birds stop to feed.

Soaring birds, such as eagles, hawks, ospreys, and vultures are particularly dependent on proper wind conditions for migration, as migrants soar on convective thermals that are generated by the differential heating of the Earth's surface. It is estimated that the normal pre-migratory fat load of 100 grams in a Broad-winged Hawk would be exhausted in only five days of flapping flight. But by spiraling among thermals, its stored fat would last 20 days, more than enough time to provide energy for its 3,000-mile journey (Lincoln et al. [26]; and Migratory Bird Center [27]).

Indirectly, weather can influence the abundance and activity of nest predators; the abundance and availability of food, which influence frequency of double-brooding, nestling survival, and hence seasonal fecundity; settlement patterns; and synchrony of settling, which, in turn, affects local density.

5 Climate change and migration

Birds are affected directly by climate; for example, they tolerate only a narrow range of temperature or rainfall. Therefore climate affects where birds live. Migratory species occupy several different areas of the planet in the course of their lives, while residents are confined to a much narrower range of climatic conditions. They are also affected indirectly—for example, through the effects of climate on their habitat and food supply (Migratory Bird Center [27]).

It is difficult to separate direct and indirect effects, but in the case of North American songbirds, January temperatures and the availability of suitable habitat determine winter distribution. Therefore as winters become warmer, bird distributions are likely to change. The implications of climate change—that is, long-term shifts in average weather—on migratory bird species have only recently begun to be addressed. There is already strong evidence that animals and plants have been affected by recent climate change. Impacts include changes in breeding performance (e.g. egg size, nesting success, etc.), changes in population distribution and size, and changes in timing of migration BOU/ECSA [28]).

Many of the changes expected in birds as a result of changing climate are subtle. One of the most common changes recorded in other parts of the world is that birds start nesting earlier. In many species, the signal to lay the first egg is temperature, as it is often a good predictor of food supplies (insects) for the young. And so, if springs become warmer, birds will breed earlier. In North America, Tree Swallows breed nine days earlier today that they did 30 years ago. In Britain, some species nest as many as 18 days earlier than 30 or 40 years ago. Climate change will also profoundly affect migration, as birds must time their flights with food supplies as they pass through multiple regions. For example, in order for the Semipalmated Sandpiper to make its flight successfully, it must take off with a tail wind and at the right time in order to coincide with the availability of its food (mud-shrimps). Its nesting grounds (Arctic tundra), wintering grounds (tropical mudflats) and migration habitat (temperate mudflats) are all susceptible to the effects of rising sea level.

Climate change is causing sea levels to rise now. It is important to note that birds have been adapting to changing climates throughout their long evolutionary history, and will no doubt continue to do so. Yet current and predicted climate changes differ in two important ways from earlier, natural changes: namely, they are faster, and they are taking place in addition to additional environmental changes, such as chemical contamination and habitat loss and fragmentation (Lincoln et al. [26]; BOU/ECSA [28]; and Migratory Bird Center [27]).

6 Climate change and pandemic influenza

6.1 Climate change, migratory species, and pandemic influenza

From the above discussion, it is abundantly clear that weather and climate profoundly affect bird migration, and likely therefore play a role in the spread of avian influenza. Fortunately, the summer and fall of 2006 were relatively 'quiet' regarding avian influenza with Africa enduring no resurgence, Europe experiencing no cases since the outbreak in Turkey, and Vietnam, a previous hot-spot for avian influenza, suffering no cases. Specialists suggest that this quiet period has resulted from public health actions, such as risk-reduction education and measures, and improved monitoring systems.

But experts caution that the H5N1 virus has not disappeared, and could, in fact, be smouldering. *Scientific American* reported on January 9th that a farmer in eastern China had contracted the H5N1 virus in December – the country's first human case of avian influenza since July, and Indonesia confirmed a death and second case in 2007 (WHO [29]).

Could warm temperatures have been playing a role in the fall quiescence? Provisional temperature data chronicle 2006 as the sixth-warmest year on record since 1850. Record-breaking temperatures occurred throughout Europe, which experienced its warmest fall in 500 years. Central England, where temperature records extend back to 1659, recorded its warmest July, September, and autumn temperatures, and Switzerland reported November and early-December temperature readings 10°C above normal (Met Office [30]; and Planetark [31]). Anecdotally, in North America, New York City experienced no snowfall in November and December for the first time since 1877. In December 2006, buds appeared on apple trees in Maryland, while crocuses pushed up through the ground in New Jersey, and frogs, which normally hibernate through the winter months, were emerging, thinking spring had come.

The British Royal Society for the Protection of Birds and leading experts forecast that with increasing winter warmth, some birds will not migrate, or will migrate later in the season. The events of 2006 would seem to support their predictions. In December, European birds, including ducks, robins, and thrushes, failed to fly south from Scandinavia because of mild temperatures, and swans, which usually arrive in Britain from Siberia in October, stopped for longer than average because of an ample food supply in countries such as Estonia.

Perhaps this fall's 'calm' before the proverbial storm has been linked, in part, to warmer temperatures, and fewer, shorter bird migrations (Met Office [30]; and Planetark [31]). Regardless, it has bought us time to prepare. Even though H5N1 virus has largely fallen off media radar screens, it has not done so for public health officials, who remain concerned that the virus may mutate and become easily transmissible among humans.

6.2 Climate change, ice, and influenza

Warming will profoundly affect Earth, causing sea level to rise, and glaciers and permafrost to melt. More immediately, the United Kingdom's Met Office predicts that 2007 may become the warmest year on record (Met Office [30]). Warmer temperatures could mean that bodies of victims of pandemics, such as the 1918 Spanish influenza, could float to the surface of the permafrost. These bodies could pose a potential risk.

If this seems unlikely, the possibility was a concern to American scientists as early as 1996. Scientists were concerned that victims of smallpox and Spanish influenza might float to the surface of the Earth with warming or erode out of riparian environments, as rivers cut new courses with climate change. Burying a body in permafrost is akin to storing it in a freezer, which perfectly preserves food, and does not allow for decomposition. Permafrost might preserve the body and the virus – and perhaps serve as a source of infection (Duncan [16]).

But ice, and particularly lake ice, may also pose a risk. Migratory birds fly south in the fall, visiting lakes along their paths, and shed influenza virus into the water. In winter, the lakes freeze, and thus preserve influenza A virus for months, years, and perhaps much longer; microbes encased in glacial ice have been shown to be viable for hundreds of thousands of years. In spring, thawing releases trapped, current and past virus into the water – and perhaps may explain the re-emergence of past influenza A viruses decades after their initial emergence.

In the short term, warm winters may delay annual bird migration, and the spread of seasonal/pandemic influenza. And in the long term, warmer temperatures may thaw bodies/ice, and release current/past strains of influenza virus.

7 Summary and challenges

The information presented here highlights the need to scientifically test the linkages between climate change and influenza. Scientific study requires overcoming methodological challenges. For example, which climatic variables should be used, as migratory birds are exposed to a range of weather systems during their annual cycle? Should local weather variables or large-scale weather patterns be used? Which measures of migration should be used—first arrival dates/last dates, fitness and population consequences of migration? Can researchers undertake meta-analyses demonstrating why some species respond strongly to climate change and others do not?

References

[1] IPCC. 2007. Climate change 2007: the physical basis. Summary for policymakers. http://www.ipcc.ch. 26/02/07.

[2] Duncan, K. 2006 a. Climate change, health, and women. Climate Change and Health Impacts Atlantic Conference 2006. St. John's, Newfoundland and Labrador, March 23-24, 2006.

[3] Duncan, K. 2006 b. Forewarned is forearmed. The 2006 Conference Board of Canada CSR Conference. Toronto, Canada, May 17, 2006.

[4] Duncan, K. 2006 c. Pandemic flu: current threat and call for ethics. *Management Ethics.* Spring, 2006.
[5] Duncan, K. 2006 d. Ethics Still Un-Addressed In Pandemic Preparedness: Possible Planning Guidelines. *Management Ethics*, Fall, 2006.
[6] Chivian, E. 1993. *Critical Condition: Human Health and the Environment.* MIT Press.
[7] McMichael, A. 2005. Modern life has brought humans and microbes closer than ever before. *The Sydney Morning Herald*, October 17, 2005.
[8] WHO. 2005. Human health under threat from ecosystem degradation. Media release. December 9 2005.
[9] IISD. 2006. Scientific seminar on avian influenza, the environment, and migratory birds. http://www.iisd.ca/ymb/ais/ymbvol123num1e.html. 9/01/07.
[10] Houghton, J., Filho, L., Callender, B. et al. 1995. *Climate Change 1995: The Science of Climate Change.* Contribution of Working Group I to the Second Assessment Report of the Intergovernmental Panel on Climate Change (IPCC). Cambridge University Press.
[11] Houghton, J., Ding, Y., Griggs, D. et al. (eds). 2001. *Climate Change 2001: The Scientific Basis.* Contribution of Working Group I to the Third Assessment Report of the Intergovernmental Panel on Climate Change (IPCC). Cambridge University Press.
[12] Cohen, S. and Miller, K. 2001. North America. In: McCarthy, J., Canziani, O., Leary, N. et al. *Climate Change 2001: Impacts, Adaptation, and Vulnerability.* Contribution of Working Group II to the Third Assessment Report of the Intergovernmental Panel on Climate Change (IPCC). Cambridge University Press.
[13] McCarthy, J., Canziani, O., Leary, N. et al. 2001. *Climate Change 2001: Impacts, Adaptation, and Vulnerability.* Contribution of Working Group II to the Third Assessment Report of the Intergovernmental Panel on Climate Change (IPCC). Cambridge University Press.
[14] Collier, L. and Oxford, J. 1996. *Human Virology: A Text for Students of Medicine, Dentistry, and Microbiology.* Oxford University Press.
[15] Hill and Knowlton, 1998. *The 1918 Project.* Hill and Knowlton.
[16] Duncan, K. 2003. *Hunting the 1918 Flu: One Scientist's Search for a Killer Virus.* University of Toronto Press.
[17] Horimoto, T. and Kawaoka, Y. 2001. Pandemic threat posed by avian influenza A viruses. *Clinical Microbiological Review* 14(1):129-49.
[18] OIE. 2004. Highly pathogenic avian influenza. International Health Code. Chap 2.7.12. 2004 Manual of Diagnostic Tests and Vaccines for Terrestrial Animals. Avian influenza. http://www.oie.int/eng/normes /MMANUAL/A_00037.htm. 30/12/06.
[19] OIE. 2006. Highly pathogenic avian influenza. http://www.oie.int/eng /maladies/fiches/a_A150.htm. 30/12/06.
[20] Liu, J., Xiao, H., Lei, F. et al. 2005. Highly pathogenic H5N1 influenza virus infection in migratory birds. *Science* 2005 Aug 19; 309(5738):1206.

[21] Chen, H., Smith, G., Zhang, S. et al. 2005. Avian flu: H5N1 virus outbreak in migratory waterfowl. *Nature* Jul 14; 436(7048):191-2.
[22] Olsen, B., Munster, V., Wallensten, A. et al. 2006. Global patterns of influenza A virus in wild birds. *Science* 2006 Apr 12; 312:384-8.
[23] FAO/OIE/WHO. 2004. Joint warning: domestic ducks could pose a new Avian influenza threat. Nov 11, 2004.
[24] FAO. 2005. Wild birds expected to spread bird flu virus further. FAO news release. August 31, 2005.
[25] FAO. 2006. FAO and IOE International Scientific Conference on Avian Influenza and Wild Birds. http://www.fao.org/ag/againfo /subjects/en/health/diseases-cards/conference/index_en.html. 8/01/07.
[26] Lincoln, F., Peterson, S., and Zimmerman, J. 1998. Migration of birds. U.S. Department of the Interior, U.S. Fish and Wildlife Service, Washington, D.C. Circular 16. Jamestown, ND: Northern Prairie Wildlife Research Center Online. http://www.npwrc.usgs.gov/resource/birds /migratio/index.htm. 10/01/07.
[27] Migratory Bird Center. 2006. The effect of climate change on migratory birds. http://nationalzoo.si.edu/Conservationandscience/Migratorybirds /Research/Climate_Change/default.cfm. 05/01/07.
[28] BOU/ECSA. 2002. *Conference Report: Climate Change and Coastal Birds.* A joint BOU/ECSA (Estuarine and Coastal Studies Association) conference, University of Hull, 22-24 March 2002.
[29] WHO. 2007. Cumulative number of confirmed human cases of Avian Influenza A/(H5N1) reported to WHO. http://www.who.int/csr/disease /avian_influenza/country/cases_table_2007_02_19/en/index.html. 23/02/07.
[30] Met Office. 2006. World weather impacts. Warmth delays bird migrations. http://www.metoffice.gov.uk/weather/impacts/200612 /18016131.html. 05/01/07.
[31] Planetark. 2006. Warm winter keeps migrating birds at home. Some European birds delay migration due to warmth. Planetark.org, Dec. 20, 2006. http://www.heatisonline.org/contentserver/objecthandlers /index.cfm?id=6193&method=full. 30/12/06.

Environmental education and the health risk question: how do we educate the educators working with this theme?

D. M. Bianchini Bonotto
Departamento de Educação, Instituto de Biociências, UNESP, Rio Claro, Brazil

Abstract

Our society is presently seeing a trend of continuous increase of risk with severe consequences, especially those linked to environmental aspects. It has obligated us to reflect on this production and its effects, either positive or negative, and, after a long reflection, to think about the adopted model of civilization and the possibilities of changing such a model. The educational institution is among the social departments responsible for this revision process, since it represents one possibility to promote a more critical vision from society, providing it with tools needed for a more responsible action. However, schools are dominated by a traditional work, which does not allow for enough and proper attention to these relevant and current questions, and which involve a critical analysis of the conceptions and values established by our civilization, resulting in the present patterns of science-technology-society relations and their influence on the environment and health. Several research works have indicated a diversity of barriers that obstruct this necessary change. Since formal education plays an important role in the education of society for this theme, in this paper the possibilities and difficulty dealing with this problem are discussed, focusing on the question of teacher education, based on investigations related to teacher education programs for environmental education. The data collected show the urgency for introducing this theme in teacher training programs, taking into account the fact that educators have their own conceptions, values and attitudes that should be considered in these programs.
Keywords: environmental education, risk literacy, health education, teacher education programs.

doi:10.2495/EHR070231

1 Introduction

In our contemporary society, the growing number of scientific and technological activities has resulted in a series of new products and growing influences that affect the entire world and our lives. For instance, recent biotechnological processes have generated genetically modified foods that play a part in farming and supermarkets in several countries. At the same time, discussions about whether enough research has been conducted to indicate that environmental or health problems derivate from these processes are presented, showing other interests involved in these researches and the social nature of scientific activity, intrinsically linked to social, economic and political influences.

Through this question, ingenuous observers or consumers believe that these products mean an unquestionable benefit to society, and with this view, they can be interpreted as a sign of progress and welfare, with total confidence in the defenders and sellers of this technology and the products derived from it. For others, in a radical opposite position, these apparent benefits presented by scientific and technological "advances" are essentially negative and must be fought off.

In fact, dealing with this specific matter and many similar others, we are presently seeing a trend of continuous increase in environmental risks, many of them having severe consequences, which have obligated our society to reflect on these productions and products, with their positive and/or negative consequences, without yielding, as Kneller [1] points out, to a superficial optimism or a frenetic hostility.

Thus, the enhancement of the human action impact allowed for the idea of environmental risk, calling for efforts towards the assessment of these risks, at a certain point predictable by modeling and interpretative techniques.

However, neither the possibilities of these technical predictions are total nor these assessment processes are a question of scientific procedures only, because, on further reflection, evaluating them and our choices are also a question of a worldview and the model of society constructed from this view. Based on this broad approach, as Jacobi [2] stresses, we must think about the adopted model of society and the possibilities of changing such a model, participating in this change at individual and collective levels.

This calls for a society prepared for this task, and the educational institution is among the social departments responsible for this process, since it represents one possibility of promoting a more critical view from society, providing it with tools needed for a more responsible action related to such task. Environmental education should develop democratic forms of popular participation, thus allowing society to learn how to collectively fight for their rights, as well as be responsible for a more balanced and healthier environment, surpassing the limitations of waiting and confidentially obey the decisions taken by specialists and government agencies [3], either acting according to influences of the media or minor interests.

In terms of official proposals and curricular documents, these aims have been presented and have been made public around the world in the last decades. In the case of Brazil, in the late 90s the Brazilian Federal Board of Education proposed the inclusion of Environment and Health among the themes to be explored at the country's schools, indicating the need to deal with these issues at all school levels and through an interdisciplinary approach.

These documents show that these themes have great community relevance and, in order to be conveniently dealt with, it should not remain restricted to a single school discipline only. They also indicate that this educative work should deal not only with knowledge and skills content but also within a broader approach, with value content too, aiming at an education for citizenship.

However, in spite of these references and documents, schools are dominated by traditional work, which does not allow for enough and proper attention to these relevant and current questions. Several researches, focusing on different subjects, aspects of the teaching and learning processes, school and curricular politics, have indicated a diversity of barriers that obstruct this necessary change.

Clément et al [4] presented some preliminary results coming from pilot tests developed during the first year of the European project "Biology, Health and Environmental Education for better Citizenship", finding that teaching/learning related to "questions vives" in Biology, Health and environmental issues is confronted to very different ways of thinking depending on the socio-economic and cultural contexts of each country. These aspects must be considered when these issues are dealt with, which means a great challenge to educators, since there is non-familiarity of the teachers to deal with the value content in education as a whole [5], something necessary to deal with these cultural dimensions.

Dawson [6] pointed out that, despite the increasing importance of biotechnology topics in our society, it is not regularly taught in schools, stressing the desirability of awareness of the development and range of student's understandings and attitudes may lead to a more appropriate use of biotechnology curriculum materials and thus improved biotechnology education in schools.

Aikenhead [7] discussed the "science for all" versus "science for an elite" dilemma that has plagued Science and Technology Education throughout 150 years of science education's formal existence. He argued that, although the last one – the traditional vision of school science – has been the status quo all these years, the first, called by him as a humanistic-cultural approach, has experienced a renaissance since the World War II. It promotes practical utility, human values, and a connectedness with personal and societal issues. According to this author over the past 40 years a considerable amount of research has accumulated that now provides solid evidence for understanding the educational needs of students. However, he stressed the tension between educational soundness and political reality,

that can force us to compromise our choices when we confront non-rational realities such as historical precedence, pressure from universities, directives from professional interest groups, and science and technology teachers who hold preconceptions at odds with humanistic-cultural approach to school science (p.12).

In accordance with this proposition, and specifically concerning the question of environmental risks, as Riechard [8], it has been pointed out that, despite the fact that the accurate perceptions of risk are necessary for the attainment of a risk-literate society, the public education system has been treated as a peripheral aspect of the risk policy process. So, practically no attention is given to the improvement of this task. It explains the findings of Vargas et al (2003), that, in a preliminary study about the productions found in the Educational Material Collection of an Environmental and Health Education Laboratory, indicated the occurrence of voids in preventive education approaches, such as the need to better integrate concerns about AIDS and reproductive health with healthy policies and actions.

Taking this situation into account, in this paper I intend to focus on the question of teacher education for environmental education (EE) in general, since the teacher is an essential element in the effective implementation of any innovation [10]. I focus on the question from data collected at two exploratory researches that investigated the teachers' learning in environmental education programs, pointing out aspects that can help those who intend to draw up proposals involving environmental risks in general and the health questions associated with them, considering that they are part of EE contents.

I agree with the authors who do not conceive of teacher education programs as limited to a transmission of knowledge and skills [11–13]. Teachers are not mere consumers of academic knowledge and proposals presented to them in pre- or in-service courses, because they are active knowledge-makers. Learning to teach is really a complex process involving affective, cognitive and ethical factors, amongst others [13]. Thus, teacher education also consists of an investigation problem, as it seeks to elucidate different aspects involved in this process. As a consequence, teacher education for a differentiated educational content, as shown in this paper, has led me into two exploratory researches, trying to find how the apprehension and incorporation of this content occurs.

These researches, in a qualitative approach [14], involved interventions carried out by myself. One intervention was directed towards a group of in-service teachers and the other towards pre-service teachers, during two teacher education programs that I carried out. In these programs, the teachers have some time to discuss basic topics of EE, using the remaining time to prepare and carry out their classes, seeking to incorporate those aspects.

My goal was to investigate the teachers' learning how to deal with basic topics of EE, and point out relevant aspects involved in apprehending and incorporating them in their classes. The data were collected from my field notes and all kinds of writing done by the teachers, such as their exercises, personal reflections and teaching plans.

After analyzing all the data, I could identify some key issues that I will now present by showing excerpts from the teachers' writing that illustrate them. In order to preserve their identity, teachers were identified by letters.

2 The novelty of the subject and the process of construction and reconstruction of knowledge about it

The teachers had, in general, a traditional naturalist and conservationist model of EE, having the basic aim at changing individual behavior, in which the structural causes of the environmental problems are presented as nonsocial or universal, and are unrelated to the underlying social forces [15].

The teachers demonstrated good acceptance of the exhibited conception of broad EE, in which the natural and cultural aspects interpenetrate in the composition of the environment, according to the following report:

The enlarged EE approach involving political, economic and social issues is clearer to me. There were some obscure aspects that I can say I understand now. For example, I did not know that social problems could be included in EE, or if it should only be treated by the Social Sciences; but I know it now (B).

Referring to the conceptions and value content of the environmental question, involving the Science-Technology-Society (STS) relations, a pre-service teacher that had reflected on the view of society-nature separation established by our present society wrote:

The [question] man-nature dichotomy has become very clear to me. I had not thought about this before (K.E.).

However, it was not easy for them to deepen their knowledge of this referential while dealing with the aspects focusing on beliefs and values involving STS relations and the environmental question. Pre-service teacher B.B. clearly explained to me his difficulty seeing the value within the general content of science classes, probably due to the fact that he was only prepared for the "traditional work" throughout his school life. In-service teacher R. identified and very clearly expressed the difficulty modifying her vision of a scientist (an unusual and special human being), according to the following report:

(...) I confess that I am still bound to the conception of a scientist as someone distant from the actual world (R).

This last report indicates a difficulty changing conceptions. Despite the fact that she understood the different conceptions, she shows us that it cannot be quickly modified by/after a discussion. A change depends on other factors and one discussion can mean only the beginning of the process.

Another moment that indicated the complexity of this process occurred when teachers prepared and developed their teaching plans. The in-service teachers exposed their difficulties leading their classes to aspects focusing the STS relations and the environmental question, as follows:

Maybe I can not yet argue when an issue on how to accommodate development and the environment is raised (...) *how to work with a society where the persons currently aim at jobs and a comfortable life so that the environment is not part of their own life proposals* (L).

So as to exemplify these difficulties, one pre-service teacher focused on a theme related to medicinal plants, considering aspects of the conflict between the use popular knowledge of medicinal teas and medicines provided by the pharmaceutical industry. That teacher included a reflection "*concerning the use of allopathic drugs and its possible replacement by home-made medicinal teas*" in her plan. She also intended to deal with "*the question of the marketing done by the big pharmaceutical companies*" as one proposed discussion (P).

Despite the fact that it was laudable to present the controversy between the medicinal homemade teas use and the companies doing marketing, I have found a "dichotomist" approach to the question of the manufactured and homemade drugs while analyzing the entire teaching plan. The teacher proposed an appreciation and valuation of the homemade drugs and their relationship with and old tradition. As for the manufactured drugs, it was suggested "*to think about their use/abuse and to recognize them as drugs*" (in a bad sense), as a clear opposition. After analyzing the plan, I pointed out this problem to the teacher who agreed with me. However, since I did not observe the teachers' classes, I cannot confirm whether this dichotomist approach was actually changed.

Considering that the subject treated in the programs is filled with conceptions and concepts that can be deepened more and more [16], I think that such learning calls for a process of continuous construction and reconstruction of knowledge. Also, considering the novelty that this subject means to teachers and taking into account its importance to our society, its study requires an urgent education effort, by introducing it into initial and permanent teacher education programs, which have a design that allows us to follow the process of teachers' learning, which is difficult to do in factual and short time designs.

3 Emergent feelings

Another aspect that was captured in these research works refers to the feelings manifested during reflections on conceptions and values of society and the educative work to deal with them. The suggestion to modify traditional practices, dealing with a changing of conceptions and values to construct a new model of society is not an easy matter for teachers.

The discussions about the relationship between the environmental question and our society's capitalist and consumption model, as well as the deep proposals to change this model, caused discouragement and feelings of disbelief for the group of in-service teachers.

In their writing, they exhibited signs of insecurity and doubts after some discussions. This mainly occurred when they reflected on the intensity of the necessary changes and how our daily actions – personal and pedagogic – are distant from those considered more appropriate in terms of the presented referential. Some teachers also referred to their own values, which they had not clearly recognized before, as the following reports suggest:

The present-day activities showed how difficult it is to change. By the way, is it possible? I saw that all these things are already part of our culture and they represent a habit acquired before birth. I particularly adore technology, new things (...) (V).

The time at which we analyzed the content of poetries made me reflect on my own values, on the things that are actually relevant to my life (E. A. S. O.).

The reflections on environmental problems and the values and choices of our present model of society necessarily promote the examination of teachers' own values, which is not an easy matter. And as Aikenhead [7] pointed out, teachers' values, beliefs and ideologies must be in harmony before a teacher teaches subjects related to these aspects.

In the group of pre-service teachers, some of them clearly exposed their fear and insecurity of having an authoritarian attitude when dealing with the value content of the environmental question, as we can see in the following statement:

The values education is a difficult task, because sometimes we do what we cannot do. The education that I received imposed opinions on me, and then it is not easy for me to do it differently. (F.A.K)

I conclude that, besides knowledge, feelings must also be considered an important content of teacher education programs, and, consequently, they must be handled with care [17], having a confidence space to be showed and worked. This is another aspect to be properly addressed in teacher education programs concerning the theme, making it possible to work the anxieties arising from the aim of favoring the intended changing process. As Gayford and Dillon [18] pointed out, a simple preoccupation with knowledge and conceptual understandings denies the role of the emotions and the wider aspects of "knowing" should involve consideration of it too.

4 The tendency to work with conceptual content

When dealing with the need to work with ethical questions and the values content of environmental problems, practically all teachers agreed on the need to work with them at school, but the question about how to do it is not easy for them. Many pre-service teachers investigated here became surprised at the discussions involving the value content in educative work, as the following statement shows us:

I had never deeply thought about the values the teacher can pass on to their students and the way such theme may be worked. (M.F.G.)

The difficulties understanding and dealing with the value content in the teaching and learning process, presented in the literature [19, 20], were clearly verified in these investigations, not only during the classes and written exercises, in which the issue was raised, but also in the teaching plans.

Practically all teaching plans had a tendency to emphasize conceptual content, and I had to indicate it to all teachers, encouraging them to look for the value content of the subjects they would teach.

When I assigned pre-service teachers a written exercise asking them to analyze their previous teaching plans (the ones they had prepared before our classes about values) and examine the value content of the subject matter they had intended to teach, some of them perceived the absence of specific propositions for this content.

They had difficulty detecting the values content of a theme, such as describing it in their plans. In some cases, concepts and understandings are presented as values, demonstrating that it is not clear for many of them what a concept, idea or fact is, and which values and valuations are linked to them. During the initial classes, pre-service teacher B.B. clearly explained to me his difficulty seeing the value within the general content of science classes, probably due to the fact he was only prepared to the "traditional work" in his school life.

Since the broader educative work that is necessary to handle the environmental question in its broad approach must deal with values subjacent to this, the difficulties teachers go through to deal with values must be considered; and teacher education programs have to place special attention to this aspect – warning teachers of the tendency for this content to be forgotten – which can allow for a better incorporation of an intentional and specific educative work with the value content.

5 Final considerations

The data collected show the urgency for introducing themes related to EE in trainee teachers programs, since the traditional school is either distant from these actual needs or focus on them improperly. Educators generally have a lack of knowledge of theses matters, and are informed about them basically through the media. On the other hand, beyond the aspect of knowledge, the teachers' conceptions, values and attitudes, beliefs and disbeliefs (the ones they will bring into their practices, although sometimes they are hidden) must be considered in any training program.

Bearing in mind that the incorporation of an innovation in teacher practices does not occur automatically, the programs cannot contain only lectures, but also activities, discussions and enough time for teachers to try bringing the innovation into their practices even during the programs.

Finally, considering that there must be several other aspects not revealed by these exploratory research works stressed here and take up the question that there are several barriers that obstruct a change of traditional education and the traditional world view, I would like to finish these considerations about EE and the environmental health risk question, pointing out the need to consider in one way the complexity of cultural changing and in another its necessity.

Without exaggerated optimism or pessimism, I consider that it is important to recognize the limitations of this task of looking for its possibilities. In terms of research in the education field, that can illuminate the understanding of educational practices to help the proposal of more effective ones, I agree with the recommendations of Aikenhead [7], indicating that *future projects, both on small-scale and large-scale, will need to manage the dynamics among research, policy, practice, and especially power".*

References

[1] Kneller, G.F. *A Ciência como Atividade Humana*. Zahar Editora e EdUSP: Rio de Janeiro, 1994.

[2] Jacobi, P. Educar na sociedade de risco: o desafio de construir. *CDRom of Anais do III EPEA*, Ribeirão Preto, p. 1-15, 2005.

[3] Bonotto, D.M.B. The environmental education and the risk literacy: an approach to a healthy and sustainable society. *Environmental Healthy Risk*, eds. D. Fajzieva, & C.A. Brebbia, WITPress: Southampton, pp. 247-256, 2001.

[4] Clémente, P.; Carvalho, G.; Abrougui, M.; Kkalil, I.; Thiaw, M.S.; Ndiaye and V.; Varga, A. Differences in values associated to biology, healthy and environmental questions among France, Portugal, Hungary, Senegal, Lebanon and Tunisia. *Proceedings XII IOSTE Symposium*, eds. S. Yoong; M. Ismail; A.N. Md. Zain; F. Salleh; F.S. Fook; L.C. Sam and M.N.L. Yan, Zillion Circle Ed.: Penang, 2006, pp.149-151.

[5] Bonotto, D.M.B. Understandings of the Science and Biology Trainee Teachers of the Value Content of Environmental Education and its Teaching. *Proceedings XII IOSTE Symposium*, eds. S. Yoong; M. Ismail; A.N. Md. Zain; F. Salleh; F.S. Fook; L.C. Sam and M.N.L. Yan, Zillion Circle Ed.: Penang, 2006, pp. 128-131.

[6] Dawson, V. An Exploration of High School (12-17 Year Old) Students' Understandings of, and Attitudes Towards Biotechnology Processes. *Research in Science Education*, **37**, pp. 59-73, 2007.

[7] Aikenhead, G. The Humanistic and Cultural Aspects of Science and Technology Education. Eds. R.M. Janiuk & E. Samonek-Miciuk, *Science and Technology Education for a Diverse World.* Maria Curie-Sklodowska University Press: Lublin, p.11-36, 2006.

[8] Riechard, D.E. Risk literacy: Is It the Missing in Environmental Education? *The Journal of Environmental Education,* v**25**, n°1, pp. 8-12, 1993.

[9] Vargas, E.; Monteiro, S.; Silva, F. and Cruz, M. AIDS and reproductive health: an analysis of the production of educational technology. *Proceedings X IOSTE Symposium*, eds. N. Bizzo; C.S. Kawasaki; L. Ferracioli and V.L. da Rosa, Foz do Iguaçu, v.1, pp. 199-208, 2002.

[10] Nóvoa, A. Formação de professores e profissão doente. Ed. A. NÓVOA, *Os professores e sua formação*, Publicações Dom Quixote: Lisboa, pp.15-33, 1992.
[11] Zeichner. *A formação reflexiva de professores: idéias e práticas*. Educa: Lisboa, 1993.
[12] Marcelo, C. *Formação de professores para uma mudança educativa*. Porto Editora: Porto, 1999.
[13] Mizukami, M.G.N.; Reali, A.M.M.R.; Reyes, C.R.; Lima, E.F.; Martucci, E.M.; Abib, M.L.V.S.; Mello, R.R. and Tancredi, R.M.S.P. A reflexão sobre a ação pedagógica como estratégia de modificação da escola pública elementar numa perspectiva de formação continuada no local de trabalho. *Anais do IX ENDIPE*, Lindóia, pp.490-509, 1998.
[14] Bogdan, R. & Biklen, S. *Investigação qualitativa em Educação: uma introdução à teoria e aos métodos*. Porto Editora: Porto, 1994.
[15] Corcoran, P.B. & Sievers, E. Reconceptualizing Environmental Education: Five Possibilities. *The Journal of Environmental Education*, v**25**, nº 4, pp.4-8, 1994.
[16] Zabala, A. *A prática educativa: como ensinar*. Artmed: Porto Alegre, 1998.
[17] Bonotto, Investigating an in-service program for elementary school teachers about the STS relations and the environmental problems, eds. R.M. Janiuk & E. Samonek-Miciuk, *Science and Technology Education for a Diverse World*, Maria Curie-Sklodowska University Press: Lublin, p. 135-144, 2006.
[18] Gayford, C. & Dillon, P. Policy and The Practice of Environmental Education in England: a dilemma for teachers. *Environmental Education research*, v**1**, nº 2, pp.173-183, 1995.
[19] Halstead, J.M. & Taylor, M.J. Learning and teaching about values: a review of recent research. *Cambridge Journal of education*, **v.30**, nº 2, p. 170-202, 2000.
[20] Levinson, R. Teaching ethical issues in Science. *Proceedings X IOSTE Symposium*, eds. N. Bizzo; C.S. Kawasaki; L. Ferracioli and V.L. da Rosa, Foz do Iguaçu, v. 2, p. 488-497, 2002.

Risk analysis of heavy metal contaminated habitats using a wolf spider, *Pardosa astrigera* (Araneae: Lycosidae)

M.-P. Jung, H. Kim, S.-T. Kim & J.-H. Lee
Department of Agricultural Biotechnology,
Seoul National University, Korea

Abstract

Using biological indicators to evaluate the healthiness of ecological habitats is increasingly important. Spiders are considered very useful candidates for this purpose, but few studies have been conducted. This study was conducted to investigate a relationship between heavy metal (cadmium (Cd) and lead (Pb)) contamination levels in soil habitats and their accumulations in a wolf spider, *Pardosa astrigera,* and to develop a bio-evaluation system for soil risk assessment of Cd and Pb using *P. astrigera.* Contents of Cd and Pb in a female adult *P. astrigera* and soil were estimated in nine sites in September, 2004 in Korea. Cd and Pb contamination levels in soil were well described by the Cd and Pb content of female adult *P. astrigera* by power functions. A bio-evaluation system is proposed for a soil risk assessment of Cd and Pb with *P. astrigera* using the amount of bioaccumulation and the lethal body concentration.
Keywords: Pardosa astrigera, heavy metal, Cd, Pb, biological indicator, bioaccumulation.

1 Introduction

The practical soil quality evaluation methodology has not been improved much because the progress in soil ecology theory has not led to practical strategies for soil evaluation [1]. One way of improving soil quality evaluation methods is to develop ecological indicator systems that can be used in soil quality assessments. Ecological indicators are useful instruments to bridge the gap between soil science and soil regulation practice [2].

WIT Transactions on Biomedicine and Health, Vol 11, © 2007 WIT Press
www.witpress.com, ISSN 1743-3525 (on-line)
doi:10.2495/EHR070241

Heavy metals (*e.g.* Cd and Pb) are commonly investigated components of soil pollution because of their toxicity and stability. Field and laboratory studies were carried out to investigate bioaccumulation and effect of heavy metals on soil invertebrates [3–10]. However, few attempts have been made to predict heavy metal contamination levels in soil by estimating bioaccumulation of heavy metals in soil invertebrates. Although direct measurement of soil for heavy metal contamination is useful, it may be costly and often incorrect because of high variation in soil contaminations within the site. In this regard, using biological indicators for evaluation of healthiness of ecological habitats for heavy metal contamination is perhaps more reliable because actively moving carnivorous arthropods can cover a relatively wide range and accumulate heavy metals by bio-concentration through a food chain as well as by direct soil contact in the habitats. Spiders are considered very useful candidates for this purpose. Ground-dwelling hunting spiders may reflect the pollution level of their habitats better than web-building spiders [11]. *Pardosa astrigera* can be a good candidate because it is a ground-dwelling hunting spider, can be easily sampled, is one of the dominant species in terrestrial ecosystems and its major diets are springtails and dipterans which inhabit soil [12–14].

Objectives of this study, therefore, are to quantify relationships between Pb and Cd levels in soil and their accumulations in a wolf spider, *P. astrigera* and to develop a bio-evaluation system for soil risk assessment of Pb and Cd using *P. astrigera.*

2 Materials and methods

2.1 Study sites and sampling methods

Five agricultural (A, B, F, H, and I), two residential (C and G), and two industrial sites (D and E) were selected according to expected differences in Cd and Pb contamination levels in soil (Figure 1). Five sites (A, B, C, D, and E) were selected along the Singil stream between Ansan and Sihueng city in Korea. Residential and industrial sites were located along the Singil stream.

Hand-collecting was used to collect female adult *P. astrigera* in each site to estimate bioaccumulation in September, 2004. Thirty individuals were collected at the same time from each site. Three topsoil samples (ca. 500g each) were taken at the area where spiders were collected.

2.2 Exposure of heavy metals and determination of heavy metal contents in *P. astrigera* and soil

Cd and Pb levels in field sampled soil and female adult *P. astrigera* were measured. For the measurement of heavy metal content in the spiders, five *P. astrigera* were grouped as one and measured. Thus, six measurements were made for each site. For measurement of soil, three measurements were made for each site. Also, dry weights of examined *P. astrigera* were measured.

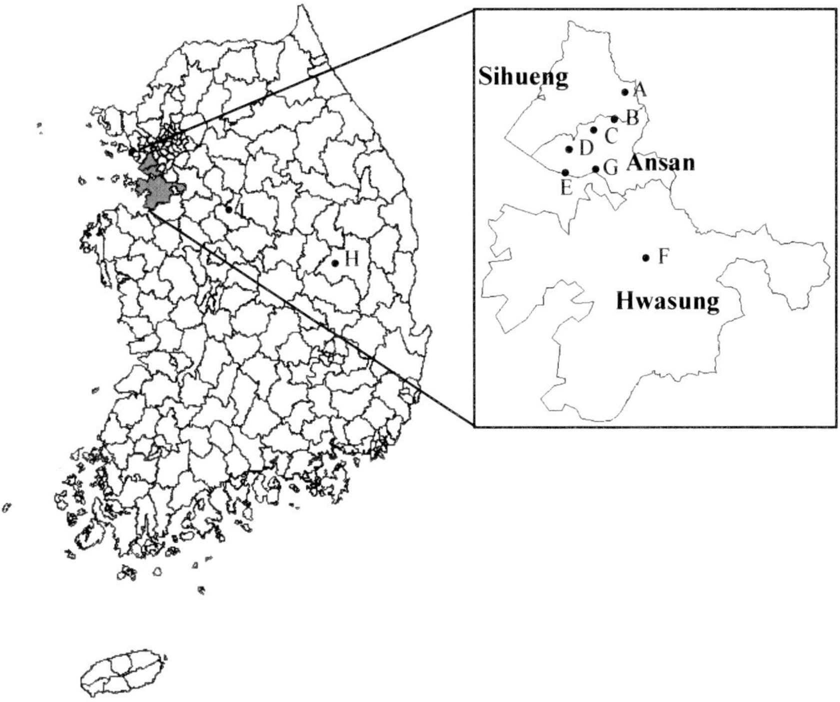

Figure 1: Map of study sites.

Female, sub adult or adult *P. astrigera* were collected from the unpolluted site and were exposed to Cd and Pb by dietary uptake in the laboratory. Adult *Drosophila melanogaster* reared by exposing Cd 10mg/kg and Pb 100mg/kg, respectively, were used as foods. Three fruit flies per day were provided to individual *P. astrigera* until *P. astrigera* died. Then, Cd and Pb levels of five *P. astrigera* were analyzed to estimate lethal body concentration. Ten replications were conducted in this experiment. Also, dry weight of examined *P. astrigera* was measured.

For the measurement of Cd and Pb, ICP (Inductively Coupled Plasma Emission Spectrometer) was used at the NICEM (National Instrumentation Center for Environmental Management) in Seoul National University.

2.3 Statistical analysis

Power functions were used to describe the relationship between bioaccumulation of *P. astrigera* and heavy metal contents in soil. The equations are:

$$y_1 = a_1 + b_1 x_1^{c1} \quad (1)$$

$$y_2 = a_2 x_2^{b2} \quad (2)$$

where, y_1 and y_2 are Cd and Pb concentration in soil, respectively. x_1 and x_2 are Cd and Pb concentration in female adult *P. astrigera*, respectively.

3 Result and discussion

3.1 Relationship of bioaccumulation of *P. astrigera* and concentration in soil of Cadmium and Lead

The lethal concentrations of Cd and Pb for *P. astrigera* in this experiment were measured. The Cd and Pb concentration in the female adult *P. astrigera* and soil varied among sites: very high in site C, E, and G (residential or industrial sites), low in site A and I (agricultural sites) (Table 1). The Cd concentration in *P. astrigera* was higher by 10-700 times than that in soil. The Pb concentration in *P. astrigera* was higher by 1-20 times than that in soil. It was reported that spiders accumulated Cd, Cu, and Zn to the concentrations greater than those present in the soil but did not accumulate Pb [11]. Like *Steatoda bipunctata* (Theridiidae) [14], *P. astrigera* may behave as a regulator for Pb, which accumulates heavy metals to a certain level and then excretes them beyond the level, but as an accumulator for Cd.

Table 1: Mean concentration of cadmium and lead in female adult *P. astirgera* and soil.

Sites	Cd (μg/g)		Pb (μg/g)	
	Female adult	Soil	Female adult	Soil
A	7.14	0.03	37.97	1.60
B	11.33	0.25	51.35	8.50
C	17.04	1.46	79.31	52.20
D	22.79	0.27	61.35	17.20
E	36.60	1.41	101.78	96.70
F	16.17	0.10	66.55	2.80
G	30.14	0.95	105.96	69.50
H	8.00	0.28	69.93	30.20
I	7.20	0.01	53.88	2.70

The relationship between bioaccumulation of female adult *P. astrigera* and heavy metal concentration in soil was well described by power functions (Figure 2). However, these models must be applied to the conditions of <2mg/kg for Cd and <120mg/kg for Pb in soil, respectively because two models were developed using *P. astrigera* collected in mostly moderately contaminated habitats. Further calibration studies may be needed in habitats of a higher contamination level.

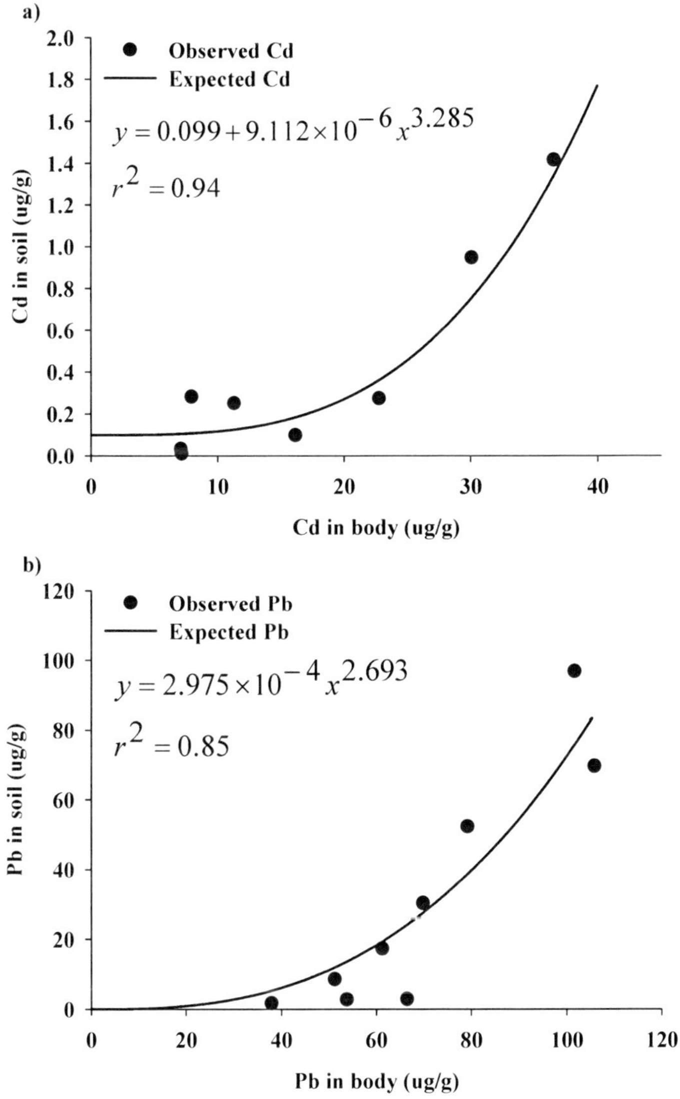

Figure 2: Relationships between heavy metal content in adult female of *P. astrigera* and soil. a: Cd, b: Pb.

3.2 Use of *P. astrigera* in risk assessment of heavy metal contamination in soil

The bio-indicator index for toxicant residues, β, as the average of the quotient of the observed residue in a species and the internal threshold concentration, and the reference system for evaluating bio-indicator index for toxicant residues (Figure 3a) were proposed by van Straalen [10]. The bio-indicator index for toxicant residues can be interpreted as the fraction of the internal threshold concentration that is occupied by the residue: *e.g.* <0.01 as negligible risk in the reference system. In our study (*i.e.* the modified reference system), the threshold of negligible risk was modified as <0.02 because the amount of bioaccumulation of *P. astrigera* was very diverse from 0mg/kg to 20mg/kg for Cd, and from 0mg/kg to 60mg/kg for Pb in uncontaminated sites. In Korea, action level for Cd and Pb contamination in soil is 4 mg/kg and 300 mg/kg in agricultural areas, respectively. The modified reference system is shown in Figure 3b.

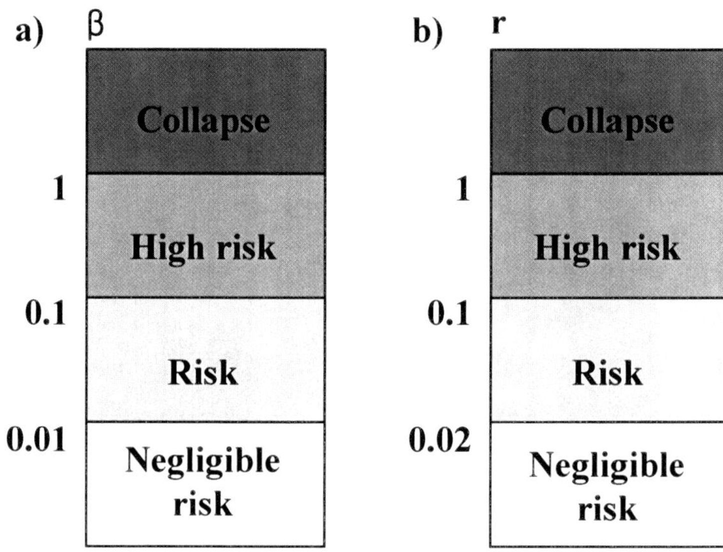

Figure 3: a) The reference system for evaluation the bioindicator index for toxicant residues, β proposed by Van Straalen [10]. b) The modified reference system for evaluation the heavy metal contamination in soil. r is risk ratio (the quotient of the observed residue in a species and the internal threshold concentration).

In the laboratory experiment, estimated lethal body concentration (mean±s.e) of *P. astrigera* for Cd and Pb was 1,050.5±18.61mg/kg and 3,122.8±35.04mg/kg, respectively. Using these values, the risk ratios (the quotient of the observed residue in a species and the internal threshold concentration) for study sites for Cd and Pb were calculated (Table 2). According to the modified reference system, for Cd, the site A, B, C, F, H, and I were characterized as a negligible risk zone, while the site D, E, and G were evaluated as a risk zone. For Pb, the site A, B, and I were evaluated as a negligible risk zone while other sites were as a risk zone. This system is highly compatible with direct measurement of soil and is applicable for evaluation of soil habitat contamination.

Further calibration and validation studies are necessary since there are some limitations in using lethal body concentration [10]: *e.g.* physiological conditions and presence of other metals in the body can affect the lethal dosage.

Table 2: Risk assessment of this nine study sites using risk ratio (r) estimated from Cd and Pb concentration in *P. astrigera*.

Sites	Cd		Pb	
	Observed residue	r	Observed residue	r
A	7.14	0.007	37.97	0.012
B	11.33	0.011	51.35	0.016
C	17.04	0.016	79.31	0.025
D	22.79	0.022	61.35	0.020
E	36.60	0.035	101.78	0.033
F	16.17	0.015	66.55	0.021
G	30.14	0.029	105.96	0.034
H	8.00	0.008	69.93	0.022
I	7.20	0.007	53.88	0.017

Acknowledgement

This work was supported by Ministry of Environment, Republic of Korea (2004-09001-0012-0) and the Brain Korea 21 program.

References

[1] Van Straalen, N.M., Assessment of soil contamination a functional perspective. *Biodegradation*, **13**, pp. 41-52, 2002.

[2] Van Straalen, N.M., The use of soil invertebrates in ecological surveys of contaminated soils (Chapter 6). *Vital Soil*, ed. P. Doelman & H. Eijsackers, Elsevier: Amsterdam, pp. 159-195, 2004.

[3] Belotti, E., Assessment of a soil quality criterion by means of a field survey. *Applied Soil Ecology*, **10**, pp. 51-63, 1998.

[4] Dallinger, R. & Rainbow, P.S., (eds). *Ecotoxicology of Metals in Invertebrates*, Lewis Publishers: Boca Raton, 1993.

[5] Heikens, A., Peijnenburg, W.J.G.M., & Hendriks, A.J., Bioaccumulation of heavy metals in terrestrial invertebrates. *Environmental Pollution*, **113**, pp. 385-393, 2001.

[6] Hussein, M.A., Obuid-Allah, A.H., Mohammad, A.H., Scott-Fordsmand, J.J., & Abd El-Wakeil, K.F., Seasonal variation in heavy metal accumulation in subtropical population of the terrestrial isopod, *Porcellio Laevis*. *Ecotoxicology and Environmental Safety*, **63**, pp. 168-174, 2006

[7] Laing, G.D, Bogaert, N., Tack, F.M.G., Verloo, M.G., & Hendrickx, F., Heavy metal contents (Cd, Cu, Zn) in spiders (Pirata piraticus) living in intertidal sediments of the river Scheldt estuary (Belgium) as affected by substrate characteristics. *The Science of the Total Environment*, **289**, pp. 71-81, 2002.

[8] Ross, S.M., *Toxic Metals in Soil/Plant Systems*, John Wiley and Sons: Chichester, 1994.

[9] Skubala, P & Kafel, A., Oribatid mite communities and metal bioaccumulation in orbatid species (Acari, Oribatida) along the heavy metal gradient in forest ecosystems. *Environmental Pollution*, **132**, pp. 51-60, 2004.

[10] van Straalen, N.M. & Krivolutsky, D.A., (eds). *Bioindicator Systems for Soil Pollution*, Kluwer Academic Publishers: Dordrecht, 1996.

[11] Marc, P., Canard, A., & Ysnel, F., Spiders (Araneae) useful for pest limitation and bioindication, *Agriculture, Ecosystems and Environment*, **74**, pp. 229-273, 1999.

[12] Im, M.S. & Kim, S.T., *Field Guide of Korean Spiders*, Konkuk University Press, Seoul, p 170, 2000 (in Korean).

[13] Miyashita, K., Seasonal Change of population Density and Some Characteristics of overwintering Nymph of Lycosa T-insignita Boes. Et STR. (Araneae: Lycosidae). *Applied Entomology and Zoology*, **4**, pp. 1-8, 1969.

[14] Nyffeler, M & Benz, G., Feeding ecology and predatory importance of wolf spiders (Pardosa spp.) (Araneae, Lycosidae) in winter wheat fields. *Journal of Applied Entomology*, **106**, pp. 123-134, 1988.

[15] Clausen, I.H.S., On the dynamics of cadmium and lead in *Steatoda bipunctata* (Araneae). *Proc. Of the 5th Int. Conf. Bioindicatores Deteriorisations Regionis*, eds. J. Bohac & Ruzicka, pp. 315-318, 1989.

Methods for calculating PNECs using species sensitivity distribution (SSD) with various hypothesis on the way to handle ecotoxicity data

P. Ciffroy
EDF Research and Development, Département Laboratoire National d'Hydraulique et Environnement, Chatou, France

Abstract

Species sensitivity distribution (SSD) methodology is currently used to determine the Predicted No Effect Concentration (PNEC) of a substance, considering chronic ecotoxicological tests on three taxonomic groups: algae, invertebrates and vertebrates (aquatic environment). However, SSD methodology raises some practical questions due to the multiple possibilities of handling the available data. In particular the following points are often discussed: (1) how to take into account the intra-species variation; (2) how to handle heterogeneous repartition of available data among the taxonomic groups; (3) could we use the information contained in acute data, and how, in the construction of SSDs; (4) when only a limited number of data is available, how is it possible to build relevant SSDs. Different approaches have been tested in answer to each of these questions: For questions (1) and (2): different methods were compared, each of them being characterized by a different way of taking into account intra-species variation and proportions of taxonomic groups (vertebrates, invertebrates and algae), as well as by the actual method of calculation of the HC5 (Hazardous Concentration) and its confidence interval. These different methods were compared for 15 substances using NOEC data available in the literature and the uncertainty associated to the data treatment was quantified. For question (3): an "Acute-to-Chronic Transformation" (ACT) function was derived and a methodology for the incorporation of acute data in the construction of SSDs was tested. This ACT method was tested on 11 substances: for each substance, the actual chronic SSD was compared to the predicted SSD derived from the incorporation of transformed acute data. For question (4): Bayesian methods were tested to build SSDs from limited datasets and the relevance of such methods was discussed. Various approaches are suggested here in answer to each of these three questions. They have been combined in a comprehensive overview to define alternative strategies according to the availability of ecotoxicological data.

Keywords: risk assessment, species sensitivity distribution, PNEC, uncertainty.

WIT Transactions on Biomedicine and Health, Vol 11, © 2007 WIT Press
www.witpress.com, ISSN 1743-3525 (on-line)
doi:10.2495/EHR070251

1 Introduction

The so-called "*Species Sensitivity Distribution*" (SSD) methodology has been used since 1996 in the European Community [1] in order to determine the "*Predicted No Effect Concentration*" (PNEC) of a substance, where chronic ecotoxological tests carried out on the substance are numerous enough (a minimum of fifteen or so). For the aquatic environment with which we are concerned, the three taxonomic groups, algae, invertebrates and vertebrates, need to be represented. This approach is based on the hypothesis that the species for which results of ecotoxicological tests are known are representative, in terms of sensitivity, of the totality of the species in the environment (e.g. see Aldenberg and Slob [2]). A likely distribution of species sensitivity is then estimated from these results, which enables a concentration that is assumed to protect a given percentage of the species in the environment to be calculated. The agreed European concentration is HC5_50%, the hazardous concentration protecting 95% of species with 50% confidence.

The SSD approach raises a number of questions (e.g. see Forbes and Calow [3]). From a practical point of view, irrespective of validation and criteria used for selecting the results of ecotoxicological tests used in SSD (criteria which we shall not discuss here), we will concentrate on the following questions:

- When the chronic ecotoxicological results are numerous enough:
  1. Should intra-species variation be taken into account? And if so, how?
  2. How do we take into account the fact that the number of available data varies from one category of species to another (between vertebrates, invertebrates and algae)?
- When chronic ecotoxicological results are limited, but acute ecotoxicological tests are numerous enough:
  3. Can acute toxicity data for a substance give us information about the chronic toxicity of the same substance and be used for building chronic SSD?
- When ecotoxicological tests are scarce (typically less than 10):
  4. is it possible to build relevant SSDs through techniques adapted for the treatment of small samples like Bayesian methods?

Various approaches are suggested here in answer to each of these questions. They have been combined in a comprehensive overview to define alternative strategies according to the availability of ecotoxicological data.

1.1 Strategies for large chronic datasets

1.1.1 Materials and methods

(1) *Taking into account intra-species variation*

In the method commonly used (European Commission [1]) for building SSDs in the case of large datasets of chronic ecotoxicological tests, the various test results that may exist for the same species (e.g. for daphnia) are averaged; as a result, a single value per species (the geometric mean) is used to determine the SSD. Because of differences in experimental conditions, strains of species, stages of development, etc, the intra-species variation between test results is frequently observed to be very high, and is sometimes equivalent to the inter-species variation. In the current methodology, this source of variability (the intra-species variation) is ignored. While it is not legitimate to ignore *a priori* intra-species variation by calculating a mean of the data, neither is it satisfactory to consider the set of data as it stands without taking into account the label "species", since one species is frequently much more abundant than the others with respect to the number of data (especially daphnia).

In order to study the effect of taking intra-species variation into account or not, Duboudin et al (2004) [4] compared three approaches that stem directly from the above discussion:

(1.1) The entire set of data available is treated as if they all belonged to different species. Intra-species variation is taken into account in the same way as inter-species variation, but there is a risk of giving too much importance to one species if the number of data we have for one species is high.

(1.2) As is done in the usual method, a geometric mean of data for each species is first calculated. In this case, intra-species variation is ignored.

(1.3) All the data are used, but each piece of data is weighted in order to give each species the same weight within the SSD. Intra-species variation is taken into account, and no species is given more importance than any other.

(2) *Taking into account the relative distribution of data among the three taxonomic groups: vertebrates, invertebrates and algae*

For the determination of an aquatic PNEC, the SSD method is based on breaking down species into three taxonomic groups: vertebrates, invertebrates and algae. In most cases, it is necessary to incorporate these three taxonomic groups into the same SSD, which then raises the question of the proportions of data taken into account for each group.

Most research uses the data available in the literature and implicitly assumes that its distribution among the three species previously described is representative of the proportions existing in the environment. However, as a general rule, the representativity of laboratory species as compared to species in the environment is not guaranteed (Forbes and Calow [3]), because lab species are chosen because they are easy to breed and they are not the result of a random sample from among all the species. Thus, letting literature references decide which proportions of data are used to construct an SSD does not seem to be very satisfactory, since these proportions vary from one toxicant to another.

Duboudin et al [4] compared three approaches to study how much effect the distribution of data among taxonomic groups has:

(2.1) As is done in the usual method, the proportions of data given in the literature are retained. Ultimately, no distinction is made between the three taxonomic groups.

(2.2) The data is balanced, in such a way that the three taxonomic groups are equally weighted in the SSD.

(2.3) The data is weighted in such a way as to respect the proportions proposed by Forbes and Calow [3]: 10%, 26% and 64% for vertebrates, invertebrates and algae respectively.

Table 1: Statistical characteristics of results associated with 63 methods of calculation of HC5 toxicant by toxicant.

Toxicant :	Deviation to the mean				Amplitude	
	min	25th percentile (q25)	75th percentile (q75)	max	q75-q25	max-min
atrazine	-0.41	-0.16	0.13	0.48	0.29	0.89
boric acid	-0.58	-0.28	0.27	0.61	0.56	1.19
butylbenzyl phthalate	-0.11	-0.05	0.04	0.19	0.09	0.30
cadmium	-0.21	-0.07	0.09	0.19	0.15	0.41
chromium	-0.27	-0.09	0.11	0.37	0.21	0.65
copper	-0.31	-0.18	0.16	0.30	0.33	0.61
dibutyl phthalate	-0.21	-0.13	0.03	0.42	0.17	0.63
dodmac	-0.35	-0.15	0.13	0.30	0.28	0.64
lead	-0.24	-0.10	0.09	0.29	0.20	0.53
lindane	-0.53	-0.37	0.31	0.54	0.68	1.07
mercury	-0.54	-0.21	0.31	0.59	0.52	1.13
nickel	-0.45	-0.17	0.15	0.50	0.32	0.95
parathion	-0.56	-0.30	0.26	0.60	0.57	1.16
pentachlorophenol	-0.38	-0.17	0.13	0.40	0.31	0.78
zinc	-0.20	-0.12	0.06	0.25	0.18	0.46

2 Results and discussion

Duboudin et al [4] have combined in a near-comprehensive experimental design the different above-indicated options to handle ecotoxicological data, yielding, from the same set of data 63 distinct ways of calculating an HC5 (different statistical methods to build SSDs were also included in their analysis – not presented in this paper). This experimental design was tested on 15 toxicants, using chronic aquatic NOEC (*No Observed Effect Concentration*) data available for these toxicants. A comparison of these various approaches was then undertaken, with a view to determining the variability of the HC5 according to the chosen assumptions and to determining the respective effect of each of the options on the calculation of the HC5.

Results are summarized in Table 1. The deviation to the mean and the amplitudes of the outputs (distances max-min and 75th percentile-25th percentile, in log base 10) are indicated to show the variability of the HC5 according to the assumptions chosen to handle data. The 'max-min' amplitude of the HCs5 calculated according to the various assumptions varies from one toxicant to another: it lies between 0.3 (in log base 10) for butylbenzyl phthalate and 1.19 (i.e. more than one order of magnitude for concentrations) for boric acid; it exceeds 0.5 (factor of 3) in 12 cases out of 15. An ANOVA analysis conducted for each toxicant showed that: (i) the parameter related to 'taxonomic distribution of data' turns out to be the preponderant parameter for variations in HC5 for 7 toxicants out of 15; (ii) the 'intra-species variation' parameter is preponderant for 5 toxicants out of 15. Thus, the ranking in order of importance of the studies parameters varies according to the toxicant and the related set of data.

2.1.1 Recommendations

The study conducted by Duboudin et al [4] showed that different methods can be separated by one order of magnitude for the same toxicant. Regardless of differences in toxicity between substances, the HC5s differ by the options used, firstly in terms of taxonomic groups and intra-species variation, and to a lesser degree in terms of the choice of distribution. In order to obtain comparable HC5 between substances, it could be recommended to use a homogeneous method, that allows one to take into account intra-species variations and constant distribution of data among taxonomic groups:

- regarding redundant data for each species, rather that using a geometric mean as done by the current method, we favor a weighted method that allows one to account for intra species variation while giving the same weight within the SSD.
- regarding the proportion of data among taxonomic groups, we favor weighted methods that allow one to conduct a homogeneous treatment for all the toxicants.

2.2 Strategies for large acute datasets

2.2.1 Materials and methods

For many substances, insufficient or even no chronic data are available. In such cases, the PNEC is based on a limited number of data and on uncertainty factors (10, 100, 1000 depending on the case [1]): only the lowest value is used to estimate the PNEC and no confidence interval can be allotted to it. However, for some of these substances, a large number of acute data may be available. Then, we are faced with the following problem: (question 3.1.) can acute toxicity data for a substance give us information about the chronic toxicity of the same substance and be used to build chronic SSDs?

Some methods were developed in the past, that are based on the transformation of type LC_{50} or EC_{50} acute toxicity data concerning one species into predicted chronic data for the same species, using an ACR (*Acute to Chronic Ratio*) (e.g. Parkurst et al [5]). However, the ACR method showed some limitations: significant differences in ACR ratios among different families of toxicants or species (e.g. Länge et al [6]; Brix et al [7]). So in order to apply this approach correctly it would be necessary to know the ACR ratios for each family of substances, and virtually for every species, which is impossible.

Duboudin et al [8] compared, for several substances, SSDs constructed from acute toxicity data with SSDs constructed from chronic data, and more specifically the *mean* and *standard* statistics of the log-normal distributions associated with both of them. They developed thus an Acute-to-Chronic Transformation method allowing one to incorporate acute data in the construction of chronic SSDs.

Table 2: Inter-distribution distances HC5s for Acute, Chronic and ACT SSDs, for 11 substances (data in log base 10). ACT = acute to chronic data transformation; A = acute and C = chronic.

Substances	Interdistribution distance[1]		HC5		
	A-C	ACT-C	A	ACT	C
cadmium	2.39	0.14	0.69	-0.23	-0.29
copper	1.23	0.06	0.99	0.22	0.22
nickel	1.89	0.12	2.55	0.87	0.80
lead	1.60	0.18	1.71	0.68	1.09
zinc	1.53	0.06	2.18	1.08	1.22
mercury	1.27	0.27	0.86	0.11	-0.53
chromium	1.67	0.16	2.09	0.93	0.97
lindane	0.49	0.02	0.74	-0.10	-0.11
atrazine	2.05	0.34	3.34	0.89	0.71
parathion	1.28	0.16	-0.31	-1.20	-1.58
pentachloro-phenol	0.69	0.26	1.36	0.48	0.90
Mean	*1.46*	*0.16*	*1.47*	*0.34*	*0.31*

[1]defined as $D(d_1,d_2) = \lim_{n\to\infty}\left[\frac{1}{n}\sum_{k=0}^{n-1}\left|\text{quantile}_{k/_{n-1}}(d_1) - \text{quantile}_{k/_{n-1}}(d_2)\right|\right]$

2.2.2 Results and discussion

Duboudin et al [8] developed relationships to transform a data sample representative of the acute toxicity of a substance on the vertebrates and invertebrates into a data sample predicted to be representative of the chronic toxicity of the same substance (ACT method). This method was tested and validated on 11 substances for which a sufficient number of chronic and acute data are available. For each of these substances, three SSDs were constructed and compared using different sets of data: (i) SSD with acute data only; (ii) SSD with chronic data only; (iii) predicted chronic SSD using acute-to-chronic transformation data (ACT SSD). Results of HC5s obtained with these methods are summarized in Table 2: the inter-distributions mean distance is 1.46 between acute and chronic data as opposed to 0.16 between ACT and chronic; for the 11 substances under consideration, while the difference in absolute values (Table 6) between acute HC5% and chronic HC5% is on average 1.16 in log base 10, it is 0.21 on average between ACT HC5% and chronic HC5%, which represents a ratio in the region of 1.6 between concentration values. These results confirm that the ACT method is successful at reproducing a distribution of chronic toxicity data from samples of acute data and predicting a chronic HC5% value, even if the quality of the prediction varies from one substance to another.

2.2.3 Recommendations

The ACT approach developed by Duboudin et al [8] thus has two main advantages over the assessment factors method: first, rather than providing a single value, it gives a distribution of vertebrate and/or invertebrate data, associated with a confidence envelope for acute-to-chronic transformation. This or these distribution(s) of predicted chronic data can be compared with real available chronic values if existent. The few available chronic values can be incorporated into the acute values after ACT transformation and thus be taken into account when constructing an SSD. Second, if completed successfully (incorporation of the three taxonomic groups into the same SSD with the wished representativeness for each one), the ACT approach provides an HC5% value associated with a confidence interval which takes into account, on the one hand, natural variation of data, and on the other, the uncertainty of the acute-to-chronic transformation.

2.3 Strategies for small datasets

For most of the toxicants, available data are scarce and, in such cases, the assessment method is applied: as previously indicated, uncertainty factors (10, 100, 1000 depending on the case [1]) are affected to the lowest ecotoxicological value to estimate the PNEC and no confidence interval can be allotted to it. In such cases, different alternative methods can be proposed to build SSDs, even with a limited set of data (see Verdonck et al [9]). Among these methods, Bayesian statistics corresponds to practical situation that end-users meet: a limited data sample is available and the uncertainty of the SSD that fits the dataset is modelled assuming that the parameters of the SSD are themselves distributed.

Aldenberg and Jaworska [10] used theoretical sets of data to compare 'classical' statistics (i.e. maximum likelihood method) and Bayesian methods to derive HC5. They provided tabulations for direct applications of Bayesian methods for the calculation of HC5s, associated with confidence intervals, as a function of the number of available tests. An extract of the table provided by Aldenberg and Jaworska [10] is proposed in Table 3. The methods allows thus to quantify the confidence interval of the HC5, that decreases when the number of data increases. Moreover, it is observed that the generation of new ecotoxicological data (e.g. from 5 to 7 data) allows reducing the conservatism of the predicted PNEC. This method has thus main advantages over the assessment factors method: it uses all the available ecotoxicological data (and not the lowest one as for the assessment factor method); it provides a confidence interval for HC5; it stimulates the generation of new data that can contribute to limit the conservatism of the predictions.

Table 3: Calculation of HC5s by the Bayesian method as a function of sample size (from Aldenberg and Jaworska [18]).

	HC5 = mean – *k*.standard_deviation		
Number of data	*k* for HC5(5%)	*k* for HC5(50%)	*k* for HC5(95%)
5	4.2	1.78	0.82
7	3.4	1.73	0.92
10	2.91	1.7	0.99
infinity	1.64	1.64	1.64

3 Conclusions

This paper summarizes previous works undertaken to improve the determination of PNEC values, using preferentially the Species Sensitivity Distribution (SSD) method. It underlines some possible strategies for calculating HC5s according to the size of data sample:

- when the number of chronic data is sufficient (e.g. more than 15 data), it could be recommended to use a homogeneous method, that allows to take into account intra-species variations and constant distribution of data among taxonomic groups;
- when the chronic dataset is limited, but acute dataset is sufficient, an Acute-to-Chronic Transformation method could be used to incorporate acute data in the construction of the chronic SSD;
- when only a few number of data is available, Bayesian techniques (already tabulated) could be used to build SSDs, with associated confidence intervals.

References

[1] European Commission. 1996. Technical Guidance Document in support of commission directive 93/67/EEC on risk assessment for new notified substance and commission regulation 5EC) No 1488/94 on risk assessment for existing substance. Part II. Office for Official Publications of the European Communities. Luxembourg. CR-48-96-001-EN-C ; CR-48-96-002-EN-C ; CR-48-96-003-EN-C ; CR-48-96-004-EN-C.

[2] Aldenberg T, and Slob W. 1993. Confidence limits for hazardous concentrations based on chronic NOEC toxicity data. *Ecotoxicology and Environmental Safety* 25:48-63.

[3] Forbes VE and Calow P. 2002. Species Sensitivity Distributions Revisited: A critical Appraisal. *Human an Ecological Risk Assessment* 8:3:473-492.

[4] Duboudin C, Ciffroy P, Magaud H, 2004. Effects of data manipulation and statistical methods on species sensitivity distribution. *Environmental Toxicology and Chemistry,* Vol. 23, No 2, 489-499.

[5] Parkurst BR, Warren-Hicks W, Cardwell RD, Volosin J, Etchison T, Butscher JB, Covington SM. 1995. Risk managing methods. *Water Environ Technol* 7:39-43

[6] Länge R, Hutchinson TH, Scholz N, Solbe J. 1999. Analysis of the Ecetoc aquatic toxicity (EAT) database. II - Comparison of acute to chronic ratios for various aquatic organisms and chemical substances. *Chemosphere* 36:1:115-127.

[7] Brix KV, Deforest DK, Adams WJ. 2001. Assessing acute and chronic copper risks to freshwater aquatic life using species sensitivity distributions for different taxonomix groups. *Environ Toxicol Chem* 20:8:1847-1856.

[8] Duboudin C, Ciffroy P, Magaud H, 2004. Acute-to-chronic species sensitivity distribution extrapolation. *Environmental Toxicology and Chemistry,* Vol. 23, No 7, 1774-1785

[9] Verdonck F, Jaworska J, Thas O, Vanrolleghem P., 2001. Determining environmental standards using bootstrapping, Bayesian and maximum likelihood techniques: a comparative study. *Analytica Chimica Acta,* Vol 446, Issues 1-2, 427-436

[10] Aldenberg T, Jaworska J, 2000. Uncertainty of the hazardous concentration and fraction affected for normal Species Sensitivity Distribution. *Ecotoxicology and Environmental Safety,* 46, 1-18.

Section 6
Social and economic issues

Khartoum 2030: towards the healthy city

A. M. Ahmad
Department of Architecture, Faculty of Engineering and Architecture, University of Khartoum, Sudan

Abstract

At Independence, in 1956, the Sudanese capital, Khartoum, ranked among the healthiest and most attractive Arab capitals. Today, five decades later, it has dropped to settle among the world's bottom capitals in the quality of its physical and socio-cultural environments. This is manifest in the persistent cropping up of squatter settlements around it, the inadequacy of surface water drainage, the poverty of sewage disposal systems, the depletion of greenery, the shortage and unacceptable quality of drinking water and the traffic chaos and all that emanates from it.

In a retarded country almost permanently in dictatorial grips so little reliable data exists that we can write about scientific issues only in general qualitative terms. Yet, I shall attempt to describe the great potential of the city, highlight the main physical environmental threats, discuss the recent positive developments, then argue that Khartoum has the potential to mature into a model *Healthy City* by, say, 2030.

Keywords: healthy city, Khartoum, environmental hazards, post-oil development.

1 Introduction

A recent 'quality of living' report has rated Khartoum fifth *from the bottom* – the 211th of 215 cities surveyed. The survey conducted by *Mercer Human Resources Consulting* in 2006 analysed '39 quality of life criteria for each city including political, economic and social factors, personal safety and health, education, transport and other public services' and ranked the cities accordingly [1].

Lower than Khartoum in ranking came only Pointe Noire (Congo), Baghdad (Iraq), Bangui (Central African Republic) and finally Brazzaville (Congo), the world's worst city to live in by Mercer's criteria. One sees at a glance that these cities, unlike Khartoum, have been or are being devastated by long civil wars –

WIT Transactions on Biomedicine and Health, Vol 11, © 2007 WIT Press
www.witpress.com, ISSN 1743-3525 (on-line)
doi:10.2495/EHR070261

which further underlines the backward state of Khartoum. Of the bottom twenty cities seventeen were African. Incidentally, the top cities were Zurich, Geneva, Vancouver and Vienna.

Even allowing some room for contesting the criteria or the procedure for ranking, the fact remains that Khartoum has a pretty dismal environment to offer its residents.

These pages will look only into the environmental health aspects of the city in light of the available information and will argue that there is still room for hope under the newly emergent conditions and that it will be possible to upgrade it to the status of an ideal *Healthy City* in the span of some 25 years.

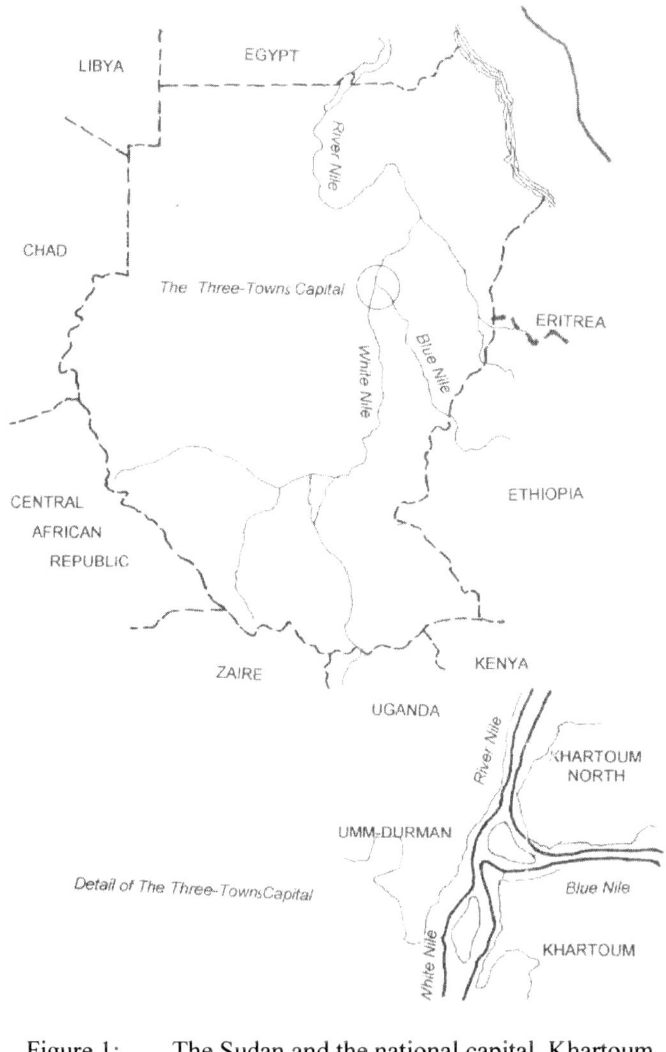

Figure 1: The Sudan and the national capital, Khartoum.

2 Background

Khartoum enjoys a distinctive location at the heart of a huge country. At its own heart the Blue Nile advancing from the south east and the White Nile from the south merge and flow jointly northwards dividing Greater Khartoum into three discrete sectors: Khartoum, Umm-Durman, and Khartoum North (fig 1). The terrain is mostly flat except in Umm-Durman where it is fairly rugged and the soil is clayey and fertile in Khartoum and Khartoum North and sandy or rocky in Umm-Durman. The city (lat 15 36' N) lies in a semi-desert zone with a hot dry season coming in two installments extending over about seven months, a two-month rainy season and a brief cool dry season lasting about three months; but the approaching desert, not yet effectively confronted, is gradually transforming the region into a typical hot dry zone. Mean air temperatures range from 27.3 to 41.9°C in May and from 15.6 to 30.7°C in January. Total annual rainfall amounts to 121 mm spread mainly over July, August and September. About twelve dust storms blow annually [2]. Today, the city is gradually being engulfed and desiccated by the critical buffer front of the advancing desert aided by harmful human activities and irresponsible government policies.

The city suffers from sprawl; it has a very low density, its buildings being predominantly single storey and with vast open spaces within its boundary. The population of Khartoum (the name now referring to the whole city) is unknown – the last census was conducted in 1993 and since then civil wars and natural disasters have caused considerable population swings with the displaced people heading mostly towards the national capital. The current official population estimate is seven million, almost a fifth of the total population of the country.

3 Environmental health risks

Let us review the major environmental health risks affecting Khartoum.

3.1 Surface water drainage

One of the disadvantages of the flat terrain is poor natural drainage. In Khartoum this is coupled with old constructed drains that, having outlived their usefulness, promptly fill up until natural evaporation empties them.

During the rainy season and with heavy rainfall on the Ethiopian highlands Khartoum urban areas are threatened by water in three forms: rainfall, river overflows every about 7 years and floodwater from outside its boundary. This has to be considered simultaneously with substandard road construction, untreated open spaces, inadequate garbage disposal and vulnerability to river flooding. A single heavy rain cripples the city for several days: vehicles are stranded, roads damaged, employees cannot be questioned about their absence when their homes are at risk of collapsing if immediate measures to get rid of the water are not taken (fig 2).

The incidence of malaria in the Sudan has been one of the highest in the Arab region but again no reliable data exist because of the selective sampling and because the whole southern region has been inaccessible for three decades. The specialized centre for malaria in Abu Usher south of Khartoum has long been closed.

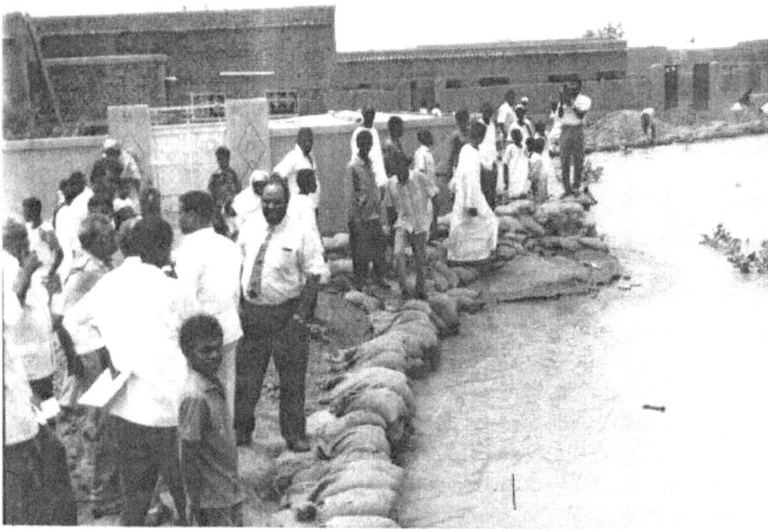

Figure 2: River overflows in suburban Khartoum.

3.2 Squatter settlements

Another disadvantage of the flat terrain is the relative ease with which illegal settlements materialise and slowly entangle the city. The successive natural and man-made disasters have resulted in millions of displaced people and refugees to neighbouring countries. Government estimates give illegal settlers as fully 50% of the total population of Khartoum i.e. about 3.5 million souls.

While it is comforting that those victims ultimately find refuge in the city, it is a tangible reality that their effect on the urban environment is detrimental. The majority of these communities are illiterate and some can hardly communicate in Arabic. They live in substandard shelter lacking safe drinking water, toilet facilities, employment opportunities and basic health, education and entertainment facilities and experience difficulties in being accepted by the original population. They live in continual contact with their domestic animals. Admittedly, they produce little waste and are competent in recycling and finding new uses for other people's waste. However, they cut down trees for fuel, fodder and home construction; their goats feed freely on any handy greenery. Some of them are engaged in crime: theft, liquor brewing, prostitution and practices approaching witchcraft. The incidence of AIDS/HIV among them is known to be higher than the city's average although no official figures are ever divulged.

3.3 Sewage disposal

The sewage network covers no more than 7% of the city. It is old dating back to the1950s with frequent nasty overflows sometimes invading the drinking water network. Part of the First and Second Class residential areas (as the colonial classification has them) are served alternatively by septic tanks and soak-away wells (about 8%). But the majority of the houses, about 85%, are served by pit latrines. Part of the squatter areas totally lacks this service [3].

Sinking wells and pit latrines is expensive especially in Umm-Durman where the soil is rocky and the first aquifer lies at depths of 20–40 metres. They also work towards polluting the soil and the ground water. In old Umm-Durman with its traditional organic layouts and narrow twisting lanes, introducing a sewage network is an enormously demanding task, technically and economically. Disposal of treated sewage used to be in the green belt, a stretch 10 kilometres long 3.5 kilometres wide south of Khartoum. This was grown in 1961, remained healthy for over a decade and then dried and devastated through official negligence and the activities of squatters already mentioned. By the late 1970s the belt had disappeared. Other green belts have been proposed in subsequent master plans but never implemented. Sewage disposal remains one of the major ailments of the city.

3.4 Traffic

Traffic problems are on the rise. They emanate less from the presence of too many vehicles than from the absence of effective planning. The number of vehicles rose progressively from 148,000 in 1984 to 380,000 in 2003 to 400,000 in 2004 to 460,000 in 2005. At present this number is increasing at the rate of 120-150 a day. This constitutes about 80% of the total vehicles in the country and 90% of these are private cars. In 2004 the number of deaths due to traffic accidents was 1306; in 2005 it was 1403 [4].

There are no statistics for the suburban traffic that enters the city in the early morning and leaves by the late afternoon. This traffic is a main 'ruralising' influence on the city due to the chaos it creates; sadly, it also has a known corrupting influence on some of the police. No segregation of vehicles by size has been planned in the streets and huge trucks coming from Port Sudan on the Red Sea keep entering the city all day long and mixing with its the normal traffic.

Traffic planning has not kept up with this increase. Private car ownership is rising; public transport is less than adequate. No attempt to plan parking in the city centre has yet been made.

Only in the last few years have official eyes turned to this field – two bridges have been constructed one across the Blue Nile and one across the White Nile; two more are under construction across the Blue Nile raising the number of bridges serving the city to eight.

Still on the drawing boards are plans for inner, middle and outer ring roads circling the three towns to reduce congestion.

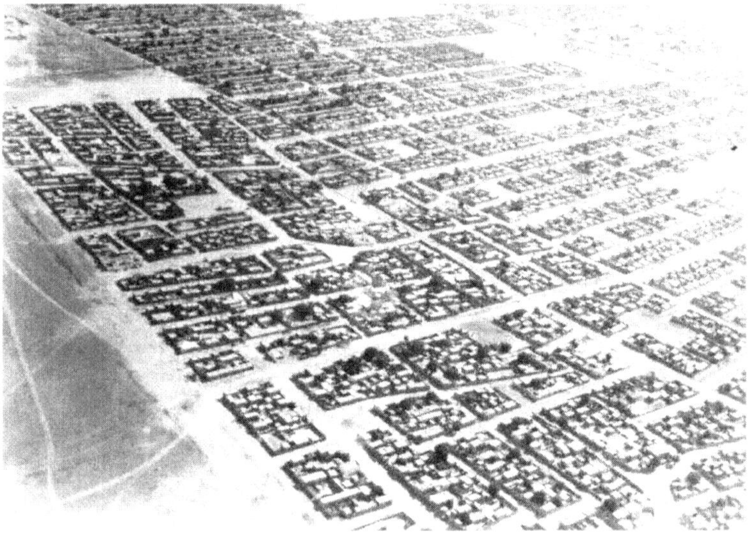

Figure 3: Low-density housing projects increase the city's sprawl and reduce its efficiency.

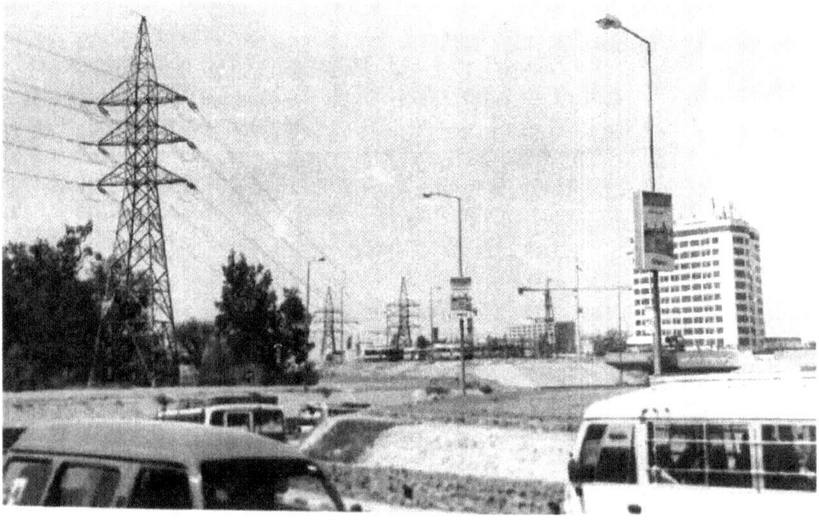

Figure 4: High voltage electricity lines crossing residential areas spread a new hazard: electro magnetic fields (EMFs).

3.5 Electromagnetic fields (EMFs)

The host of urban hazards constantly within our visual, auditory and olfactory fields has been joined lately by more subtle newcomers: electromagnetic fields (EMFs).

These fields are known to impair human health through their emission of waves penetrating the body, the EM energy absorbed is then converted to heat within its cells causing brain cancer and leukemia, with the youth and children being its most vulnerable group (fig 4).

Khartoum is being invaded by two sources of EM fields: high tension electricity lines and mobile base stations. No attempts have been made to maintain recommended safe distances, given as 150m, from residential areas and some officials keep shamelessly dismissing the EM hazard as grossly exaggerated.

4 Recent positive developments

A bright side has recently emerged due to three potentially positive, inter-related developments in the country forcing developmental, economic goals finally to take priority over political ones.

First, oil exports started in July 1999. Since then the exported quantity has risen to 450,000 barrels a day, an official figure disputed by opposition leaders who regard it as deliberately played down and is nearer 800,000 barrels a day [5]. The price has mounted from $25 then to over $60 a barrel. Total oil reserves are estimated by the government at 5 billion barrels. Eyes worldwide started as a consequence to get set on the Sudan.

Secondly, a peace agreement was concluded in 2005 which ended a 21-year civil war in the south. Two of its consequences are of direct relevance to our subject. One is the saving of a daily $2 million allegedly spent by the government in the war. The other is that the peace should trigger counter migration of southern displaced people from the national capital back to their abandoned home provinces; at least a million people are expected to quit Khartoum by early 2008, the time set for launching the fifth population census.

Thirdly, the country suddenly became a magnet for Arab, Western and Asian (mainly Chinese) investors and sizable projects are now in the making. Foreign investments have so far (in February 2007) reached $6 billion [6]. The economy is currently one of the fastest growing in Africa – the International Monetary Fund (IMF) expects Sudan's GDP to grow by 13% in 2007. And of these revenues the national capital will inevitably get the lion's share.

As I was finalising this text the government declared that all drugs for malaria will henceforth be given free as well as HIV/AIDS tests.

Two new industrial areas are being constructed at the fringes of the city and when part of the existing factories and workshops move out to them a relieving effect on the related traffic volume and flow and on air quality will be felt.

The Marawi Dam, presently under construction 350 km north of Khartoum is calculated to produce 1259 MW and drastically reduce the frequent power cuts suffered by the city.

5 Towards the healthy city

Most of the ingredients for a 'healthy city' exist in Khartoum. The time seems ripe to exploit them and the expected benefits are certain to outweigh the costs: a favourable physical setting, plentiful water resources, fertile soil, available capital, available professional expertise and the fact that most of the foregoing environmental problems are still at an early manageable stage.

The achievement of a 'healthy city' by 2030 is by no means a wild dream. Yet turning Khartoum into a sustainable healthy city requires more than solving the problems within its boundaries. It requires immediate implementation of the decentralisation policy officially adopted in 1971. That should create a dynamic series of provincial capitals and an effective hierarchy of settlements over the country and thus help in reaching distant regions and stemming the migration tide to the national capital.

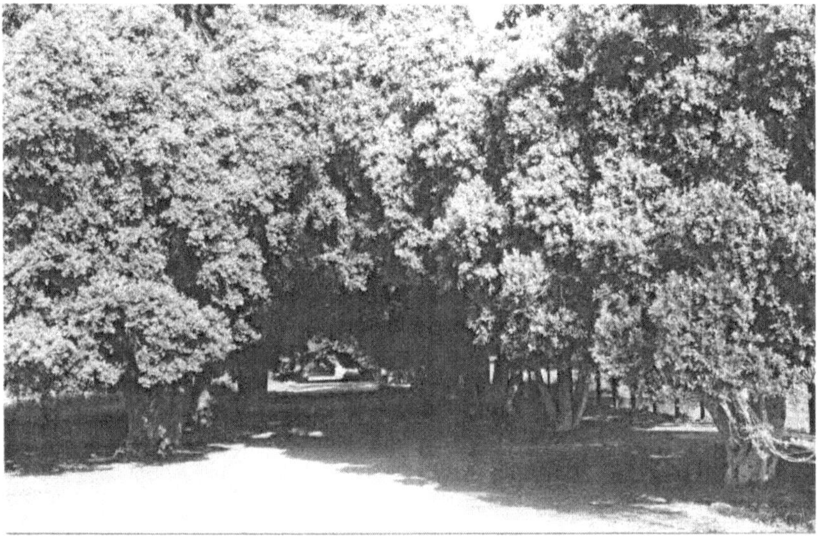

Figure 5: Some parts of Khartoum have retained their old dense greenery.

It also requires drastic measures against the city's own sprawl and for increasing the present low densities. This will improve the physical environment and reduce the crippling inefficiency of the city, reduce journeys to work and atmospheric pollution (fig 4).

It requires efforts to 'green' the city once again – 'green' not in the superficial sense of restoring and consolidating its visible greenery but in the deeper sense of making the city more ecologically responsive, stopping trespassing on agricultural land and natural parks by converting them to residential uses for quick cash, reclaiming some of the lost parks and open spaces, reducing the ecological footprint of the city by exploiting its fertile banks and abundant fresh water for food and fuel production, moving harmful elements such as brick kilns well outside the urban boundary and so on (fig 5).

The coming of an oil culture if not expertly handled can be detrimental to the Sudanese society – not unlike the current 'Islamist' rule imposed on this multicultural, multiethnic society. The symptoms are already in the horizon: calling Khartoum the Dubai of East Africa, being obsessed with a stereotypical western 'image' to attract foreign investors and a readiness to ignore the failures of this stereotype and shun the centuries-old accumulated knowledge. In my view, taking the Arab Gulf or Saudi Arabia as a model is a step in the wrong direction. To the educated Sudanese 'Gulf' conjures up an image of 'false' and for authenticity we may need to study, for example, the Brazilian, Indian, Malaysian or Mexican experience in architecture and urban development.

It is imperative for a genuine quantum leap that the whole approach to handling the environment be utterly transparent and scientific. Environmental Impact Assessments, for example, have been undertaken only when pressure was applied by the press or by such bodies as the *Sudanese Environment Conservation Society*. Such assessments should become standard practice and a proper data base should urgently be built to facilitate them.

The project will need detailed feasibility studies, time schedules, cost analyses, etc, which are beyond the scope of this brief review and will require sustained multidisciplinary team work. But before this, what is needed for this project to materialise is political will.

Acknowledgements

This is a shortened version of an unpublished report. Part of the data has been collected by M. Sc. (Physical Planning) students: Dalal Suliman, El Amin Awad, Fadl el Mula Abdel Basit, Loai Khalafalla, Mai Abdel Raouf, Mohamed el Ghazali, Nahla Omer, Reem Mohamed Seif, Salwa Awad, Sawsan Badi, Shereen Mohamed. However, they are not responsible for any views or criticisms expressed in this paper.

References

[1] BBC News. *World's Worst Cities*. Microsoft Internet Explorer. 2006.
[2] Government of the Sudan. Ministry of Interior Affairs. Meteorological Department. *Climatic Normals (1970-2000)*
[3] Interviews with officials in the Khartoum Municipality (Arabic). *As-Sudani* Newspaper. Khartoum, January 18, 2007.
[4] An interview with Major Muhammad Abdel Mageed El Tayyib, Director General of Khartoum Traffic Administration (Arabic). *Ash-Sharq Al-Awsat*. London. June 27, 2006.
[5] Edward Leeno: The Government is hiding half the oil production. (Arabic). *As-Sahafa*. Khartoum January 24, 2007.
[6] Minister of Finance: Foreign investment reaches $6 billion apart from petrol. (Arabic). *Al-Ayyam* Newspaper, Khartoum, February 21, 2007.

Comparative study of environmental regulations in Latin America

G. Rincón[1,2], L. Cremades[2], U. Ehrmann[1] & A. Peña[1]
[1]*Universidad Simón Bolívar, Dpto. Procesos y Sistemas, Venezuela*
[2]*Universitat Politècnica de Catalunya, Spain*

Abstract

Air quality regulations describe the quality level enforced by the regulating authority. These regulations have been established as an attempt to reduce and control the negative impact of air pollution upon the environment and human health. They are based upon the concentration levels of pollutants that are considered non-hazardous for each individual, including the more vulnerable population like children and the elderly. This study presents an analysis of current environmental regulations for permitted PTS, PM_{10}, $PM_{2.5}$, CO, NO_2, SO_2, and O_3 concentration levels in thirteen Latin-American countries (LACs), and their comparison with similar regulations established by the United States Environmental Protection Agency (US EPA) and the World Health Organization (WHO). Most LACs reproduce US EPA standards, regardless of their specific regional circumstances; however, they do not update these standards at the frequency the US EPA does. Few regulations follow WHO recommendations. Concerns are raised regarding LACs capabilities to effectively monitor air quality and enforce compliance.
Keywords: air quality, Latin American standard regulations, WHO, US EPA, criteria pollutants, compliance.

1 Introduction

Air Quality regulations describe the maximum allowed pollution levels enforced by the regulating authority [1]. The upper threshold values established by the standard regulations correspond to those limits below which no harmful effects due to air pollution are expected. The aim of these regulations is to protect the citizens' health.

WIT Transactions on Biomedicine and Health, Vol 11, © 2007 WIT Press
www.witpress.com, ISSN 1743-3525 (on-line)
doi:10.2495/EHR070271

While designing regulations, local factors such as race related health risk, available technologies, social factors, economics, degree of development, capability to implement these regulations and control compliance, should ideally be considered [2]. This implies that each country should establish its own regulations, based on internationally accepted health risk studies, but adapted to local factors and circumstances revealed through site specific scientific and epidemiological evidence.

In most of the developed world, environmental regulations are revised periodically in response to new scientific evidence and feedback experiences. Also, there is a general awareness among citizens, actual air quality information can be easily accessed, and has become an issue of public interest.

The objective of the present study is to compare air quality regulations in force among Latin American Countries (LACs). Issues such as site specificity, local health risk assessment, revision periods and comparison with air quality standards in force in developed countries will be addressed.

For this purpose, we analyzed the air quality regulations of thirteen LACs, and compared them with each other, and with those regulations recommended by the World Health Organization (WHO) in their Air Quality Guidelines (AQGs) [2], and those established by United States Environmental Protection Agency (US EPA) in their National Ambient Air Quality Standards (NAAQS) [3].

2 Scope of the study

In the present study, six from the seven US EPA NAAQS criteria pollutants were considered; that is, particulate matter with an aerodynamic diameter less than or equal to 10 microns (PM_{10}), particulate matter with a diameter less than or equal to 2.5 microns ($PM_{2.5}$), carbon monoxide (CO), nitrogen dioxide (NO_2), ozone (O_3), and sulfur oxides (SO_x). In addition, total suspended particles (TSP) were included because most LACs regulate their concentration. For each contaminant, the two most frequently regulated averaging periods (AP) were considered.

3 Description and impact of each pollutant

3.1 Particulate matter

Particulate matter (PM) is the term used for any substance, except water, that is suspended in the atmosphere as solid particles or liquid droplets under normal conditions. Their size is microscopic, but above molecular dimensions. These particles originate from diverse sources such as mechanical disruption processes (crushing, grinding, abrasion), power plants, industrial processes, and diesel trucks, and may be formed in the atmosphere by transformation of gaseous emissions. According to their size, PM is classified into PTS, PM_{10} (coarse particles) and $PM_{2.5}$ (fine particles).

Several epidemiological studies have linked PM with premature mortality, respiratory diseases, respiratory emergencies, and lung cancer [4–6]. PM enters the respiratory system by inhalation. There, PM_{10} deposits in the upper respiratory tract, while $PM_{2.5}$ is capable to penetrate the alveolar region. Because $PM_{2,5}$ penetrates deeper into the lungs and its composition includes more toxic substances, these particles pose a much higher health risk than the PM_{10}. Therefore, the WHO and US EPA establish more stringent maximum allowed limits for $PM_{2.5}$.

The averaging period (AP) considered in this study for TSP, PM_{10} and $PM_{2.5}$ correspond to 24 hours and annual arithmetic mean. Those are also the APs established by the US EPA and WHO regulations for PM10 and $PM_{2.5}$.

3.2 Carbon Monoxide

Carbon monoxide (CO) is a colorless, odorless and poisonous gas produced by incomplete burning of carbon in fuels. When CO enters the bloodstream, it reduces the delivery of oxygen to the body's organs and tissues. Health threats are most serious for those who suffer from cardiovascular disease, particularly those with angina or peripheral vascular disease. Exposure to elevated CO levels can cause impairment of visual perception, manual dexterity, learning ability and performance of complex tasks.

APs considered for CO in this study are 8 hours and 1 hour, similarly to US EPA and WHO.

3.3 Nitrogen Dioxide

Combustion processes generate NO as sub-products. In the troposphere, NO rapidly oxidizes to NO_2, which is toxic at concentration levels above $200\mu g/m^3$. In the presence of hydrocarbons, NO_2 initiates free radical chain reactions that produce tropospheric ozone and nitrite aerosols, which contribute to PM2.5 and photochemical smog [2].

APs considered for NO_2 throughout this study are the same recommended by the WHO (1 hour and annual mean) whereas US EPA only considers the annual arithmetic mean.

3.4 Sulfur Dioxide

Like NO_2, SO_2 results from combustion processes; in this case, they originate from sulfur compounds present in fossil fuels. Therefore, atmospheric SO_2 concentration levels are higher in those countries where fuel sulfur content is not regulated. Besides being toxic by itself, SO_2 produces sulfate particles in the atmosphere. Chronic SO_2 and sulfate particle exposure correlates with increased premature mortality due to respiratory and cardiovascular diseases [7].

APs considered in this study are similar to those regulated by US EPA; that is, 24 hours and annual mean. Due to its acute toxicity, WHO recommends SO_2 APs of 10 minutes and 24 hours.

3.5 Ozone

Ozone is a secondary pollutant that results from sunlight induced photochemical chain reactions of nitrogen oxides (NO_x) and volatile organic compounds

(VOCs). Ozone is a powerful oxidant that causes severe respiratory tract irritations. Several studies have revealed associations between O_3 and hospital admissions or emergency visits for respiratory conditions, diminished lung function, and more recently, acute effects on mortality in large cities [8].

Again APs considered in this study coincide with those established by US EPA (1-h and 8-h); while WHO only suggests APs of 8 hours.

3.6 Sample of Latin-American Countries (LACs) studied

Among the twenty-two Latin-American countries, a sample of thirteen was selected. These are Mexico, Brazil, and Chile [9–11] which have highly polluted mega cities; El Salvador, Costa Rica, Nicaragua and Panama [12–15] which are small Central American countries, but their capital cities exhibit significant air pollution; and Argentina, Bolivia, Colombia, Ecuador, Peru and Venezuela [16–21], six South American countries with no significant air pollution problems reported. For comparative purposes, US EPA's NAAQS and WHO's AQGs were selected as reference standards.

It is necessary to point out that all the information regarding LAC, US EPA and WHO air quality regulations was obtained from official government Web sites [12–21].

4 Latin American air quality regulations

Following, each contaminant considered in this study is discussed in a separate section. Comparisons of the maximum allowed concentration levels for each contaminant are represented in bar graphs, with US EPA and WHO reference values displayed as horizontal lines. Empty spots for a given country in the bar graphs indicate that the particular pollutant and/or AP are not regulated in that country.

4.1 Particulate matter

In spite of the fact that US EPA's NAAQS, based upon epidemiologic evidences, since 1987 no longer regulate TSP but PM_{10}, and discriminate between PM_{10} and $PM_{2.5}$ since 1997, most LAC still regulate TSP regardless of their size, and without taking into consideration the severe health risks associated with the smaller particles.

Figure 1 displays the TSP for 24 hour and annual mean APs. It reveals that regulations for most countries are similar for both APs. With the exception of Colombia and Panama, all 24 hour standards correspond to values between 240 and 260 $\mu g/m^3$, and all annual mean standards correspond to values between 75 and 80$\mu g/m^3$. Colombia has less stringent regulations whereas Panama has more stringent regulations. Argentinean air quality regulations do consider an AP of one month for TSP (150 $\mu g/m^3$), instead of 24-h and annual mean APs. Chile and Peru are the only LAC in the sample that do not regulate TSP anymore.

On the other hand, five out of the thirteen LAC do not regulate PM_{10}, (Argentina, Colombia, Ecuador, Venezuela, and Panama), ignoring the relatively increased health risk of the smaller particles. Argentinean and Colombian air quality regulations have last been updated before US EPA began to differentiate between TSP and PM_{10} (1973 and 1982 respectively;) amazingly, these countries have not revised their regulations more recently to include particulate matter discrimination according to its size. Even more surprisingly, the other three countries, whose last air quality revisions occurred after 1987 (Ecuador, 1999; Venezuela, 1995 and Panama, 1998), neither included particle size considerations in their regulations.

It is important to point out that since the late 1980s is well known that the health risk associated with TSP is not relevant in comparison with the risk associated with the smaller particles (PM_{10} and $PM_{2.5}$). Therefore, neither US EPA nor WHO regulate TSP anymore; whereas PM_{10} and specially $PM_{2.5}$ are so harmful that, until 2005, the WHO AQGs considered that there was no safe upper threshold.

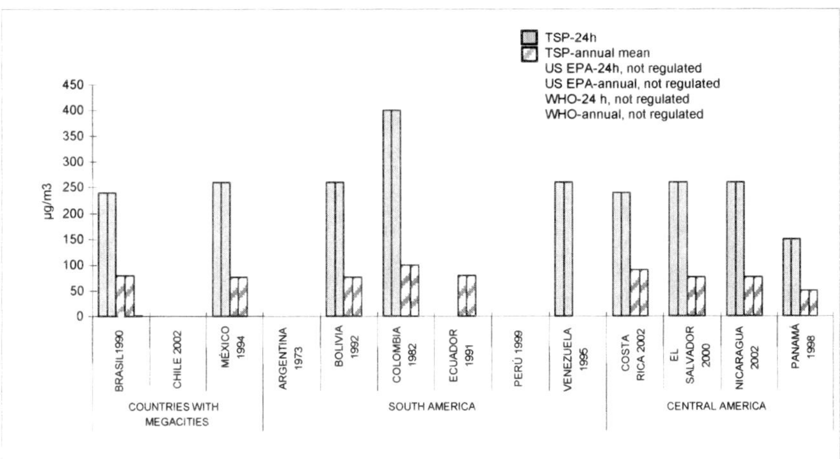

Figure 1: TSP-24h and TSP-annual regulations.

Figure 2 reveals that eight of the LAC studied regulates PM_{10} for 24-h AP and seven additionally regulate the annual mean. All 24-h regulations establish the same upper threshold value than US EPA since 1987. Similarly, six of the LAC establishes the same upper threshold value for the annual mean than US EPA used to until 2006. Only Costa Rica sets a higher upper limit value. Interestingly, Chilean PM_{10} regulations, in force since 2002, coincide completely with US EPA's 2006 revision.

Regarding $PM_{2.5}$, only El Salvador has regulated this pollutant since 2000. The upper threshold values are similar to those established by US EPA since 1997 until 2006 (65µg/m^3 and 15µg/m^3). El Salvador is a very small Central American country with high population density, high degree of deforestation, and many obsolete vehicles with no emission control. Actual WHO recommended values are more stringent than US EPA standards.

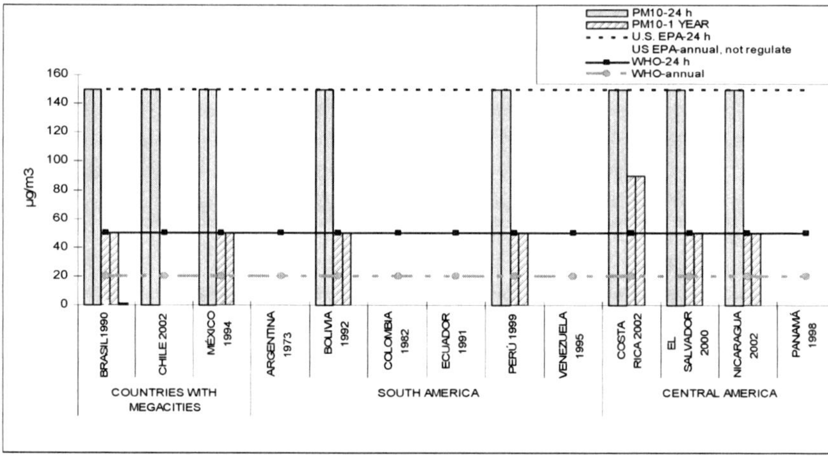

Figure 2: PM_{10}-24h and PM_{10}-annual mean regulations.

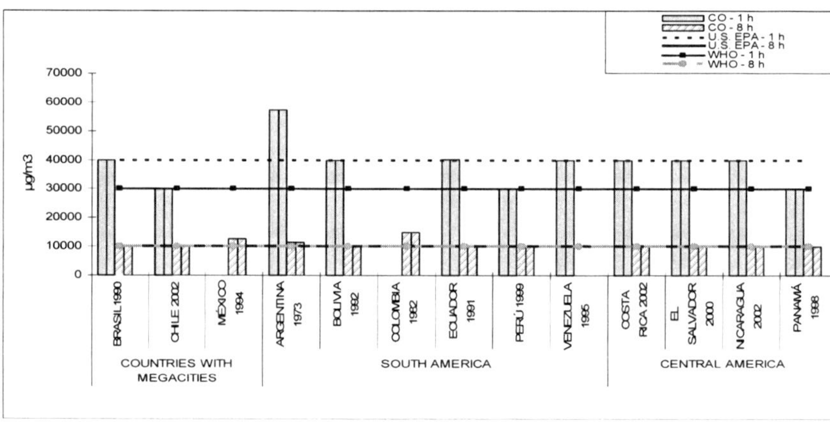

Figure 3: CO-1h and CO-8h regulations.

4.2 Carbon monoxide

Figure 3 compares CO regulations for 1 hour and 8 hour APs. It shows that twelve of the LACs regulate this pollutant. For 1-h AP, seven of these countries establish the same upper threshold limits than US EPA (40 mg/m^3), three of them establish the more stringent WHO recommended limits (30 mg/m^3), while once again, Argentina permits much higher concentrations; perhaps because this country has not revised their air quality standards since 1973. Neither Mexico nor Colombia regulate 1-h atmospheric CO concentrations.

Regarding APs of 8-h, maximum allowed CO limits of US EPA AAQS, WHO AGGs and most LACs that regulate this pollutant, are similar (10 mg/m^3). Mexico and Colombia allow slightly higher 8-h CO concentrations, while Venezuela does not regulate CO for 8-h AP.

4.3 Nitrogen dioxide

Figure 4 shows that all LACs in the sample have some kind of NO_2 regulations (Venezuelan regulations are not displayed in figure 4 because they only consider 24-h APs). Mexico, Argentina and Bolivia only consider 1 hour APs, Colombia, Ecuador, El Salvador and Panama consider only annual mean concentrations (similarly to US EPA), and Brazil, Chile, Peru, Costa Rica, and Nicaragua regulate both, 1 hour and annual mean APs.

Except for Peru, all upper NO_2 limits for 1 hour AP are well above WHO recommended guidelines (320-400 vs 200 $\mu g/m^3$). US EPA standards, usually more flexible than WHO's guidelines, do not include 1-h AP. Once again, Argentina stands out for its flexible regulations.

All LACs that regulate annual mean AP for NO_2 use the same standard than US EPA, which is more than twice the WHO AQG recommended limit.

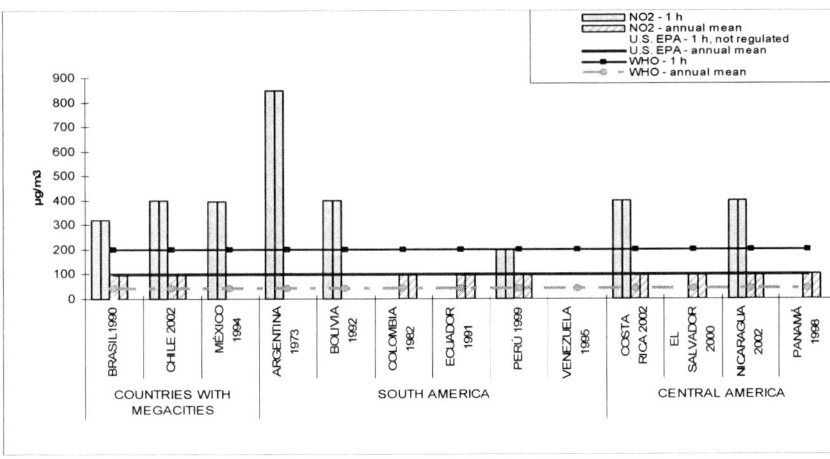

Figure 4: NO_2-1h and NO_2 annual mean regulations.

4.4 Sulphur dioxide

In spite of studies that evidence severe acute SO_2 toxicity over short time periods (10 min), neither US EPA nor any of the LACs in the sample regulate this pollutant for similar APs. WHO recommends upper threshold values of $500\mu g/m^3$ for a 10 minute AP. Figure 5 reveals that all LACs except Argentina regulate atmospheric SO_2 concentration either for 24-h AP, annual mean AP, or both. Argentina does not show standard values in figure 5, because its regulated AP is one month (150 $\mu g/m^3$). All permitted annual SO_2 concentrations are similar, and coincide with US EPA ($80\mu g/m^3$). For a 24-hour AP, most standards are also similar to those established by the US EPA (~365 $\mu g/m^3$). Chile and Mexico have slightly more strict regulations. It is worth noting that 2005 WHO recommend SO_2 concentrations limits are approximately 18 times lower than the US EPA limits.

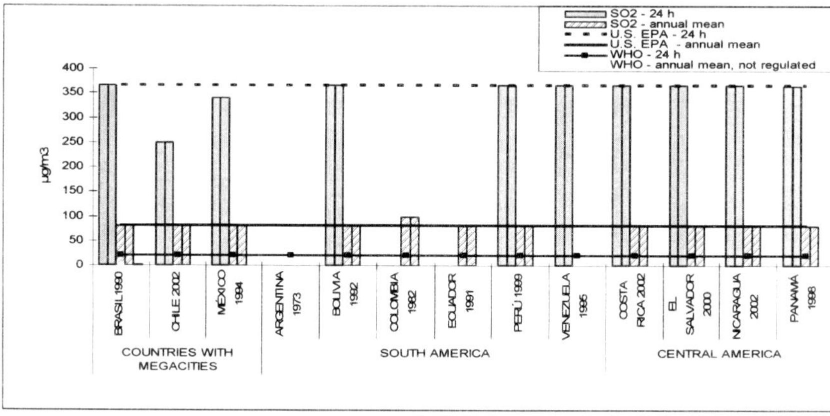

Figure 5: SO_2-24h and SO_2 annual mean regulations.

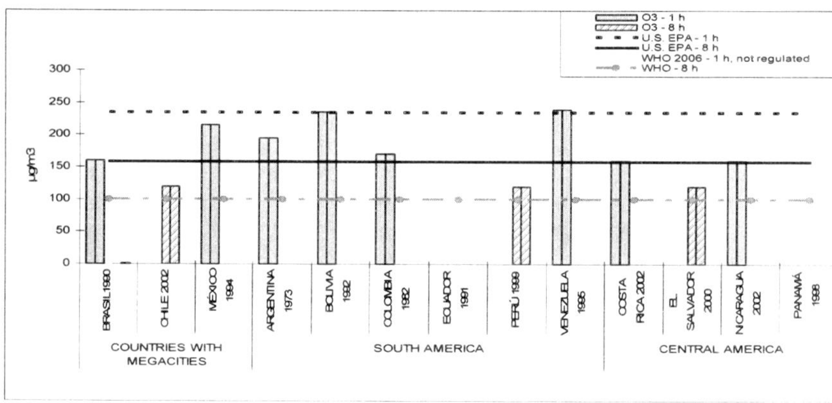

Figure 6: O_3-1h and O_3-8h regulations.

4.5 Ozone

Figure 6 shows that overall, O_3 regulations among LACs are the least uniform of all criteria pollutants. Most LACs regulate O_3 for a 1 hour AP. Except for Bolivia and Venezuela, their standards, including Argentina, are more stringent than the US EPA standards. WHO does not regulate this AP.

Only three countries consider 8 hour APs (Chile, Peru, El Salvador). Surprisingly, their standards are similar the WHO recommended AQS value (100µg/m^3), and significantly lower than the upper limit value established by the US EPA (157 µg/m^3).

5 Examination and compliance

The success of environmental regulations depends on the regulating agent's capability to enforce their compliance. In this study, we tried to locate in the

Web public information regarding criteria pollutant concentrations of the LACs studied. These type of reports are easily available for developed countries. For example, Web AirNow continuously displays actual air quality indexes for major US cities [22]. On the contrary, similar reports for the LACs were not easily available. Up to our knowledge, only Mexico, Brazil and Chile publish continuously updated reports that reveal effective air quality control programs.

For the remaining LACs no similar information was located in the Web, which indicates that, in best of circumstances, this information is not easily accessible by the LAC's citizens. Scarce public information regarding LAC air quality raises concerns about their monitoring and control programs, and consequently their compliance.

6 Final remarks

By far, most LAC air quality regulations reproduce those US EPA standards in force at the time the countries design their own regulations, regardless of site specific factors, regional epidemiologic studies, or capability to control compliance.

Only in a few cases, WHO guidelines are considered; even though this is the organization that cares for human health worldwide, and is constituted by members of all nations, including those LACs studied herein.

Moreover, environmental regulations do not seem to be subjected to regular revision periods since most regulations have not been updated in more than 5 years. That is, they reproduce US EPA standards, but they do not actualize them according to US EPA AAQS or to proper scientific evidence. Consequently, maximum allowed pollutant concentrations are not adjusted adequately to protect public health. For instance, failure to regulate PM_{10} and $PM_{2.5}$ instead of TSP reveal little concern for timely updates to ensure public health.

It is worth to note that most LACs are developing countries that lack of well-organized administrative systems capable to pursue efficient air quality control programs and thus, ensure compliance. Indeed, only the most industrially countries exhibit evidence of systematic air quality control. No regulation will protect human health if its compliance is not ensured. Since air pollution has global impact, efforts to develop effective regional surveillance systems should be international.

References

[1] World Heath Organization. Guidelines for Air Quality: WHO/SDE/OEH/ 00.02.2000.

[2] World Heath Organization. Guidelines for Air Quality for particulate matter, ozone, nitrogen, nitrogen dioxide and sulphur dioxide: WHO/SDE/ PHE/06.02.2005.

[3] US Environmental Protection Agency. National Ambient Air Quality Standards, 2006.

[4] Ostro B. & Chestnut L., Assessing the Health Benefits of Reducing Particulate Matter Air Pollution in the United States, *Environmental Research*, Section A, 76, pp. 94-106,1998.

[5] Dockery D.W., Pope, C., Xu X., Spengler J., Ware J., Fay M., Ferris B. & Speizer F., An Association between Air Pollution and Mortality in Six US Cities T*he New England Journal of Medicine*, 329(24), pp.1753-1759, 1993.

[6] Pope C.A., Schwartz J. & Ramsom M.R., Daily mortality and PM10 pollution in Utah Valley. *Arch Environ Health*, 47(3), pp. 211-217, 1992.

[7] Sánchez J., Romieu I., Ruiz S., Pino P. & Gutierrez M., Efectos agudos de las partículas respirables y del dióxido de azufre sobre la salud respiratoria en niños del área industrial de Puchuncaví, Chile. *Rev Panam Salud Publica/Pan Am J Public Health,* 6(6), pp.384-391, 1999.

[8] Knowlton, K.; Rosenthal, J. E.; Hogrefe, C.; Lynn, B.; Gaffin, S.; Goldberg, R.; Rosenzweig, C.; Civerolo, K.; Ku, J. and Kinney P. L. Assessing Ozone-Related Health Impacts under a Changing Climate. *Environ Health Perspect*, 112(15), pp.1557–1563, 2004.

[9] Normativa Oficial Mexicana, NOM-020-021-022-023-024-025- SSA1-1993, 18/08/94.

[10] Consejo Nacional de Medio Ambiente (CONAMA) N° 3, Valores Nacionales de la Calidad del Aire, Brasil. 28/06/90.

[11] Diario Oficial de La República de Chile N° 110, 112, 113, 114, 115, 59(98, Norma Primaria de la Calidad del Aire, 06/08/02.

[12] Casa Presidencial de El Salvador, Norma de Calidad de Aire Ambiente, 31/05/2000.

[13] Gaceta Oficial de Costa Rica. Nª 30221-S, Artículo 5, 21/03/2002.

[14] República de Nicaragua, NTON 05 012-02, Nª 5, Límites Máximos de Inmisión de Contaminantes en el Aire, 2002.

[15] Gaceta Oficial de Panamá, Decreto N° 158, Normas de Calidad del Aire Ambiente, 1998.

[16] Ley Nacional 20.284 "Contaminación atmosférica", Buenos Aires 16/04/1973, Boletín Oficial 03/05/1973.

[17] Ley de Medio Ambiente 1333, 27 de abril 1992, Gaceta Oficial de Bolivia, 15/07/1992.

[18] Ministerio de Salud, Niveles de Contaminantes del Aire, Colombia. 1982.

[19] Registro Oficial N° 726, Reglamento de las Normas de Calidad del Aire, Ecuador,15/07/1991.

[20] Comisión Nacional del Ambiente (CONAM), Estándares Nacionales de la Calidad del Aire, Perú, 1999.

[21] Decreto 638. "Norma sobre calidad del aire y control de la contaminación atmosférica". Gaceta Oficial de Rep. Venezuela, Número 4899, Mayo, 1995.

[22] AirNow, http://airnow.gov/ February 2007

Reducing the environmental health risk of the vulnerable group in a developing country: a case study of metropolitan Lagos

I. Nwokoro
Department of Urban and Regional Planning, University of Lagos, Nigeria

Abstract

The household, workplace, outdoor and transportation environments pose risks to health in a number of different ways, from the poor quality of the air many people breathe to the hazards we face as a result of climate change. This problem is exacerbated by the high population growth rate of Metropolitan Lagos. This puts a lot of pressure on existing infrastructural and social services which further degrade the environment. Unfortunately, the poor are the most vulnerable to these health and environmental hazards. This paper focused on the social and environmental health risk factors associated with vulnerable groups in Metropolitan Lagos. Specifically, this paper reports how these factors affect the health conditions of these groups of people. Metropolitan Lagos is stratified into various neighbourhoods according to income level and density. Three low income/high density areas were selected for study. The direct observation, administration of questionnaire and Focus Group Discussion (FGD) methods of data collection were employed in addition to the use of secondary based facility data. Information were sought on environmental risk variables like the quality of water, sanitary conditions, refuse disposal types, drainage conditions, sources and intensity of air pollution and sources of energy for cooking. These variables were correlated against health indexes like morbidity and mortality. Results show a strong association between environmental factors and the health status of people especially the poor in the study area.
Keywords: environmental health factors, metropolitan Lagos, vulnerable group, health hazards, mortality, low income communities, air pollution, Bariga, Agege, Ajegunle.

www.witpress.com, ISSN 1743-3525 (on-line)
doi:10.2495/EHR070281

1 Introduction

The environment is a composite of behavioral settings which greatly affects our health. Environmental factors that affect health are in turn linked to underlying pressures on the environment. These pressures are a result of intense urbanization witnessed by most developing countries especially, Metropolitan Lagos. In a recent United Nations Development Programme (UNDP) [1] study, Metropolitan Lagos is presently estimated to be 16.86 and is expected to hit the 24.5 million population mark and thus be among the ten most populous cities in the world by the year 2015. This is indeed frightening, considering the small size of the state put at 300sqkm and the type of density just stated, the weak infrastructural base to support such a huge population and, the current economic growth rate which is below 13%. This is strongly supported by the WHO/UNICEF Global Water Supply and Sanitation Assessment [2]. Exposure prevalence study which concluded that, overall, 99.8% of deaths associated with risk factors are in developing countries, and 90% are deaths of children.

However, these hazards have changed from the traditional factors often caused by poverty and insufficient development, and include lack of safe drinking water, inadequate sanitation and waste disposal methods to more modern hazards which are more global. These include; lack of coordinated health and environmental safeguards, air pollution, over-consumption of natural resources, widespread water pollution, population sprawl, intensive industrial development, climate change, and stratospheric ozone depletion. Each of these environmental hazards is associated with a variety of economic and social determinants of health. Unfortunately, air pollution has remained a major problem in Metropolitan Lagos. Major sources such as automobiles and diesel-fired electricity generators contribute to the choking air plagued by daily smog shrouding the skyline of the central city. Studies carried out by the Federal Environmental Protection Agency (FEPA) [3] show a moderate-to-high concentration of pollutants such as carbon monoxide, sulphur dioxide, nitrogen oxides, organic acids and hydrocarbons in the atmosphere, the majority of which come from rickety and un-serviced automotive engines and industries. At the same time, however, irregular power supply in Lagos has prompted residents to turn to diesel-fired electricity generators, which add to the air pollution with their thick, dark smoke when they start operating in the event of the frequent power cuts. In addition to this is indoor air pollution which comes mostly from soot from the burning of wood, dung, crop residues and coal for cooking and heating. A study by Iwugoh et al [4] shows that water resources in Lagos for domestic, industries and commercial is becoming scarce as a result of pollution of water bodies by wastewater, which contains heavy metals, bacteria (pathogenic) etc. Closely associated with this is flooding which is a serious problem in Lagos metropolis caused by poor drainage systems, the relatively high water table and the flat topography which retards the flow of surface water run-off and prevents rapid discharge into the sea. The aim of this paper, therefore, is to identify and evaluate most of the environmental health risk factors that affect the vulnerable group in Metropolitan Lagos with a view to finding solutions to ameliorate them.

2 The setting

The Lagos metropolitan area comprises 88.7 % of Lagos state, a total of 19.87 sq. km. Presently, the population density in the built-up Metropolitan area is 20,000 persons/sq km as reported in Lagos State Economic Summit [5]. The population of Lagos metropolitan area earlier stated is about 11.2% of Nigeria's overall population. However, based on its high urbanization rates and its dense population, the poverty level in Metropolitan Lagos is very high. Records from the Federal Office of Statistics [6] indicate that about 53% of the population lives below the poverty line. Similarly, in Lagos Metropolis, there is a direct relationship between poverty and household size.

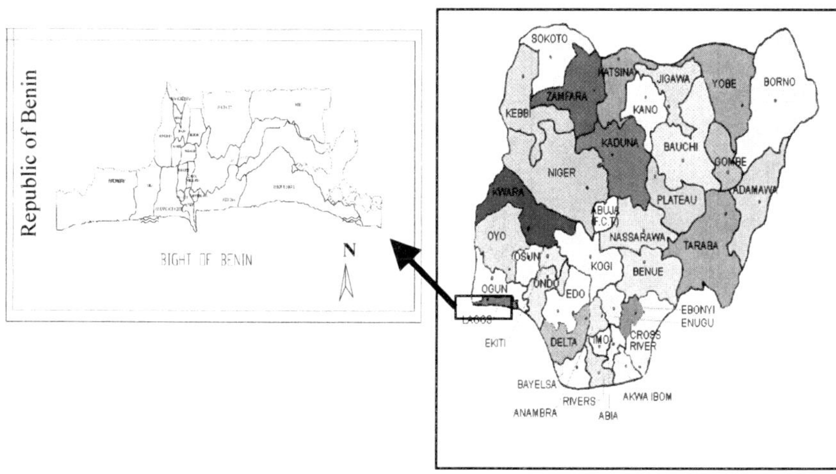

Figure 1: Map of Nigeria showing Metropolitan Lagos.

Lagos metropolis is stratified into various neighbourhoods according to income levels. The income indicators used include some socio-economic characteristics of the neighbourhoods, for example, type of accommodation (duplex, bungalow, Flat, rooming), quality of buildings(good, dilapidated), monthly income of household etc. The Income groups identified include; Low income/high density, Medium income/medium density and high income/low density. Based on this, three low income neighbourhoods were randomly selected for study. They are Bariga, Agege and Ajegunle. These low income communities are among the nine urban blighted areas in Metropolitan Lagos. The NPC 1991 population figures for the different slum areas are Bariga 90,839, Agege 19,741 and Ajegunle, 191,430. They have similar characteristics which include very low average monthly income of between N7,500 to N15,000 ($60 - $120), one room per household who are mostly tenants sharing housing facilities like bathroom, kitchen and toilet. The average household sizes are 7, 6 and 10 for Bariga, Agege and Ajegunle respectively. In terms of infrastructural facilities, most of their roads are not tarred, with blocked drainages and surroundings littered with refuse dumps. These often exacerbate flooding conditions especially in Bariga and Ajegunle areas.

3 Literature review

According to United States Agency for International Development (USAID) [7] study, natural environmental resources and the quality of its air, water, and study soil are severely threatened. The report found that increasing poverty, high population growth and migration, especially into urban areas, and political/institutional constraints are the underlying causes for environmental degradation in the country. These combinations of expanding population and increasing poverty puts increasingly severe demand upon the natural environment, the institutional structures and the resources available to manage them. These are all epitomized in Metropolitan Lagos.

The greatest degradation of the urban environment in the Third World is not merely pollution, erosion, mismanagement of waste, and the depletion and deterioration of resources, but rather it is the degraded and immensely impoverished quality of life, particularly for the majority of urban dwellers. According to the World Resources Institute (WRI)[8] about two billion hectares of soil—equal to 15 percent of the Earth's land cover—is already degraded..

Unfortunately, the poor are the most vulnerable to health and environmental hazards. Poor people are forced to overuse environmental resources to survive, and this impoverishing of the environment again threatens their survival. Accordingly, World Bank Report [9] defined poverty as 'increased vulnerability to environmental degradation or loss of access to natural resources, to employment scarcity, to property loss, to disease and ill health". Factors of vulnerability are for example poverty, illness and disabilities, age, gender, and limited access to resources.

Brundtland [10] noted the six major classes of environmental risks to include inadequate access to safe drinking water, poor hygiene and sanitation, inadequate water resource management, air pollution (indoor and outdoor), chemical hazards and unintentional injuries.

He further reports that in 2000, an estimated 1.1 billion people lacked access to an improved water source. Presently, around 2.4 billion people around the world do not have access to any type of improved sanitation facilities and that mosquitoes and worms are often the result of inadequate water resource management. Brundtland, also notes that air pollution, whether indoors from fuel consumption or tobacco smoke or outdoors from traffic and industrial pollution, is a serious risk factor for respiratory disease, a major contributor to ill-health among children around the world. Chemical hazards in the form of pollutants from unregulated industries, heavy traffic or toxic waste sites compound the hazards children are exposed to. Chronic exposure to certain chemicals has been linked to damage to the nervous system and may harm reproductive function and child development. Lastly, unintentional injuries comprising traffic injuries, poisonings, falls, burns and drowning all pose grave risks to children.

Similarly, air pollution has become a serious risk factor for respiratory disease and a major contributor to ill-health among children around the world.

Environmental factors that affect health are in turn linked to underlying pressures on the environment, which are determined by such driving forces as: Poverty and economic mobility, population dynamics, threat of violence to children in all environments, urbanization: density and transportation, social and cross-cultural diversity, science and technology education, or lack of household wastes, fresh water land use and agricultural environment, Industrialization: external and internal, energy consumption and productions patterns, economic development and globalization of industry.

Akhtar [11], Adedoyin and Watt [12] and Egunjobi [13] have shown strong evidences of a direct relationship between the human environment and health. The World Health Organization has estimated that diseases carried by air and water affect more than 700million people a year. In cities, these diseases are exacerbated by poor sanitation and infrastructure. Biological pathogens have the most serious impact on human health. Crowded conditions, poor sanitation, inadequate water supplies, poor facilities for preparing and storing food, and inadequate hygiene contribute to biological pathogen-induced ill-health.

Brundtland [10] further noted that WHO studies show that around 2 million children die each year from acute respiratory infections alone, with indoor air pollution from cooking and heating putting them at serious risk. And diarrhea, a disease related to inadequate water and sanitation, is the second biggest child killer, claiming about 1.3 million children each year. Together, diarrhea, acute respiratory infections and malaria, all associated with environmental risk factors, kill more children worldwide than any other disease. Global warming will also increase the risks and danger of exposure to heat stress, especially in urban areas, which act as local heat traps because of their interference with air flow patterns, greater reflective surface area and local heat generation.

However, there are few studies that have tried to combine the traditional and modern environmental hazards as they affect the health of the poor in Nigeria. This paper attempts to fill this hiatus in knowledge

4 Methodology

The choice of the three communities within Metropolitan Lagos has been discussed earlier. Collection of data involved direct observation method, administration of questionnaires and Focus Group Discussions (FGD). Secondary sources of data include health records especially on the cases of prevalent diseases in the Metropolitan Lagos sourced from the Lagos State Ministry of health, the Health Departments of the various local government areas where the communities belong to and one hospital (private or government owned) randomly selected from each of the communities within the study area.

To get a good and unbiased representation of the study area, all the streets in each of the communities were numbered. The average number of streets in each community is 40. Thereafter, 10 streets from each community were randomly selected using the table of random numbers. Again in each community, all the houses belonging to the 10 selected streets were enumerated for sampling. 5 houses were randomly selected for sampling on each street. This means 50 questionnaires were administered in each community. In each selected building, all the households were numbered and one household selected using the table of random numbers. The questionnaire was administered to the head of the selected household.

Hypothesis to be tested is

Ho = There is no relationship between environmental factors and health conditions of individuals.

Hi = There is a relationship between environmental factors and health conditions of individuals.

Variables of environmental factors (for example, lack of good drinking water, poor sanitation, drainage conditions etc.) were correlated against health conditions (for example, ill-health, and mortality). The Spearman Rank (Product Moment Rule) was used to test the level of significance at 95% (0.05) level.

5 Research results

The research results are discussed under three broad sections showing the association of environmental conditions and health of the residents of the low income communities. These include environmental conditions, pollution, disease pattern and relationship between environmental and health conditions.

5.1 Environmental conditions

The environmental variables considered were water quality measured by the sources of water, sanitary conditions measured by toilet types, drainage condition measured by availability of drainage facilities and refuse disposal methods also measured by the type and availability.

Table 1: Source of water supply (if 1-3 = good, otherwise, poor).

		Bariga		Agege		Ajegunle	
	Sources	No	%	No	%	No	%
1	Piped water	2.0	4.2	3.0	6.7	1.0	2.3
2	Borehole	4.0	8.3	5.0	11.1	3.0	6.8
3	Spring	0.0	0.0	0.0	0.0	0.0	0.0
4	Well	9.0	18.8	11.0	24.4	10.0	22.7
5	Water vendors	33.0	68.8	23.0	51.1	26.0	59.1
6	Stream/pond	0.0	0.0	3.0	6.7	4.0	9.1
Total		48.0	100.0	45.0	100.0	44.0	100.1

Table 1 shows that the most predominant source of water for the three communities is water vendors. These are private people who sell water in water tankers. 68.8%, 51.1% and 59.1% of respondents in Bariga, Agege and Ajegunle respectively patronize these vendors. The next major source of water is well (both deep and hand dug). The quality of these sources of water does not meet the World Health Organization (WHO) standards. They are often contaminated during the process of distribution. It is worrisome that only 4.2%, 6.7% and 2.3% of respondents in Bariga, Agege and Ajegunle have access to piped water. The few existing water piped mains are broken and lie inside dirty drainage channels. In summary only 12.5%, 17.8% and 9.15% of respondents in Bariga, Agege and Ajegunle respectively, have access to good sources of water. Poor water sources are often associated with water-borne diseases like cholera and diarrhoea which often lead to infant mortality as earlier corroborated in section 3.

Table 2 shows that a sizeable proportion of the low income communities in Metropolitan Lagos still defecate in the bush, near refuse dumps and along water bodies. The most common type of toilet facility used by residents in these areas is the pit latrine which is very unhygienic. The water closet system is almost non-existent because of the absence of in-house water connection to flush the toilets.

Table 2: Types of toilet facilities (if 1-2 = good, otherwise poor).

	Bariga		Agege		Ajegunle	
Sources	No	%	No	%	No	%
1 WC + Septic	2	4.2	5	11.1	3	6.8
2 Pour Flush	13	27.1	15	33.3	12	27.3
3 Pit Laterine	28	58.3	21	46.7	25	56.8
4 Bush/Refuse Dump	5	10.4	3	6.7	2	4.5
5 None	0	0.0	1	2.2	2	4.5
Total	48	100.0	45	100.0	44	100.0

In summary, only 31.3%, 44.4% and 34.1% of the respondents in Bariga, Agege and Ajegunle respectively have access to good toilet facilities.

An average of 80% of the total number of respondents in all the areas studied do not have access to good drainage facilities as corroborated by figure. Even where there are drainage channels, most of them are uncovered and blocked with refuse, sand and stagnant water which are fast breeding grounds for mosquitoes, the major cause of malaria.

In terms of refuse disposal facilities, an average of 70% of the respondents in the three communities patronize the local truck pushers who in turn dump the refuse indiscriminately on the roads or near water bodies. These local truck pushers collect refuse from individual households for a paltry sum and carry away the refuse uncovered thereby, allowing some debris to drop on the roads. The result of this is an unsightly environment littered with refuse and causing very offensive odour.

5.2 Pollution

The major types of pollution identified in the study area are air and water pollution. The major sources of air pollution as shown in figure 2 are fumes from rickety vehicles, smoke from neighbourhood and foul smell from surroundings. These occur in very high intensities. The three communities show the same pattern of occurrence and intensities. The atmosphere is rarely clean.

Another type of pollution identified is indoor air pollution. Sources of energy for cooking were used to measure this type of pollution. Results from table 3 show that 56.1%, 46.6% and 63.6% of respondents in Bariga, Agege and Ajegunle respectively still use poor sources of energy for cooking. Soot from the burning of wood, dung, crop residues and coal for cooking and heating are very irritating and can lead to very acute respiratory diseases especially among women and children. Cooking is done inside the living rooms and this is very hazardous. The situation is worsened by lack of ventilation in the buildings. Lung cancer has also been associated with indoor pollution.

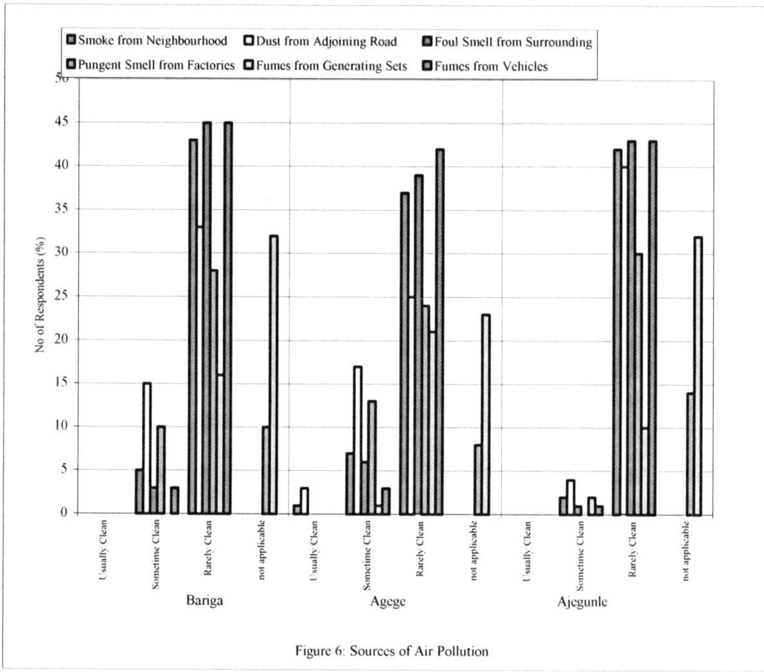

Figure 2: Major sources of air pollution and intensity.

Table 3: Sources of energy for cooking (if 1-2 = good, otherwise poor).

	Bariga		Agege		Ajegunle	
Sources	No	%	No	%	No	%
1 Gas	3	6.3	4	8.9	1	2.3
2 Kerosene	18	37.5	20	44.4	15	34.1
3 Charcoal	20	41.7	20	44.4	23	52.3
4 Firewood	5	10.4	1	2.2	3	6.8
5 Others	2	4.2	0	0.0	2	4.5
Total	48	100.0	45	100.0	44	100.0

Water pollution from waste water, solid waste dumps and effluents from industrial sources have been found to be a major health threat to residents of the study area. This is exacerbated by flooding of most areas of Lagos metropolis usually caused by a combination of human and natural factors. The human factors are as a result of poor wastewater disposal and other sanitation practices while the natural factors include rainfall, flat topography and poor infiltration. All the factors described above are associated with various environmental health diseases as discussed in the next section.

5.3 Disease pattern in the study areas and their relationship to environmental conditions

The most prevalent disease in all the communities is malaria, closely followed by diarrhoea. This was reported more by the women and children. Figure 3 describes the situation in the three communities. These are diseases associated with bad environmental conditions. Similarly, deaths related to environmental conditions recorded more than 60% in each of the communities. Questions asked on child mortality (children below 5 years) confirmed that malaria and diarrhoea were the major killer diseases. Records from each of the three hospitals sampled corroborated results from the primary data.

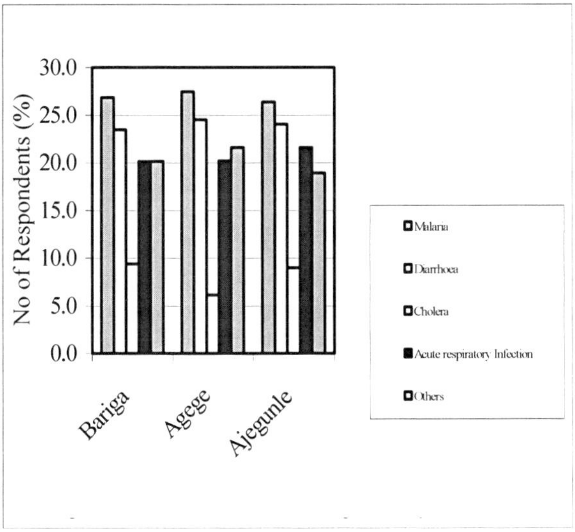

Figure 3: Prevalent diseases in the past one year.

The correlation analysis done to see the relationship between environmental conditions and health of residents show a significant association, therefore, Hi is accepted at 95% significant level. Table 4 shows the correlation matrix. There is a significant relationship between death in the past one year and quality of water and drainage facilities. The relationship between mortality and all the environmental factors is negative. Another correlation matrix between environmental factors and prevalent diseases show a high correlation between malaria and diarrhoea with environmental factors.

The summary of all the above results confirm that low income communities where most of the poor live suffer from environmental health hazards. It has also shown that women and their children are most vulnerable.

Table 4: Relationship between environmental factors and health conditions.

Correlation Matrix

	Death in the past one year	Good source of water	Bad source of water	Good toilet facilities	Poor toilet facilities	Good drainage	Poor drainage
Death in the past one year	1.000	-.809	.809	-.332	.332	-.995	.995
Good source of water	-.809	1.000	-1.000	.823	-.823	.863	-.863
Bad source of water	.809	-1.000	1.000	-.823	.823	-.863	.863
Good toilet facilities	-.332	.823	-.823	.1000	-1.000	.423	-.423
Poor toilet facilities	.332	-.823	.823	-.1000	1.000	-.423	.423
Good drainage	-.995	.863	-.863	.423	-.423	.1000	-1.000
Poor drainage	.995	-.863	.863	-.423	.423	-.1000	1.000

3 observations were used in this computation.

6 Conclusion

This study has identified both the traditional and modern environmental health risk factors faced especially by residents of low income communities in Nigeria as epitomized in Metropolitan Lagos. The following are some of the policy implications or recommendations of this paper.

Though effective and enforceable environmental policies are difficult to develop and implement in many sub-Saharan countries including Nigeria, it appears a major factor if the country must be environmentally secure. The state government should enforce the banning of importation of used vehicles for over five years. This will reduce the menace of air pollution. The production capacity of the Lagos State water Corporation (LSWC), the sole organization in charge of water supply should be increased to make potable water available to more users. The three communities studied have already been selected for upgrading. The implementation of this plan has become apt and it is hoped that the drainage, refuse disposal and flooding problems will be taken care of.

There is a need to prepare a good plan which will ensure that resources will be managed well and urban residents will breathe cleaner air, drink purer water, and lead healthier lives. Such a good plan should involve a clear understanding of problems; improved regulation; participation of all stakeholders; the use of suitable technologies; and realistic financing options

It has been established that the poor are the ones mostly environmentally at risk Investments in the human capital of the poor can also strengthen their ability to combat environmental degradation of which they are victims. Healthcare facilities should be made accessible to the vulnerable group. The Primary health care efforts of the federal, state and local governments should be intensified. This will make health care affordable to the poor.

However, while the policies mentioned above are desirable, there are some inexpensive strategies that can be employed to combat these threats. Washing hands with soap or ash before preparing food, before meals and after defecating significantly reduces the risk of diarrhea, even when the overall quantity of water available is limited. Ensuring safe sanitary facilities and the use of separate latrines for boys and girls encourages latrine use and reduces disease transmission. Proper waste management and the relocation of waste dumps away from human settlements protect children from scavenging and exposure to hazards. Safe water storage in the home and simple treatment when water quality is in doubt leads to proven health benefits. Good ventilation in homes, improved cooking stoves and clean household fuels decrease indoor air pollution and the incidence of acute respiratory infections. Screening doors, windows and eaves, along with the use of insecticide-treated mosquito nets is very effective protection against malaria.

Finally, environmental education should be a must in the curriculum of schools from post primary level.

References

[1] United Nations Development Programme (UNDP). *Human Development Report: Nigeria 2000/2001 Millennium Edition.* UNDP, Abuja.2001.

[2] World Health Organization (WHO) Water, Sanitation and Hygiene links to Health: facts and figures. 2004. http://www.who.int /water_sanitation_health/en/factsfigures04.pdf

[3] Federal Environmental Protection Agency. *Nigeria Country Analysis Brief: Environmental issues.* http://www.eia.doe.gov/cabs/nigenv.html. 2003.

[4] Iwugoh, K.O., Arcy, B.O. & Andoh, R., *Aspects of land-based Pollution of an African coastal Mega-city of Lagos.* Diffuse Pollution Conference Dublin Poster Papers, *pp. 14-123, 2003.*

[5] Lagos State Government. *Report of the Second Lagos State Economic Summit, Ehingbeti.* Ministry of Economic Planning and Budget, Ikeja, Lagos. 2001.

[6] Federal Office of Statistics, Abuja, Nigeria. 2001.

[7] United States Agency for International Development (USAID) *The challenges and possibilities facing the Nigerian environment.* 2002.

[8] World Resources Institute [WTI] *World Resources 2000-2001.* Washington DC. http://pubs.wti.org/pubs_pdf.cfm

[9] World Bank. Nigeria: Poverty in the midst of plenty: the challenge of growth with inclusion. *Report No. 14733.* 1996

[10] Brundtland, H. G., A paper delivered at the launch of World Health Day, New Delhi, India. 2003.
[11] Akhtar, R., Introduction (chapter1). *Health and Disease in Tropical Africa*, ed. Akhtar, R Harwood Academic Publishers: London, Paris New York, pp. 1-6, 1987
[12] Adedoyin, M., & Watts, S., Child health and child care in Oke-ile: An Indigenous area of the city of Ilorin, Nigeria. *Social Science and Medicine*. 29(12) pp.133-34, 1989.
[13] Egunjobi, T.O., Environmental Health Situation in Ibadan City (chapter 14) ed. Akhtar, R., *Urban Health in the Third World.* A. P. H Publishing Corporation: New Delhi, pp.301-317, 2002.

Author Index